# DRUGS
# VITAMINS
# MINERALS

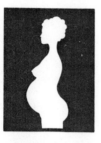

# PREGNANCY

Ann Karen Henry, Pharm.D.
Jil Feldhausen, M.S.,R.D.
Foreword by Glade Curtis, M.D., Ob-Gyn

# FISHER
# BOOKS

Publishers:    *Bill Fisher,*
               *Helen Fisher*
               *Howard Fisher*
               *Tom Monroe, P.E.*

*Chief Editor:*    *Judith Schuler*
*Editor:*    *Joyce Bush*
*Art Director:*    *Josh Young*

*Published by Fisher Books*
*P.O. Box 38040*
*Tucson, AZ 85740-8040*
*(602) 292-9080*

Library of Congress
Cataloging-in-Publication Data

Henry, Ann Karen, 1955-
   Drugs, vitamins, minerals in pregnancy.

   Includes index.
   1. Pregnancy—Nutritional aspects—
Popular works. 2. Pregnancy, Complica-
tions of—Popular works. 3. Fetus—Effect
of drugs on—Popular works.
I. Feldhausen, Jil, 1956- . II. Title.
RG525.H46    1989    618.2    88-33434
ISBN 1-55561-017-X

©1989 Fisher Books

Printed in U.S.A.
Printing 10 9 8 7 6 5 4 3

# Contents

Medications and Nutrients by Class . .iii
An Obstetrician's View on
  Pregnancy and Drugs . . . . . . 1
Introduction . . . . . . . . . . . 7
Guide to Chart Use . . . . . . . 9
Medications . . . . . . . . . . 15
Vitamins, Minerals & Supplements . 281
Other Substances . . . . . . . . 345
Miscellaneous Food Items . . . . 363
Selected Food Additives . . . . . 366
Recommended Diet . . . . . . . 370

Appendix 1
  Food Sources of Nutrients . . . . 375
Appendix 2
  Calcium & Magnesium Content
  of Drugs or Supplements . . . . 379
Appendix 3
  Caffeine in Foods, Beverages
  & Drugs . . . . . . . . . . 381
Poison-Control Centers . . . . . . 383
Brand Names . . . . . . . . . . 390
Glossary . . . . . . . . . . . 398
Index . . . . . . . . . . . . . 403

## Medications and Nutrients by Class

### Analgesics and anti-inflammatory agents

| | | | | |
|---|---|---|---|---|
| Acetaminophen | 16 | Meclofenamate | 166 |
| Aspirin | 40 | Methadone | 174 |
| Codeine | 82 | Naproxen | 184 |
| Diflunisal | 98 | Oxycodone | 196 |
| Fenoprofen | 126 | Salsalate | 240 |
| Hydrocodone | 136 | Sulindac | 250 |
| Ibuprofen | 138 | Tolmetin | 266 |
| Indomethacin | 142 | | |

### Anticoagulants

| | | | |
|---|---|---|---|
| Heparin | 134 | Warfarin | 278 |

### Anticonvulsants

| | | | |
|---|---|---|---|
| Carbamazepine | 52 | Phenobarbital | 204 |
| Clonazepam | 78 | Phenytoin | 211 |
| Divalproex | 106 | Primidone | 218 |
| Ethosuximide | 124 | Trimethadione | 270 |
| Mephobarbital | 168 | Valproic acid | 276 |
| Paramethadione | 198 | | |

### Antidiabetic agents

| | | | |
|---|---|---|---|
| Anti-diabetic agents (oral) | 38 | Insulin | 146 |

### Anti-infectives

| | | | |
|---|---|---|---|
| Acyclovir | 18 | Doxycycline | 114 |
| Amoxicillin | 28 | Erythromycin | 120 |
| Ampicillin | 30 | Ethambutol | 122 |
| Cefoxitin | 56 | Isoniazid | 150 |
| Ceftriaxone | 58 | Lindane | 158 |
| Cephalexin | 60 | Metronidazole | 178 |
| Cephradine | 62 | Miconazole | 180 |
| Clindamycin | 76 | Nitrofurantoin | 186 |
| Clotrimazole | 80 | Nystatin | 190 |
| Dicloxacillin | 96 | | |

## Anti-infectives, continued

Penicillin . . . . . . . . . . . . . 200
Pyrethrins . . . . . . . . . . . . . 231
Rifampin . . . . . . . . . . . . . 236
Streptomycin . . . . . . . . . . 244
Sulfamethoxazole . . . . . . . . 246
Tetracycline . . . . . . . . . . . 256
Trimethoprim . . . . . . . . . . 272

## Asthma medications

Albuterol . . . . . . . . . . . . . 20
Aminophylline . . . . . . . . . . 22
Cromolyn . . . . . . . . . . . . . 84
Epinephrine . . . . . . . . . . . 118
Isoetharine . . . . . . . . . . . 148
Isoproterenol . . . . . . . . . . 152
Metaproterenol . . . . . . . . . 172
Prednisone . . . . . . . . . . . 216
Terbutaline . . . . . . . . . . . 252
Theophylline . . . . . . . . . . 258

## Cold and allergy products

Ammonium chloride . . . . . . . 26
Atropine . . . . . . . . . . . . . 44
Belladonna . . . . . . . . . . . 46
Brompheniramine . . . . . . . . 48
Chlorpheniramine . . . . . . . . 66
Clemastine . . . . . . . . . . . 74
Cyproheptadine . . . . . . . . . 88
Dextromethorphan . . . . . . . 92
Diphenhydramine . . . . . . . 104
Ephedrine . . . . . . . . . . . . 116
Guaifenesin . . . . . . . . . . . 130
Pheniramine . . . . . . . . . . 202
Phenylephrine . . . . . . . . . 207
Phenylpropanolamine . . . . . 209
Pseudoephedrine . . . . . . . 228
Pyrilamine . . . . . . . . . . . 232
Terpin hydrate . . . . . . . . . 254
Tripelennamine . . . . . . . . 274

## Contraceptives

Oral contraceptives . . . . . . 191
Spermicides . . . . . . . . . . 243

## Medications for psychiatric disease

Amitriptyline . . . . . . . . . . 24
Chlordiazepoxide . . . . . . . . 64
Chlorpromazine . . . . . . . . . 68
Desipramine . . . . . . . . . . 90
Diazepam . . . . . . . . . . . . 94
Doxepin . . . . . . . . . . . . 112
Fluphenazine . . . . . . . . . 128
Haloperidol . . . . . . . . . . 132
Imipramine . . . . . . . . . . 140
Lithium . . . . . . . . . . . . . 162
Nortriptyline . . . . . . . . . . 188
Oxazepam . . . . . . . . . . . 194
Prochlorperazine . . . . . . . 221
Promethazine . . . . . . . . . 224
Thioridazine . . . . . . . . . . 260
Thiothixine . . . . . . . . . . . 262
Trifluperazine . . . . . . . . . 268

## Minerals

Calcium . . . . . . . . . . . . 284
Chromium . . . . . . . . . . . 288
Copper . . . . . . . . . . . . . 290
Fluoride . . . . . . . . . . . . 292
Iodine . . . . . . . . . . . . . 297
Iron . . . . . . . . . . . . . . 299
Magnesium . . . . . . . . . . 302
Manganese . . . . . . . . . . 304
Molybdenum . . . . . . . . . 304
Phosphorus . . . . . . . . . . 310
Potassium . . . . . . . . . . . 312
Selenium . . . . . . . . . . . 322
Sodium . . . . . . . . . . . . 324
Zinc . . . . . . . . . . . . . . 342

## Miscellaneous medications

Isotretinoin . . . . . . . . . . 154
Ritodrine . . . . . . . . . . . . 238
Sulfasalazine . . . . . . . . . 248

## Miscellaneous substances

Alcohol . . . . . . . . . . . . 346
Aspartame . . . . . . . . . . . 350
Caffeine . . . . . . . . . . . . 352
Cigarettes . . . . . . . . . . . 354
Cocaine . . . . . . . . . . . . 356
Fiber . . . . . . . . . . . . . . 357
Herbs . . . . . . . . . . . . . 359
Marijuana . . . . . . . . . . . 362

## Products for stomach and intestinal complaints

| | | | |
|---|---|---|---|
| Antacids | 32 | Meclizine | 164 |
| Anthraquinone laxatives | 36 | Metoclopramide | 176 |
| Bulk laxatives | 50 | Mineral oil | 182 |
| Castor oil | 54 | Phosphorated carbohydrate | 214 |
| Chlorpromazine | 68 | Prochloperazine | 221 |
| Cimetidine | 72 | Promethazine | 224 |
| Cyclizine | 86 | Ranitidine | 234 |
| Dimenhydrinate | 100 | Simethicone | 242 |
| Dimethylmethane laxatives | 102 | Sodium bicarbonate | 324 |
| Docusate | 110 | | |

## Thyroid medications

| | | | |
|---|---|---|---|
| Levothyroxine | 156 | Propylthiouracil | 226 |
| Liothyronine | 160 | Thyroid | 264 |

## Vitamins

| | | | |
|---|---|---|---|
| Biotin | 282 | Thiamine | 326 |
| Folate | 294 | Vitamin A | 328 |
| Niacin | 306 | Vitamin $B_{12}$ | 331 |
| Pantothenic acid | 308 | Vitamin C | 333 |
| Prenatal vitamins | 314 | Vitamin D | 335 |
| Pyridoxine | 318 | Vitamin E | 338 |
| Riboflavin | 320 | Vitamin K | 340 |

# Dedication

This book is dedicated to our families, Michael and Daniel, Britt, Evan and Emilee, and to all the little ones who make this information so important to all of us.

# Acknowledgments

We thank everyone who helped with this book, especially Joyce Bush, whose patient assistance has been so valuable. Our technical consultants, Glade Curtis, M.D. and James E. Thomasson, M.D. were enormously helpful.

We owe special thanks to Winter Griffith, M.D., for allowing us to use the superb chart format he developed for his own extremely informative books on drugs, medical tests, symptoms, and vitamins and minerals. He also graciously provided the brand-names list for vitamins and minerals and the icons from his book *Complete Guide to Vitamins, Minerals and Supplements,* ©1988 Fisher Books.

# About the Authors

Ann Karen Henry, Pharm.D., received a Bachelor of Science degree in Pharmacy from the University of Kentucky in 1977. In 1981, she completed a Doctor of Pharmacy degree from the same institution and a Clinical Pharmacy Residency from Albert B. Chandler Medical Center. Since then, she has served on the faculty at the University of Arizona. She works primarily with the Family Medicine Residency in the College of Medicine as a Clinical Consultant. A major challenge in her work has been to assist physicians in safely treating pregnant and lactating women.

Jil Feldhausen, M.S., R.D., received a degree in Dietetics from the University of Arizona in 1979. She completed an internship in Clinical Dietetics in 1981 and received a master's degree in Nutrition in 1982 from the University of Arizona. She was selected Young Dietitian of the Year in 1987. She has served on the faculty at the University of Arizona since 1982. She works with Family Medicine residents and medical students, teaching clinical nutrition.

While this book was being written, Emilee was born to Jil Feldhausen and Daniel was born to Ann Karen Henry. The pregnancies and births increased the authors' personal dedication to make this book accurate and useful to other mothers-to-be who are concerned about the health and well-being of their children and themselves.

# An Obstetrician's View on Pregnancy and Drugs

The physical and mental *in utero* development of a baby is an incredible process. In recent years, we have learned much to help you make your pregnancy and delivery a safer, more enjoyable experience. Medical advances have made it possible for women who might not be able to have children because of chronic illness or poor health to give birth safely. A good example is the diabetic woman who previously might not have been able to carry a pregnancy to term without risk of serious health complications. Today, with careful monitoring and insulin therapy, she may have many successful, safe pregnancies.

Many conditions related to pregnancy can now be treated and cured. For example, ritodrine treatment to stop premature labor and premature delivery is a major medical advance. It stops labor that begins before the fetus is mature enough to survive outside the womb. This avoids birth of a premature baby who would need intensive care and weeks or months in the hospital.

Your physician and other health-care providers have the responsibility to pass this information on to you—the pregnant woman. But part of the responsibility lies with you. Communicate with your doctor, and tell him or her about any problems you have or what your concerns are.

Once advice is given or prescriptions are written, you are responsible for following the prescribed care. If you suspect you're pregnant, notify your doctor, particularly *before* starting any course of medication. It's easy to give advice about medications before they're taken. It's more difficult to deal with with the situation when a woman says, "I'm pregnant. Will that medicine you gave me last week hurt my baby?"

This book cannot provide you with absolute answers about particular medications you may need to take. It is certainly *not* meant to replace your physician or health-care provider. So be sure to consult your physician about any concerns you have after reading the information in this book.

Pregnancy produces many symptoms. It's a time of great change in your body. Many of these changes may make you feel uncomfortable. Unfortunately, we can't always prescribe a pill or medicine to make it better.

## Preparing for Pregnancy

When discussing pregnancy and lactation, we divide the time into different periods—prepregnancy, pregnancy and lactation. In the past, few women gave much thought to the prepregnancy period and preparation for pregnancy. But today, many women are becoming concerned about their bodies before they become pregnant! When planning for pregnancy, you *can* improve the quality of the environment for your soon-to-be growing fetus. You can prepare for pregnancy and continue your practices during pregnancy.

It's important to coordinate your care with your doctor and to communicate with him or her early in your pregnancy. If possible, see your doctor for a checkup *before* you get pregnant. Ask if there are things you can do to prepare yourself for pregnancy, such as possibly changing, decreasing or stopping medications or improving your nutritional health.

One guideline is to seek general good health before you become pregnant. This includes practicing good nutrition, getting the right kind of exercise, watching your weight and avoiding chronic use of drugs, including alcohol and tobacco. However, don't stop taking *any* medication necessary for your well-being. When you make the decision to become pregnant, talk to your doctor about any medications you must take. He or she will determine a course of treatment for you and your baby.

Many medications are necessary for your continued good health, even in pregnancy. One example of a necessary drug for your health and well-being is thyroid medicine. This drug should not be stopped during pregnancy. In fact, doing so may lead to difficulty in becoming pregnant or problems carrying a pregnancy to term. On the other hand, isotretinoin (Accutane®) is something you *must* discontinue, page 154. A fetus can be seriously harmed if you continue taking Accutane during pregnancy.

If you take oral contraceptives, ask your doctor when and how to stop taking them. You need to know how much time to allow before attempting a pregnancy. This may apply to other methods of birth control, such as the IUD (intrauterine device) or gels and foams you might use. If you've been using a form of contraception and think you might be pregnant, it's important to have a pregnancy test. Then you'll know if you should continue contraception or not.

Today, there is even evidence the drugs your baby's father takes or the substances he uses before conception can affect your child! We know alcohol is associated with a long list of abnormalities. Researchers believe heavy intake by the father-to-be before conception may cause a decrease in the baby's birth weight.

### How Long Does Pregnancy Last?

The average length of a pregnancy (calculated from the first day of the last normal menstrual period) is 280 days or 40 weeks. We divide pregnancy into three equal parts called *trimesters*. Each trimester is slightly more than 13 weeks long, about 3 calendar months. Some people prefer the more precise use of weeks of pregnancy. They might say, "you are 17 weeks pregnant," or about 4 months.

Pregnancy is divided into three trimesters because fetal development and problems of pregnancy seem to fall into these time periods. For instance, most

miscarriages occur during the first trimester. Or (until recently) if a baby was born before the third trimester, it had little chance for survival.

For many, the period of "pregnancy" does not end with the birth of the baby. For different lengths of time, maternal support is continued to the infant through breast-feeding.

These time categories are useful in considering drugs during pregnancy. Specific events in fetal development occur at different stages of pregnancy; the same drug may affect development in different ways.

Organ development (heart, brain and other organs) occurs early in pregnancy. Later in pregnancy, these organ systems mature while the fetus grows and gains weight at a very rapid rate. A drug taken in the early weeks of pregnancy may have a dramatic effect on organ development. If the same medication is given during the latter part of pregnancy, it may have no effect at all. Other medications may be associated with considerable risk of toxicity at the end of pregnancy but are fairly safe during the second trimester.

### Should You Take Medications While You're Pregnant?

A *medication* is any substance used in the prevention, diagnosis, alleviation, treatment or cure of disease. This includes prescription medications and non-prescription or over-the-counter (OTC) preparations.

Pregnancy brings about many physical and emotional changes. You may be nauseated in the early stages of pregnancy. Or you may have episodes of heartburn or constipation. You can't go through your pregnancy without some discomfort. Because of the discomfort, you may be tempted to take some medication to alleviate them.

In this way, pregnancy may actually cause an increase in the amount of medications you take. This could expose your unborn baby to a number of medications and chemicals while it is developing and growing in the safety of your womb.

Giving you a medication when you're pregnant presents unique problems. Your reaction and the desired result must be considered along with the well-being of your fetus, who is also a recipient of any medication. Should you stop taking all medications during pregnancy so your baby won't be harmed? Not necessarily. As I've already said, some medications are beneficial during pregnancy—others are required for your good health. But some medications should be avoided. Before deciding about any medications or preparations you use, talk to your doctor. He or she knows your medical history and can make an informed, knowledgeable decision about your care.

You and your doctor must work together to make decisions about dealing with any discomfort you experience. In the past, most attention was directed to the pregnant woman and relief of her symptoms. Today, we recognize the importance of protecting the fetus from potentially harmful medications and providing a safe environment for development. You and your doctor must weigh the benefits of a medication for you against the risk to your growing baby.

It's also important to recognize the benefits to your developing baby from treatment of your medical problems. A good example is diabetes—successful treatment is *essential* for mother and child. From the beginning of fetal growth, your blood-sugar levels must be controlled as much as possible. Careful monitoring is important to the fetus because maternal diabetes increases risk of spontaneous miscarriage, malformations and even fetal death. Newborns have fewer complications if blood pressure is controlled.

If you take medications to treat or control a medical condition and you're considering pregnancy, consult your doctor before pregnancy. If this is not possible, consult him or her as soon as possible when you suspect you're pregnant.

The medical profession has changed its attitudes about prescribing medication for your discomfort during pregnancy. One example of our change in attitude is treatment for relief of morning sickness. Bendectin® was prescribed for pregnant women for many years to relieve symptoms of morning sickness. It was usually prescribed during the first trimester, but sometimes a woman took it her entire pregnancy.

Today, Bendectin is not available because of legal pressures. There were some reports in non-medical publications of fetal malformations, which suggested the cause was Bendectin. Lawsuits were filed, in spite of several controlled medical studies that indicated Bendectin was not the cause. The medication was removed from the market and is no longer available.

Today, we use medication less often to treat morning sickness. Psychological support, adequate rest, higher carbohydrate intake and frequent, small meals are non-medical therapies that may be helpful in treating your morning sickness. Medications that are less well-studied than Bendectin are prescribed *only* for severe nausea and vomiting that lead to dehydration and starvation.

## Medications and Other Substances

When possible, discuss medications with your doctor before you take them or even before you become pregnant. Some medications and substances are known to cause fetal malformations or adverse effects in *every* exposed pregnancy. Others cause malformations or other adverse effects in only *some* exposures. In this complicated situation, asking your doctor after you take something can be very unfortunate.

One of the more publicized episodes involving medication in pregnancy concerned prescribing thalidomide to pregnant women as a sleeping pill. Thalidomide had been shown safe in animal studies and was thought to be a useful medication for pregnant women. The medication was prescribed for several years. During those years, thousands of malformed babies were born before a cause-

and-effect relationship could be established. Nearly one-third of all women who took thalidomide during the early part of pregnancy gave birth to infants with birth defects.

Medications you take in pregnancy can pass from you to your fetus through the placenta. Your baby is at the highest risk during the entire first trimester (the first 13 weeks) and the first part of the second trimester of pregnancy. The most susceptible time seems to be around the fifth week after conception, a time of incredible development called *organogenesis.* During these important weeks of organ formation, the fetus matures very quickly and may be more susceptible to outside influences, such as medications.

Researchers believe many medications you take while you are pregnant pass to the infant in some degree. Even medications that don't pass through the placenta are important because their effects on you may be transmitted to the fetus in other ways. Animal experiments and some unfortunate human accidents have given us some understanding of medication effects on an unborn fetus. Unfortunately, even this understanding is not always complete, as the effects of thalidomide demonstrated.

Birth defects, also called *anatomic malformations* or *bodily defects,* are often believed to be a result of taking a medication at a critical time during pregnancy. The amount (dose) and time the medication is taken during pregnancy influence the result.

Tetracycline was considered safe and given routinely until the early 1960s. At that time, a 2-year-old child was found to have normally formed "baby" teeth that were stained bright yellow. After investigating various substances the mother took during pregnancy, it was narrowed down to tetracycline. Your baby's first teeth begin to calcify between the 20th and 24th weeks of pregnancy. Today, we know using tetracycline after this time causes later staining of your child's teeth.

Medications may also indirectly affect the fetus by how they impact on *your*

body. They may interfere with nutrients passing through the placenta to your baby. Other harmful effects to the fetus may not be evident immediately after birth. These include behavioral problems and learning problems that are hard to identify. Such problems may not become apparent until several years after birth or when your child starts school.

A clear cause-and-effect relationship may not be demonstrated between a medication and a result (good or bad) in pregnancy. Risks and benefits from a medication must be evaluated for each individual case. A woman with a chronic illness, such as diabetes or asthma, can now have a relatively normal pregnancy and give birth to a healthy baby. This can be accomplished through careful monitoring during pregnancy, with changes made as necessary as the pregnancy progresses. If you have asthma and take theophylline, page 258, it is very important to take the correct dosage. Your requirements may change during pregnancy, and you may need an adjustment of your medication. It's important to have the oxygen the fetus needs available in your blood so it can be transferred to the placenta.

If you have diabetes, your blood-sugar level can change, especially during the latter part of your pregnancy. Insulin, page 146, may be adjusted, or it may need to be started as you progress in your pregnancy. Following the care suggested by your doctor is essential for the good health of you and your baby.

## Over-the-Counter Medications and Preparations

Prescription medications are not the only ones that can affect your unborn baby. Many medications are available over-the-counter (OTC). Often people don't really consider them as medications when in fact they are! Vitamins, minerals, medicinal herbs, hemorrhoidal preparations, cough-and-cold remedies, diet supplements, weight-loss aids, medicinal creams and lotions, nasal sprays—this is a short list of many "medications" you may not be aware you're taking!

There are side effects in taking any of the substances listed above. Your unborn baby is exposed to these medications, too. Antihistamines and aspirin should be avoided at certain times during pregnancy, if not entirely. Avoid over-the-counter diet aids or sleeping pills. Tobacco use and alcohol consumption are not considered taking medications, but both of these substances have components that pass to the fetus.

Ask your doctor about these and any other medications you may take. It's incorrect to tell your doctor you're not taking "anything" (meaning no prescription medications) when you take ibuprofen (available over the counter) 4 times a day for arthritis, page 138.

While you're pregnant, consult your health-care provider before taking *any* medication to "treat yourself." Many over-the-counter products are safe, but it's always easier to make a decision and give an answer about taking a medication *before* you take it!

## Vitamins and Minerals

Often, people who are very careful about the medications and prescription medications they take overconsume vitamins, minerals, medicinal herbs and various other "natural" substances. They believe these substances are harmless because no prescription is needed for them. They are wrong!

Excess intake can cause various types of problems. For example, excessive amounts of vitamin A, which is stored in the body, has been associated with a number of birth defects. Recently a synthetic form of vitamin A, sold under the brand name Accutane®, has been shown to be *very* harmful! See page 154.

Vitamin and mineral deficiencies can also be the cause of some problems in pregnancy and in babies born with malformations. Studies of cause-and-effect relationships on vitamins and minerals are not as extensive as those on medications because these substances do not have to undergo the same testing before they are sold to the public.

Prenatal vitamin-mineral preparations are usually prescribed when you're pregnant or breast-feeding. Along with a well-balanced nutrition plan, your prenatal vitamin assures you receive an adequate amount of the nutrients you and your baby need.

Be sure to check with your doctor *before* you take any additional vitamins or minerals. In excessive quantities, these are *not* innocuous substances.

Many medications actually originated as medicinal herbs. These substances may be very powerful and toxic. Herbs are also unpredictable in terms of strength. This depends on how the herb is grown, harvested and stored. If you self-medicate with herbs, tell your doctor!

## Breast-feeding

Today, about half of all newborn babies are breast-fed. This is a 50% increase over the number of breast-fed babies 20 years ago. This increase is related to nutritional and immunological benefits of breast-feeding. This has been demonstrated in research comparing breast-fed to formula-fed infants.

When you nurse, you transmit medications to your newborn through your breast milk. Nearly all medications appear in your breast milk to some degree, depending on the specific qualities of the medication and the amount you take. Even if you take what you might consider a "harmless" medication, like aspirin, then nurse your baby, the baby will get some of the aspirin. Aspirin has been shown to alter the baby's bilirubin level. This effect is important in the early newborn period.

The increase in breast-feeding has also brought an increase in questions for those providing health care to breast-feeding mothers about medications they may take. Specific answers about particular medications may be very difficult to find.

We do know most medications you take pass into your breast milk and therefore to your baby. The concentrations of any medication and the result of your baby receiving it are difficult to measure. The American Academy of Pediatrics has established guidelines for medication use during lactation based on known medication concentrations in breast milk and reports of problems in babies. For many medications, there is little or no information about the effects on breast-fed infants. Your baby's doctor must weigh the relative necessity of the medication for your well-being against other factors, such as potential effects on your baby.

When there is no data from human studies, we must use research from animal studies. As more information is gathered about medications, some of our questions will be answered.

Your nutritional habits also affect your breast milk. If your nutrient intake is inadequate, the quality and quantity of your milk will decrease. If you breast-feed, you need to continue to eat a high-nutrient diet. Many of your nutrient requirements increase during breast-feeding. It's standard practice to continue taking your prenatal vitamins while breast-feeding. Rapid weight loss is not recommended while you breast-feed.

Occasionally the foods you eat may affect your baby, especially if your family or husband's family has a history of food allergies. Usually the only way to determine if this is a problem is to eliminate any suspected foods. If your baby's symptoms improve, the food may have been the cause of the problem. Sometimes babies outgrow the problems without any change in the mother's diet.

Alcohol, nicotine and caffeine also pass into your breast milk. Although the quantity of each substance that reaches the baby is decreased, they can still affect your baby. A baby's liver is unable to metabolize medications as rapidly as yours, so substances can accumulate. Our best advice to you is to moderate your intake during breast-feeding.

**Glade Curtis, M.D.**

# Introduction

Pregnancy is a time of hope and excitement. The hope for a healthy baby is a primary concern of every pregnant woman. Many factors effect the outcome of pregnancy. Environmental and genetic factors are important, as is your health.

The purpose of this book is to describe the benefits, risks and special medical concerns associated with use of medications, vitamins, minerals and other substances during pregnancy and lactation. Some substances may be beneficial or harmful if used before pregnancy, so special concerns for women planning pregnancy are also included.

Many vitamins and minerals are necessary for the growth and development of a healthy baby. Too little or too much may have a significant impact on the development of the fetus. Deficiency of some minerals during pregnancy can impact on the mother's health years later. This book addresses these concerns and many others. Planning a healthy diet for pregnancy and lactation is important to you and your baby. Guidelines in this book help you put your doctor's suggestions to work.

Half of all pregnant women use non-prescription medications. Most of this use is without the knowledge or recommendation of their doctor or nurse. Many women consider these medications to be safe because they can be purchased without a prescription. In some cases, there is considerable risk to the mother or her baby from the use of these products. This book provides information about some of these medicines.

Prescription medicines are also included to supplement information from your doctor. Do not consider any medication *entirely* safe. Many medications have been proved to be unsafe for use. Many others have limited risks from which much benefit can be derived in pregnancy. It is necessary to weigh risks and benefits with your doctor or nurse. The information in this book is intended to help you do that.

We have also included substances that have little or no supplemental or therapeutic use. Marijuana, alcohol, cocaine and tobacco (cigarettes) are substances in this category. Many women have questions and concerns about the use of any and all of them.

Information sources for this book are varied. Whenever possible, scientific evaluations of medication, vitamin or mineral use in humans have been cited. *Human studies* can provide information about risk of adverse effects in the mother, fetus or newborn compared to people who were not exposed to the substance. Information about incidence of a particular adverse effect in untreated women with the same disease can also be obtained from some studies. Risks from disease can then be separated from risk of treatment. Benefits of treatment to the mother and fetus can be determined.

For some medications, and many vitamins and minerals, scientific evaluations of human experience are not available. It is necessary to rely on observations of physicians and other health-care providers that are published in *case reports*. A report of the birth of a healthy baby after an exposure does not imply anything about the next baby exposed. A report of an adverse effect does not prove the reported exposure caused the problem. Case reports raise a concern that a substance is not entirely safe. Caution is necessary.

If no case reports or human studies are available, *animal studies* have been used. This is often the case with vitamins and minerals. They are classified as "foods" and are not required to undergo testing before approval for human consumption. If animal studies are used, it is indicated in the text. Animal studies are not always good predictors of problems in human use. In many cases, substances that did not produce malformations in animals proved to be the cause of serious malformations in babies. If no human experience is available, the presence of malformations in animals indicates a substance should only be used if it is absolutely necessary.

There is a great deal of controversy in medical publications about the use of some substances included in this book. Where controversy exists, the charts indicate conflicting reports.

All recommendations in the book are based on a balanced assessment of the information available. No recommendation in this book is intended to stand alone. Every pregnant woman should consult with her doctor or health-care provider *before* making any decisions about the use of any substance.

96 to 98% of all pregnancies result in the birth of a normal, healthy baby. Of the 2 to 4% with malformations, 90% have no identifiable cause. Only a small number can be traced to use of medications or other substances. This book will help you make informed decisions with your doctor or nurse.

# Guide to Chart Use

Information in this book is presented in easy-to-read charts similar to the sample chart shown on page 11. Charts are arranged in three sections—*medications, vitamins, minerals and supplements,* and *other substances.* The Index includes a number of different names for each chart. For complete instruction on use of the charts, refer to the descriptions of the numbered sections on the following pages and the sample chart.

## 1. Generic name

Each chart is titled by the most common generic name. Most charts cover commonly used medications, vitamins or minerals. However, some substances are included that do not have a medical or supplemental use. These charts are titled by the most common descriptive term. Examples are the generic name *phenobarbital* and the substance *cigarettes.* Each chart name is indexed.

There are hundreds of prescription and non-prescription medications, vitamins and minerals. All of them could not be included. Substances were selected for inclusion in this book based on the likelihood you need to know about them during pregnancy or lactation.

## 2. Definition and description

The most common uses of each medication, vitamin or mineral are described. There is also a simple description of the agent's action in the body. Chemical processes in the body are often very complex. The description of medication or substance action does not provide every detail but is designed to give an overview. If you have more specific questions, ask your doctor, nurse, pharmacist or dietitian.

## 3. Other names

Additional generic names and brand names are listed in this section. Each of these names is also indexed. For example,

vitamin C is the generic name on the chart, however you can find it also listed under ascorbic acid in the Index.

Brand names for combination products are listed when the most common form prescribed or used is a combination of two or more products. A list of brand names begins on page 390. Read the chart for each component to determine the action of all the products. Some ingredients may be harmless, but another could endanger you or your baby. If all active ingredients are not indicated as safe, *don't* use the product unless your doctor tells you to. If you don't find the product name from your container, check individual ingredients in the Index. Ingredients are listed on the container or you can ask your pharmacist.

There are many brand names for each generic drug. Products are continuously reformulated, and new products are introduced every year. Some are not listed in this book. Inclusion of a particular product does *not* imply endorsement.

## 4. Dosage

The dosage section includes requirements (for vitamins and minerals only), usual safe adult dose and usual toxic doses. Special dose for pregnancy is included when known.

## 5. Requirements

Requirements are established by the Committee on Dietary Allowances of the Food and Nutrition Board of the National Research Council. They are also called Recommended Dietary Allowances (RDAs). These were established on the basis of available scientific knowledge to meet known nutritional needs of nearly all healthy persons. Recommendations are updated periodically based on newly acquired scientific findings. Many experts believe RDAs are not optimal levels. However, RDAs are the only official guide to

safety. They have been carefully calculated and are a good reference point.

RDAs are recommendations for healthy
people. Special needs may arise for which
RDAs are inadequate. If any pertain to
pregnancy or lactation, they are discussed
in the chart.

## 6. Safe dosage

Safe doses for vitamins and minerals include the Estimated Safe and Adequate Intake for nutrients that have no established
RDAs and safe supplemental doses of
other nutrients. The safe supplemental
dose is the highest level considered safe
and beneficial to health.

Safe dosages for medications include
the usual range of doses for adults for the
most common uses. Your own dose of a
particular substance may be larger or
smaller than the doses listed. Do *not*
change your dose based on doses listed in
any chart. Your doctor has selected the
dose most appropriate for your medical
management, taking into consideration
your size, medical condition and personal
risks for adverse effects. Your medication
may need to be changed or discontinued
during pregnancy. Be sure to notify your
doctor as soon as you suspect you might
be pregnant.

Do not exceed dosage recommendations on the package of products purchased without a prescription, regardless
of the safe dosage range listed in the
chart. Dosage requirements vary with intended use. Each package lists the dose
needed for the intended use of the product. Exceeding the dose on the package
may produce unnecessary adverse effects.

Occasionally, your doctor will recommend a non-prescription medicine at a
higher or lower dose than recommended
on the package. Follow your doctor's
recommendations.

Adverse effects may be noted within
the usual range. Some serious adverse
effects are not related to dose. If you
develop adverse effects while using a
dose listed as safe in this section, contact
your doctor or nurse.

## 7. Toxic dosage

Toxic doses are included when exceeding a particular dose is likely to produce
dangerous symptoms or adverse effects.
Using doses less than the toxic dose does
not protect against adverse effects that are
unrelated to dose. However, staying under
these dosage levels does provide a margin
of safety for overdose symptoms. Toxic
dosages may be influenced by your size
and medical condition. Toxicity can occur
after a single, large dose (overdose) or
after smaller doses taken too frequently.

The toxic dosages represent guidelines
and should not be considered absolute.
Special warnings are included if indicated.
If you develop adverse effects or overdose
symptoms while using a dose less than the
toxic dose listed, contact your doctor or
nurse. If you think you may have exceeded the minimal toxic dose, contact your
doctor or your nearest poison-control
center. A list of U.S. and Canadian poison-
control centers begins on page 383.

## 8. Possible benefits

Possible benefits is divided into five
sections—Benefits before pregnancy,
Benefits to mother, Benefits to fetus and
Benefits during lactation. An additional
section, Benefits to newborn, is included
when appropriate.

## 9. Benefits before pregnancy

This section describes the expected
desired effect from use of a medication,
vitamin, mineral or other substance. For
example, phenobarbital is expected to
prevent seizures. It also prevents
complications of seizures, such as injury
or death during seizures. Both the direct
effect (preventing seizures) and the indi-
rect effect (preventing injury or death) are
included. Effects on fertility are discussed
when information is available.

## 10. Benefits to mother

If you are expected to derive a special
benefit from using a substance during
pregnancy, it is described in this section.
In some cases, benefits before and during

# Chart Guide

To find information about a specific medication, vitamin, mineral, supplement or substance, look in the easy-to-read charts starting on page 16. Charts like the sample below appear alphabetically by generic name.

Each section is explained, using the numbers on the chart as reference (pages 9 to 14). All charts are organized similarly, making it easy to make comparisons.

A generic name is the official chemical name. A medication, vitamin, mineral or supplement listed by generic name may have many brand names. Brand names for the United States and Canada are in a section starting on page 390.

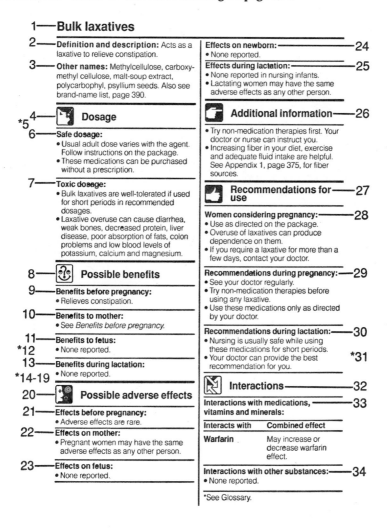

1—Bulk laxatives

2—Definition and description: Acts as a laxative to relieve constipation.

3—Other names: Methylcellulose, carboxymethyl cellulose, malt-soup extract, polycarbophyl, psyllium seeds. Also see brand-name list, page 390.

*5 4—⬛ Dosage

6—Safe dosage:
• Usual adult dose varies with the agent. Follow instructions on the package.
• These medications can be purchased without a prescription.

7—Toxic dosage:
• Bulk laxatives are well-tolerated if used for short periods in recommended dosages.
• Laxative overuse can cause diarrhea, weak bones, decreased protein, liver disease, poor absorption of fats, colon problems and low blood levels of potassium, calcium and magnesium.

8—⬛ Possible benefits

9—Benefits before pregnancy:
• Relieves constipation.

10—Benefits to mother:
• See Benefits before pregnancy.

11—Benefits to fetus:
*12 • None reported.

13—Benefits during lactation:
*14-19 • None reported.

20—⬛ Possible adverse effects

21—Effects before pregnancy:
• Adverse effects are rare.

22—Effects on mother:
• Pregnant women may have the same adverse effects as any other person.

23—Effects on fetus:
• None reported.

Effects on newborn: ————24
• None reported.

Effects during lactation: ————25
• None reported in nursing infants.
• Lactating women may have the same adverse effects as any other person.

⬛ Additional information——26
• Try non-medication therapies first. Your doctor or nurse can instruct you.
• Increasing fiber in your diet, exercise and adequate fluid intake are helpful. See Appendix 1, page 375, for fiber sources.

⬛ Recommendations for——27 use

Women considering pregnancy:————28
• Use as directed on the package.
• Overuse of laxatives can produce dependence on them.
• If you require a laxative for more than a few days, contact your doctor.

Recommendations during pregnancy:——29
• See your doctor regularly.
• Try non-medication therapies before using any laxative.
• Use these medications only as directed by your doctor.

Recommendations during lactation:——30
• Nursing is usually safe while using these medications for short periods.
• Your doctor can provide the best *31 recommendation for you.

⬛ Interactions————32

Interactions with medications,——33 vitamins and minerals:

| Interacts with | Combined effect |
| --- | --- |
| Warfarin | May increase or decrease warfarin effect. |

Interactions with other substances:——34
• None reported.

*See Glossary.

*Item not on sample chart, but in location indicated when information given.

11

pregnancy are the same. In other cases, there is a particular benefit to your health from using a substance during pregnancy.

Most of the benefits from vitamin and mineral supplementation is the prevention of deficiency. Deficiencies are described in the following major section. If there are benefits beyond that, they are described in this section.

## 11. Benefits to fetus

This section describes the benefit to your developing fetus from treatment with a substance. Descriptions of vitamin-and-mineral benefits are provided when applicable.

## 12. Benefits to newborn

Occasionally there are benefits to newborn infants from the mother's use of a substance during pregnancy. These benefits are described here. In the some cases, this section may also describe special uses of a substance in the newborn. For example, Vitamin K is given to newborns to prevent excessive bleeding. This section is only included in a few charts where it applies.

## 13. Benefits during lactation

This section describes the benefits to your baby from your use of a substance while you are nursing.

## 14. Possible effects of deficiency

This section is included *only* under vitamins and minerals. It is divided into five sections that complement the benefits section. They include Deficiency before pregnancy, Deficiency in mother, Deficiency in fetus, Deficiency in newborn and Deficiency during lactation.

Occasionally the phrase "none reported" is used. This may mean the deficiency does not exist. However, it may also mean there is a risk of deficiency, but at this time there have been no reports of complications that can be specifically attributed to that nutrient or deficiency.

## 15. Deficiency before pregnancy

Sometimes deficiencies that are present before conception can have profound effects on the outcome of a pregnancy. An example is folate deficiency and the occurrence of neural-tube defects.

## 16. Deficiency in mother

If you are expected to suffer any adverse effects from a deficiency of a nutrient during pregnancy, it is described in this section. In many cases, effects before and during pregnancy are the same.

## 17. Deficiency in fetus

This section describes the effects of a deficiency on your developing fetus. There is very little information for most nutrients. Most of the information we have is from unfortunate periods of malnutrition in human populations.

## 18. Deficiency in newborn

This section describes additional effects of a deficiency on your baby after he or she is born. For example, severe iron-deficiency anemia in the mother may cause iron-deficiency anemia in the newborn. Often this information is similar to the information under Deficiency in fetus.

## 19. Deficiency during lactation

This section describes the effects of a deficiency on you and your baby. In addition, the effect an agent has on your ability to breast-feed or the quality or quantity of breast milk is discussed when applicable.

## 20. Possible adverse effects

The discussion of possible adverse effects is divided into five sections that complement the benefits section. They include Effects before pregnancy, Effects on mother, Effects on fetus, Effects on newborn and Effects during lactation. "Effects" refer to human studies whenever possible. Animal studies are used only when studies on humans are nonexistent or limited.

Occasionally the phrase "none

reported" is used. This may mean a substance is safe to use. However, it can also mean there is a risk but at this time there are no studies to confirm or refute the theoretical risk. The Recommendations section will clarify the intent.

### 21. Effects before pregnancy

Effects before pregnancy describes possible adverse effects to you from use of a medication, vitamin, mineral or other substance. For example, alcohol intake before pregnancy can adversely affect menstrual cycle, fertility and pregnancy outcome. Common or serious adverse effects of medications are also provided.

### 22. Effects on mother

If you are expected to suffer any adverse effects from using this substance during pregnancy, it is described in this section. In some cases, effects before and during pregnancy are the same. Some substances increase obstetrical risks. For example, cigarette smoking increases the risks of placental tears, hemorrhages and increased bleeding after delivery.

### 23. Effects on fetus

This section describes the adverse effects to your developing fetus from your use of this substance. Adverse effects may be a result of excessive consumption of a substance or possible risk at the dosage level necessary for treatment. Keep in mind that sometimes the risk to you or your baby of not treating a condition is greater than the risk of adverse effects to the fetus from the therapeutic agent. When this is the case, it is clearly stated in the Additional information section. See the phenobarbital chart for an example.

### 24. Effects on newborn

Occasionally there are adverse effects on your newborn infant from your use of an agent. For example, cigarettes increase the risk of sudden infant death syndrome (SIDS) and breathing problems in newborn infants. Infants of mothers who are addicted to narcotics are likely to suffer from narcotic withdrawal.

### 25. Effects during lactation

This section describes the effects to your baby from your use of this substance while nursing. In addition, the effect an agent has on your ability to breast-feed or the quality or quantity of your breast milk is discussed when applicable.

### 26. Additional information

This section provides important information about medical conditions treated with a medication. It is not included in every chart. It is included when information is extremely important to assist you in understanding the importance of a decision to use or not to use a medication.

If an illness is associated with birth defects or other pregnancy-related problems, this section will include an explanation of risks of the illness and benefits of treatment.

Occasionally special information about medications, vitamins or minerals is also included. Primidone, page 218, is converted to phenobarbital in the body. Both substances are found in the blood and tissue if you take primidone. The primidone chart refers you to phenobarbital because effects of phenobarbital can also be found if you take primidone.

### 27. Recommendations for use

This section is divided into three categories: Women considering pregnancy, Recommendations during pregnancy and Recommendations during lactation. Rarely, Recommendations for newborn is also included. This section is intended to be a guideline and should be used to supplement your health-care provider's recommendations. Do *not* change medication without consulting your health-care provider.

### 28. Women considering pregnancy

Recommends steps to take before pregnancy to provide the optimal conditions for your health and your baby's health. Your doctor or nurse should be an active participant in carrying out these suggestions. Your doctor knows your circumstances and will modify recommendations to meet your personal needs.

If you have a chronic medical condition, consult your doctor *before* you become pregnant. Planning ahead can reduce risks to you and your baby.

## 29. Recommendations during pregnancy

Steps to take to provide optimal conditions for your health and the health of your baby during pregnancy. See your doctor or nurse regularly during pregnancy to help you carry out these suggestions. Your doctor knows your circumstances and will modify these recommendations to meet your personal needs. For example, some nutrients, such as iron, are needed in greater amounts during the second and third trimester. If you have problems with morning sickness and iron supplementation in the first trimester, the current recommendation is to delay iron supplementation until the second and third trimester unless you have iron-deficiency anemia. Only your doctor or nurse can determine if you have anemia.

## 30. Recommendations during lactation

If use of a substance warrants special care during lactation, recommendations are in this section. When no information is available on which to base recommendations, the decision to breast-feed requires careful consideration from you and your doctor.

In cases where there is a known risk, breast-feeding may be acceptable with careful attention from your doctor or nurse. This information is also provided. For a few substances, the chart merely states breast-feeding is safe. It is important to pay careful attention to the cautions in this recommendation section.

This section also provides information on vitamins and minerals. If the information is available regarding the effects of too much or too little nutrient, a recommendation is provided.

## 31. Recommendations for newborn

If special problems are expected in the newborn, you will find recommendations in this section.

## 32. Interactions

Interactions is divided into two sections—Interactions with medications, vitamins and minerals, and Interactions with other substances.

## 33. Interactions with medications, vitamins and minerals

Interactions that specifically apply to pregnancy and lactation are included in this section, along with many interactions that apply at other times. For example, phenobarbital decreases the effectiveness of oral contraceptives, increasing the chance of accidentally becoming pregnant. This interaction is listed in the chart.

The term "blood level" is often used in this section. This is the amount of the substance measured in the blood by a specific blood test. An effect on blood level may mean there is more or less of a substance in the body. Or a substance may have changed level in the blood but not in the body. If there is a known significance to the change in blood levels, that significance will be described in this section.

## 34. Interactions with other substances

Interaction with a variety of substances is included in this section. For example, taking some vitamins, minerals or medications with food may decrease effectiveness. Using others with alcohol alters activity.

# Medications

During pregnancy, every substance you take has some effect on you and your growing baby. During lactation, many medications you take pass in some strength to your nursing baby. You must be aware of the effects medications can have on both of you during this time of growth and development. Some effects are beneficial; others are not. This section provides you with information about the various medications you might take during pregnancy and lactation. Be sure to discuss all medications you take—whether prescription or over-the-counter (non-prescription)—with your doctor before you make any decisions.

*Not* taking a medication can cause more harm than continuing to take what your doctor has prescribed. The decision about continuing or discontinuing a medication is one that must be made by you and your doctor together, as a team.

# Acetaminophen

**Definition and description:**
Reduces pain and fever.
**Other names:** Tylenol®; also see brand-name list, page 390.

 **Dosage**

### Safe dosage:
- Usual adult dose—325-650mg every 4 to 6 hours for pain or fever.

### Toxic dosage:
- Exact toxic adult dose cannot be predicted. Severity of toxicity is determined by acetaminophen blood level.
- Serious toxicity can occur after a single large dose or after frequent smaller doses.
- Acetaminophen toxicity causes liver failure and death. Prompt treatment of overdose is important.
- Contact your doctor, poison-control center or emergency room if you think you have taken an overdose.

 **Possible benefits**

### Benefits before pregnancy:
- Relieves pain and fever.

### Benefits to mother:
- See *Benefits before pregnancy.*

### Benefits to fetus:
- Decreasing fever in mother reduces risk of birth defects in the fetus.

### Benefits during lactation:
- Dehydration due to fever may decrease milk production. Treating fever helps reduce this problem.

 **Possible adverse effects**

### Effects before pregnancy:
- Adverse effects are infrequent. Rash, itching, hives*, fatigue, bleeding or bruising, jaundice* and changes in urination may occur.
- Severe liver damage and death can occur from a single large dose or frequent use of moderate doses.
- Daily use for long periods can cause kidney damage.
- Notify your doctor of any adverse effects.

### Effects on mother:
- Pregnant women may have the same adverse effects as any other person.
- Call your doctor if you develop any adverse effects.

### Effects on fetus:
- Most evidence does not indicate an increased risk of birth defects after use of acetaminophen.
- Overdose during pregnancy has variable effects on the fetus. After treatment of the mother, some pregnancies have carried to term with no adverse effects on the fetus. Other fetuses have died. Premature delivery has also occurred. Early treatment of toxic doses is very important for the mother and fetus.
- Kidney failure has been reported in a fetus exposed to high doses throughout pregnancy.

### Effects on newborn:
- None reported.

### Effects during lactation:
- Acetaminophen is found in breast milk.
- Newborns cannot eliminate this medication as well as adults.
- Lactating women may have the same adverse effects as any other person.

# Acetaminophen, continued

 **Recommendations for use**

## Women considering pregnancy:

- Use only recommended doses of acetaminophen.
- Use this medication only when needed.
- Contact your doctor, emergency room or poison-control center immediately if you think you have taken a toxic dose.

## Recommendations during pregnancy:

- See your doctor regularly.
- Use this medication only as directed by your doctor.
- Avoid unnecessary use of this medication during pregnancy.
- Contact your doctor, emergency room or poison-control center immediately if you think you have taken a toxic dose.

## Recommendations during lactation:

- Nursing is usually safe when using this medication in recommended doses.
- Your doctor or your baby's doctor can provide the best recommendation for you.

 **Interactions**

### Interactions with medications, vitamins and minerals:

| Interacts with | Combined effect |
| --- | --- |
| **Metoclopramide** | Increases absorption rate of acetaminophen. |

### Interactions with other substances:

- Use with alcohol may increase risk of liver damage.

*See Glossary.

# Acyclovir

**Definition and description:** Acts as an antiviral to treat genital herpes*. It may also be used for treatment of other viral infections.

**Other names:** Zovirax®.

 ## Dosage

### Safe dosage:
- Usual adult dose for first episode— 200mg 5 times/day for 10 days.
- Dose to suppress recurrent genital herpes*—200mg 3 times/day for up to 6 months.
- Intermittent therapy of recurrent genital herpes*—200mg 5 times/day for 5 days.
- Also available as an ointment or injection for management of other infections. Topical use is less effective than use by mouth. Injectable form is reserved for serious herpes* infections.
- No safe dose has been established for pregnancy.

### Toxic dosage:
- Exact toxic dose cannot be predicted.
- Decreased kidney function has been reported after overdose.

 ## Possible benefits

### Benefits before pregnancy:
- Shortens duration of symptoms of inital genital herpes* infection.
- Decreases recurrence frequency of genital herpes*.
- Acyclovir does *not* cure genital herpes*.

### Benefits to mother:
- See *Benefits before pregnancy.*

### Benefits to fetus:
- None reported.

### Benefits during lactation:
- None reported.

 ## Possible adverse effects

### Effects before pregnancy:
- Adverse effects during short-term use include nausea, vomiting, headache, diarrhea, loss of appetite, dizziness, swelling and rash.
- During long-term suppression therapy, joint pain, fatigue, fever, irregular heartbeat, muscle cramps, menstrual irregularities, swollen lymph glands* and depression have been reported.
- Serious kidney damage has rarely occurred.
- Central-nervous-system toxicity has occurred.
- Notify your doctor of any adverse effects.

### Effects on mother:
- Pregnant women may have the same adverse effects as any other person.
- Call your doctor if you develop any adverse effects.

### Effects on fetus:
- Safety or risk has not been established.
- No adverse effects or malformations were reported in a small number of infants after use late in pregnancy. All mothers received intravenous* injections for life-threatening infections.
- There is no experience with use of acyclovir during early pregnancy.

### Effects on newborn:
- None reported after exposure before birth.
- Newborns treated with injectable acyclovir may develop kidney damage and other adverse effects.

### Effects during lactation:
- There is limited experience with this medication during nursing.
- Acyclovir is found in low levels in breast milk.
- Lactating women may have the same adverse effects as any other person.

## Additional information

- Herpes* infections can be transmitted to your baby during birth or after rupture of your bag of waters. Herpes* infections in the newborn are serious and possibly life-threatening. Prenatal care can decrease the likelihood of transmitting herpes* infections to your baby. Under some circumstances, your doctor may recommend a Cesarean delivery to avoid transmission of infection to your baby.

## Recommendations for use

### Women considering pregnancy:

- Notify your doctor if you plan to become pregnant. Possible risks to you and your baby must be considered on an individual basis.
- Do not begin using acyclovir if you think you may be pregnant.
- Your doctor can provide the best information regarding the risks of genital herpes* infections. Ask your doctor for advice *before* you become pregnant.
- *Discontinue unnecessary use before pregnancy.*

### Recommendations during pregnancy:

- See your doctor regularly.
- Avoid unnecessary use of acyclovir.
- Treatment of life-threatening herpes* infections in women with decreased immune function is *necessary*.
- Treatment of initial episodes of genital herpes* or suppression of recurrent genital herpes* is *unnecessary* treatment in pregnancy.
- Report fluid discharge from your vagina to your doctor.

### Recommendations during lactation:

- Safety or risk has not been established.
- Your doctor can provide the best recommendation for you.

## Interactions

### Interactions with medications, vitamins and minerals:

| Interacts with | Combined effect |
| --- | --- |
| **Probenecid** | Decreases acyclovir effect. |

### Interactions with other substances:

- None reported.

*See Glossary.

MEDICATION

# Albuterol

**Definition and description:** Acts as a bronchodilator to treat asthma*, chronic bronchitis* and emphysema*.

**Other names:** Salbutamol, albuterol sulfate, Proventil®, Ventolin®.

 ## Dosage

### Safe dosage:
- Albuterol can be taken by inhalation, ingestion or injection.
- Dose is determined by the person's size and route of administration.
- Usual adult dose by inhalation—2 puffs every 4 to 6 hours.
- Usual adult dose by mouth—2 to 4mg, 3 or 4 times a day.

### Toxic dosage:
- Toxic dose is influenced by the person's condition, size and age.
- Exact toxic doses cannot be predicted.
- Deaths have occurred from excessive use by inhalation. See *Effects before pregnancy.*

 ## Possible benefits

### Benefits before pregnancy:
- Relieves symptoms of asthma*, chronic bronchitis* and emphysema*.

### Benefits to mother:
- See *Benefits before pregnancy.*

### Benefits to fetus:
- Severe asthma* may have detrimental effects on the fetus. Albuterol relieves asthma* symptoms and improves oxygen exchange in the mother.
- Premature infants of mothers who take this medication may be less likely to develop lung disease associated with prematurity.
- This medication has been used to treat premature labor. This use is not approved by the FDA*. Other similar medications are preferred. See Ritodrine, page 238, and Terbutaline, page 252.
- Initial doses for premature labor may be

higher than normal doses with asthma*. Initial therapy for premature labor is usually an intravenous* infusion. Treatment with oral doses may be necessary after contractions have been stopped.

### Benefits during lactation:
- None reported.

 ## Possible adverse effects

### Effects before pregnancy:
- Adverse effects include tremor, headache, increased heart rate, unusual heart rhythm, insomnia* or drowsiness, nausea, vomiting, sweating or muscle cramps. Chest pain (angina*), high blood pressure and nervousness have been reported.
- Notify your doctor of any adverse effects.
- Albuterol has rarely worsened asthma* symptoms.
- Deaths have been reported from overuse of inhaled bronchodilators.

### Effects on mother:
- Adverse effects during treatment for premature labor include fast heart rate, high blood sugar, low blood potassium, low blood pressure, nausea and fluid in the lungs. Chest pain (angina*) has been reported. Abnormal heart rhythms have been reported. See *Additional Information.*
- Death has rarely occurred in women treated for premature labor.
- Pregnant asthmatic women may have the same adverse effects as any other person.
- Call your doctor if you develop any adverse effects.

### Effects on fetus:
- Malformations have not been reported. However, experience in early pregnancy is limited.
- Safety or risk in early pregnancy has not been established.
- During treatment of premature labor, fetal heart rate and blood sugar are increased.

### Effects on newborn:
- Infants exposed to high doses when mother is treated for premature labor may have low blood sugar.

### Effects during lactation:
- None reported. It is unknown if albuterol enters breast milk.
- Lactating women may have the same adverse effects as any other person.

 ## Additional information

- Pregnancy may affect asthma*. About 50% of pregnant asthmatic women have no change in symptoms during pregnancy, 30% improve and 20% worsen. If symptoms worsen during one pregnancy, they are more likely to worsen in other pregnancies.
- Premature delivery, low birth weight, stillbirth, newborn deaths and maternal deaths are more likely to occur in women with asthma*. Treatment of asthma* improves outcome.
- Premature delivery is associated with a high infant-mortality rate. For each 2 weeks a fetus remains in the uterus between the 25th and 37th week of pregnancy, newborn mortality is cut in half.
- Premature delivery is associated with blindness, mental retardation and severe lung disease.
- Benefits to the baby from medication use often outweigh the risks of using medication. Your doctor will select the best medication for you.
- This medication is eliminated from the body more rapidly in pregnant women than other persons. Your doctor will select the best dose for you.

 ## Recommendations for use

### Women considering pregnancy:
- Notify your doctor if you plan to become pregnant. Risks to you and your baby must be considered on an individual basis.
- Do not exceed the dose recommended by your doctor.
- Notify your doctor if symptoms worsen while using this medication.
- If you have frequent asthma* attacks, it is important to work with your doctor to control your asthma* *before* pregnancy.
- Your doctor can provide the best recommendation for you. Do *not* change your medications unless your doctor tells you to do so.

### Recommendations during pregnancy:
- See your doctor regularly.
- Do not exceed the dose recommended by your doctor.
- Notify your doctor if symptoms worsen while using this medication.
- If your asthma* improves, your doctor may decrease your medication.
- If your asthma* worsens, your doctor may increase your medications.
- Do not adjust your dose without medical supervision.
- Avoid exposure to anything that worsens your asthma*.
- Carefully follow your doctor's instructions for treating premature labor.

### Recommendations during lactation:
- Your doctor or your baby's doctor can provide the best recommendation for you.
- If nursing is attempted, taking albuterol by inhalation produces lower levels of albuterol in your blood and possibly in your breast milk.

 ## Interactions

**Interactions with medications, vitamins and minerals:**

| Interacts with | Combined effect |
| --- | --- |
| Adrenergic stimulants* | Increases heart rate. |
| Beta-adrenergic blockers* | Decreases albuterol effectiveness. |

**Interactions with other substances:**
- None reported.

*See Glossary.

# Aminophylline

**Definition and description:** Acts as a bronchodilator* to relieve and prevent symptoms of asthma* and reversible symptoms of chronic bronchitis* and emphysema.* Aminophylline is converted to theophylline in the body.

**Other names:** See brand-name list, page 390.

 Dosage

### Safe dosage:
- Usual adult dose—600 to 1,600mg/day. Your doctor will use blood levels to determine correct dosage.
- The dose needed may be higher or lower than the range specified.

### Toxic dosage:
- Exact toxic dose cannot be predicted.
- Overdose can cause life-threatening symptoms.
- Toxic symptoms include nausea, vomiting, diarrhea, convulsions, fainting, fever and dehydration.
- Death may occur after severe overdose.
- Call your doctor, poison-control center or emergency room if you think you have taken an overdose.

 Possible benefits

### Benefits before pregnancy:
- Prevents or relieves asthma* symptoms.

### Benefits to mother:
- See *Benefits before pregnancy.*
- The incidence of pre-eclampsia* is decreased in women with asthma* who use theophylline compared to those who are left untreated. See *Additional information* and Theophylline, page 258.

### Benefits to fetus:
- Severe asthma* may have detrimental effects on the fetus. Aminophylline relieves symptoms of asthma* and improves oxygen supply in the mother and fetus.

### Benefits to newborn:
- May decrease hyaline membrane disease* in premature infants.
- Treats apnea* in newborns. Apnea* is a cause of infant deaths.

### Benefits during lactation:
- None reported.

 Possible adverse effects

### Effects before pregnancy:
- Adverse effects include nausea, vomiting, loss of appetite, dizziness, headache, nervousness, sleeplessness, agitation, fast heartbeat, flushing, unusual heart rhythm, fast breathing and rash.
- Notify your doctor of any new or unusual adverse effects.

### Effects on mother:
- Pregnant women may have the same adverse effects as any other person.
- Call your doctor if you develop any new adverse effects or if adverse effects worsen during pregnancy.
- Late in pregnancy, blood levels may increase, causing adverse effects. Call your doctor if you develop toxic symptoms. See *Toxic dosage.*

### Effects on fetus:
- Available evidence does not indicate an increase in malformations.

### Effects on newborn:
- Theophylline toxicity has been reported in some infants exposed to aminophylline before birth. Symptoms include jitteriness, vomiting and irritability. These infants had theophylline blood levels in the therapeutic range for newborns. See *Additional information.*
- Newborns convert theophylline to caffeine in the liver. See *Additional information* and Caffeine, page 352.
- Infants treated with aminophylline may develop restlessness, stomach upset and poor feeding. Serious toxicity may occur with overdose.

## Effects during lactation:

- Theophylline is found in breast milk. See *Additional information*.
- Irritability was reported in a nursing infant exposed to theophylline.
- Lactating women may have the same adverse effects as any other person.

 ## Additional information

- Because aminophylline is converted to theophylline in the body, theophylline blood levels are used to adjust dosage.
- Pregnancy may affect asthma*. About 50% of pregnant asthmatic women have no change in symptoms during pregnancy, 30% improve and 20% worsen. If symptoms worsen during one pregnancy, they are more likely to worsen in other pregnancies.
- Premature delivery, low birth weight, stillbirth, newborn deaths and maternal deaths are more likely to occur in women with asthma*. Treatment of asthma* improves outcome.

 ## Recommendations for use

### Women considering pregnancy:

- Notify your doctor if you plan to become pregnant. Possible risks to you and your baby must be considered on an individual basis.
- Use this medication as directed by your doctor.
- If you have frequent asthma* attacks, it is important to work with your doctor to control your asthma* *before* pregnancy.
- Your doctor can provide the best recommendation for you. Do *not* change your medications unless your doctor tells you to do so.

### Recommendations during pregnancy:

- See your doctor regularly.
- Blood levels should be checked often during pregnancy and for a few weeks after delivery to balance adverse effects and effectiveness of medication.
- Your doctor may want to adjust medication dosage during and after pregnancy. Follow your doctor's instructions carefully.

- Avoid anything that worsens your asthma* symptoms.

### Recommendations during lactation:

- Nursing is usually safe with close medical supervision.
- Your baby's doctor may want to check your baby's theophylline blood levels.
- Notify your baby's doctor if your baby develops irritability, sleeplessness or poor feeding.

 ## Interactions

### Interactions with medications, vitamins and minerals:

| Interacts with | Combined effect |
| --- | --- |
| Barbiturates | Decreases aminophylline effect. |
| Beta-adrenergic blockers* | Inhibits aminophylline action. Decreases aminophylline elimination. |
| Carbamazepine | Decreases aminophylline effect. |
| Cimetidine | Increases aminophylline toxicity. |
| Ephedrine | Increases sleeplessness and nervousness. |
| Erythromycin | Increases aminophylline toxicity. |
| Lithium | Decreases lithium effect. |
| Phenytoin | Decreases aminophylline effect. |
| Ranitidine | May increase aminophylline toxicity. |
| Rifampin | Decreases aminophylline effect. |
| Verapamil | Increases aminophylline effect. |

### Interactions with other substances:

- Smoking deceases aminophylline effect.

*See Glossary.

# Amitriptyline

**Definition and description:** Acts as an antidepressant to relieve symptoms of depression. Amitriptyline is converted to nortriptyline in the liver.

**Other names:** Elavil®, Elegen-G®, Endep®.

 ## Dosage

**Safe dosage:**
- Usual adult dose—50 to 150mg/day.

**Toxic dosage:**
- Exact toxic dose cannot be predicted.
- Overdose has produced serious, life-threatening toxicity.
- Symptoms include confusion, hallucinations*, drowsiness, decreased or increased body temperature, muscle rigidity, dangerous heart rhythm, dilated pupils, low blood pressure and loss of consciousness.
- Death may occur after severe overdose.
- Contact your doctor, poison-control center or emergency room if you think you have taken an overdose.

 ## Possible benefits

**Benefits before pregnancy:**
- Controls symptoms of depression.

**Benefits to mother:**
- See Benefits before pregnancy.

**Benefits to fetus:**
- None reported.

**Benefits during lactation:**
- None reported.

 ## Possible adverse effects

**Effects before pregnancy:**
- Adverse reactions include low blood pressure or (less often) high blood pressure, rapid heart rate, unusual heart rhythm, altered mental state, tingling, staggering, ringing in ears, seizures, dry mouth, blurred vision, constipation, difficulty urinating, rash, hives*, sensitivity to sunburn, low blood-cell count, nausea, vomiting, diarrhea, jaundice*, dizziness, headache and drowsiness.
- Notify your doctor of any new or unusual adverse effects.

**Effects on mother:**
- Pregnant women may have the same adverse effects as any other person.
- Call your doctor if you develop any new adverse effects or if adverse effects worsen during pregnancy.

**Effects on fetus:**
- Most evidence indicates no increased rate of malformations. However, some controversy exists concerning limb malformations.
- Ask your doctor to review the evidence with you.

**Effects on newborn:**
- Use of a similar medication late in pregnancy produced withdrawal symptoms in newborns, including irritability, rapid heart rate, sweating and seizures. See Imipramine, page 140.
- Inability to urinate was reported in one infant.

**Effects during lactation:**
- Amitriptyline and nortriptyline are found in breast milk after use of amitriptyline. See Additional information.
- Lactating women may have the same adverse effects as any other person.

 ## Additional information

- Amitriptyline is converted to nortriptyline in the liver. Both amitriptyline and nortriptyline are active as antidepressants. See Nortriptyline, page 188.
- Pregnancy may be complicated by development or recurrence of a serious mental disorder. Treatments other than medication should be tried first. If the risks of mental illness are considered serious, use of medications to treat your illness is important.
- Depression during pregnancy may threaten you or your fetus if you are suicidal, unable to eat or if you have impaired judgment.

• Your doctor will determine if medication is necessary.

## Recommendations for use

### Women considering pregnancy:
• Use amitriptyline as directed by your doctor.
• Do not exceed the dose recommended by your doctor.
• Notify your doctor if you plan to become pregnant. Possible risks to you and your baby must be considered on an individual basis.
• Your doctor can provide the best recommendation for you.

### Recommendations during pregnancy:
• See your doctor regularly.
• Use amitriptyline as directed by your doctor.
• Do not exceed the dose recommended by your doctor.
• Avoid use near the time of delivery, if possible.

### Recommendations during lactation:
• Nursing is usually safe while using this medication.
• Your doctor or your baby's doctor can provide the best recommendation for you.

## Interactions

### Interactions with medications, vitamins and minerals:

| Interacts with | Combined effect |
| --- | --- |
| Amphetamines | Increases amphetamine toxicity. |
| Anticholinergics* | Increases toxicity of both. |
| Barbiturates | Decreases antidepressant effect. |
| Cimetidines | Increases antidepressant toxicity. |
| Clonidine | Increases blood pressure. |
| Debrisoquin | Increases blood pressure. |
| Epinephrine | Increases blood pressure. |
| Guanethidine | Increases blood pressure. |
| Isoproterenol | May cause abnormal heart rhythm. |
| Methyldopa | Increases blood pressure. |
| Monoamine oxidase (MAO) inhibitors | Causes fever and seizures. |
| Phenothiazines | Increases toxicity of both. |
| Phenylephrine (intravenous*) | Increases blood pressure. |
| Phenytoin | Increases phenytoin toxicity. |
| Warfarin | Increases risk of bleeding. |

### Interactions with other substances:
• Use with alcohol increases drowsiness and slows reaction time.
• Smoking may decrease amitriptyline effectiveness.

*See Glossary.

MEDICATION

# Ammonium Chloride

**Definition and description:** Acts as an expectorant to promote removal of secretions from airways. Also acts as a urine acidifier to increase acidity in the urine.

**Other names:** See brand-name list, page 390.

 ## Dosage

**Safe dosage:**
- Usual adult expectorant dose—300mg every 2 to 4 hours, as needed.
- Higher doses may be used for acidifying urine.
- This medication can be purchased without a prescription. It is also found in products requiring a prescription.

**Toxic dosage:**
- Exact toxic dose cannot be predicted.
- Low doses have caused severe poisoning in some persons.
- Contact your doctor, poison-control center or emergency room if you think you have taken an overdose.
- Symptoms of toxicity include change in consciousness, tremor and exaggerated reflexes.

 ## Possible benefits

**Benefits before pregnancy:**
- May help remove secretions from airways.

**Benefits to mother:**
- See *Benefits before pregnancy.*

**Benefits to fetus:**
- None reported.

**Benefits during lactation:**
- None reported.

 ## Possible adverse effects

**Effects before pregnancy:**
- At high doses, acidosis* has been reported.

**Effects on mother:**
- Acidosis* has been reported in women who were exposed near the time of delivery.
- Pregnant women may have the same adverse effects as any other person.
- Discontinue use and call your doctor if you develop any adverse effects during pregnancy.

**Effects on fetus:**
- Some malformations have been reported after use of this medication, including hernias*, cataracts* and benign tumors*.
- Cough mixtures and expectorants, as separate groups, are each associated with an increased risk of eye and ear abnormalities. Ammonium chloride is found in cough mixtures and expectorants.

**Effects on newborn:**
- Acidosis* has been reported in infants exposed near the time of delivery.

**Effects during lactation:**
- Lactating women may have the same adverse effects as any other person.

 ## Additional information

- The FDA* does not classify ammonium chloride as effective in removing secretions from airways. Increasing fluid intake to 6 to 8 glasses of water a day may be as effective.
- This medication does not cure or shorten the course of an illness. It provides relief for symptoms, but otherwise it offers no benefit.
- Viral illnesses and fever have been implicated as a cause of birth defects. Ammonium chloride is often used to relieve symptoms of viral illnesses. Contact your doctor if you have a fever.
- This medication is often used in combination with other medications. Most studies did not study persons using it alone. It is difficult to determine if ammonium chloride caused any malformations.

**Recommendations for use**

## Women considering pregnancy:

- Use medication as directed on the package.
- Do not exceed the suggested dose.
- Use only when needed.
- Adequate fluid intake may make this medication unnecessary.
- This medication works better with adequate fluid intake.
- Drink 6 to 8 large glasses of water each day.

## Recommendations during pregnancy:

- Safety or risk has not been established.
- See your doctor regularly.
- Adequate fluid intake may make this medication unnecessary for loosening secretions.
- Drink 6 to 8 large glasses of water each day.
- Avoid unnecessary use during pregnancy. Use only if directed by your doctor.
- This medication is not clearly effective as an expectorant, so even minimal risks outweigh benefits for that use.

## Recommendations during lactation:

- Safety or risk has not been established.
- Your doctor or your baby's doctor can provide the best recommendation for you.

 **Interactions**

### Interactions with medications, vitamins and minerals:

| Interacts with | Combined effect |
|---|---|
| **Aspirin** | Increases blood aspirin levels. |
| **Chlorpropamide** | Increases chlorpropamide effect. |
| **Ephedrine** | May decrease ephedrine effect. |
| **Methadone** | Decreases methadone effect. |
| **Para aminosali-cylic acid (PAS)** | Causes crystals in urine. |
| **Phenylpro-panolamine** | May decrease phenylpropanolamine effect. |
| **Pseudo-ephedrine** | May decrease pseudoephedrine effect. |
| **Spironolactone** | Increases risk of acidosis*. |

### Interactions with other substances:

- None reported.

*See Glossary.

# Amoxicillin

### Definition and description:
Antibiotic of the penicillin class. Treats susceptible bacterial infections.

**Other names:** See brand-name list, page 390.

 ## Dosage

### Safe dosage:
- Usual adult dose—250 to 500mg every 8 hours by mouth.

### Toxic dosage:
- Penicillin antibiotics are well-tolerated. Adverse effects increase with increasing dose.
- Exact toxic dose cannot be predicted.
- Life-threatening allergic reaction has occurred after use of amoxicillin.
- Contact your doctor or emergency room immediately if you have difficulty breathing or swelling of the face, mouth or throat. Hives* sometimes precede serious reactions.

 ## Possible benefits

### Benefits before pregnancy:
- Cures susceptible bacterial infections.

### Benefits to mother:
- Some bacterial infections may be very serious to the mother. This medication can cure susceptible infections.

### Benefits to fetus:
- Some bacterial infections in the mother may increase risk to the fetus. This medication can cure susceptible infections.

### Benefits during lactation:
- None reported.

 ## Possible adverse effects

### Effects before pregnancy:
- Adverse effects include nausea, vomiting, diarrhea, rash, hives*, itching, difficulty breathing, anemia* and decreased blood-cell count.
- Fatal allergic reactions have occurred rarely.
- Notify your doctor of any adverse effects.

### Effects on mother:
- Decreased urinary estriol excretion may affect some laboratory tests. Your doctor can select alternative tests that are not affected.
- Pregnant women may have the same adverse effects as any other person.
- Call your doctor if you develop any adverse effects.

### Effects on fetus:
- Penicillin antibiotics are usually considered safe for the fetus.

### Effects on newborn:
- None reported in infants exposed before birth.
- Diarrhea and thrush* may occur in newborns treated with amoxicillin.

### Effects during lactation:
- Amoxicillin is found in low levels in breast milk.
- Thrush* and diarrhea were reported in infants exposed to a similar medication. See Ampicillin, page 30.
- Lactating women may have the same adverse effects as any other person.

 ## Additional information

- Some doctors believe exposure to penicillins during breast-feeding may be associated with allergy to penicillins. There is no supporting evidence.
- Some bacterial infections may be very serious to the mother or the baby. It is important to treat these infections.
- Risks from infection or medication must be considered on an individual basis. Your doctor can advise you.
- Blood levels of amoxicillin are lower in pregnant women than other women given the same dose. Your doctor will select the best dose for you.

**Recommendations for use**

### Women considering pregnancy:

- Use this medication as directed by your doctor.
- Notify your doctor of any adverse effects.
- Ask your doctor for advice if you use oral contraceptives while taking amoxicillin.

### Recommendations during pregnancy:

- Use this medication as directed by your doctor.
- Notify your doctor of any adverse effects.
- Contact your doctor if symptoms continue.

### Recommendations during lactation:

- Nursing is safe when using this medication.
- Notify your doctor or your baby's doctor if you notice white patches in the baby's mouth or if your baby has diarrhea.

 **Interactions**

### Interactions with medications, vitamins and minerals:

| Interacts with | Combined effect |
| --- | --- |
| Atenolol | Decreases atenolol effect. |
| Chlor-amphenicol | Decreases chloram-phenicol effect. |
| Methotrexate | Increases methotrexate toxicity. |
| Oral contraceptives | Decreases contraceptive effect. |
| Tetracycline | Decreases penicillin effect. |

### Interactions with other substances:

- Taking amoxicillin with food decreases effectiveness.

*See Glossary.

# Ampicillin

**Definition and description:** Antibiotic of the penicillin class. Treats susceptible bacterial infections.

**Other names:** Ampicillin sodium, ampicillin trihydrate. Also see brand-name list, page 390.

 ## Dosage

### Safe dosage:
- Usual adult dose—250 to 500mg every 6 hours by mouth.
- Larger doses given by injection may be required for serious infections.

### Toxic dosage:
- Penicillin antibiotics are well-tolerated. Adverse effects increase with increasing dose.
- Exact toxic dose cannot be predicted.
- Life-threatening allergic reactions have occurred after use of ampicillin. Contact your doctor or emergency room immediately if you have difficulty breathing or swelling of the face, mouth or throat. Hives* sometimes precede serious reactions.

 ## Possible benefits

### Benefits before pregnancy:
- Cures susceptible bacterial infections.

### Benefits to mother:
- Some bacterial infections may be very serious to the mother. This medication can cure susceptible infections.

### Benefits to fetus:
- Some bacterial infections in the mother may increase risk to the fetus. This medication can cure susceptible infections.

### Benefits during lactation:
- None reported.

 ## Possible adverse effects

### Effects before pregnancy:
- Adverse affects include nausea, vomiting, diarrhea, rash, hives*, itching, difficulty breathing, anemia* and decreased blood-cell count.
- Fatal allergic reactions have rarely occurred.
- Notify your doctor of any adverse effects.

### Effects on mother:
- Pregnant women may have the same adverse effects as any other person.
- Call your doctor if you develop any adverse effects.
- Decreased urinary estriol excretion may affect some laboratory tests used in pregnancy. Your doctor can select alternative tests that are not affected.

### Effects on fetus:
- Penicillin antibiotics are usually considered safe for the fetus.

### Effects on newborn:
- None reported in infants exposed before birth.
- Diarrhea and thrush* may occur in newborns treated with ampicillin.

### Effects during lactation:
- Ampicillin is found in low levels in breast milk.
- Thrush* and diarrhea were reported in one infant.
- Lactating women may have the same adverse effects as any other person.

## Additional information

- Some doctors believe exposure to penicillins during breast-feeding may be associated with allergy to penicillins. There is no supporting evidence.
- Some bacterial infections may be very serious to the mother or the baby. It is important to treat these infections.
- Blood levels of ampicillin are lower in pregnant women than other women given the same dose. Your doctor will se
- e lower in pregnant women than other women given the same dose. Your doctor will select the best dose for you.

 ## Recommendations for use

### Women considering pregnancy:
- Use this medication as directed by your doctor.
- Notify your doctor of any adverse effects.
- Ask your doctor for advice if you use oral contraceptives while taking ampicillin.

### Recommendations during pregnancy:
- Use this medication as directed by your doctor.
- Notify your doctor of any adverse effects.
- Contact your doctor if symptoms continue.

### Recommendations during lactation:
- Nursing is safe when using this medication.
- Notify your doctor or your baby's doctor if you notice white patches in the baby's mouth or if your baby has diarrhea.

 ## Interactions

**Interactions with medications, vitamins and minerals:**

| Interacts with | Combined effect |
| --- | --- |
| Atenolol | Decreases atenolol effect. |
| Chlor-amphenicol | Decreases penicillin effect. |
| Methotrexate | Increases methotrexate toxicity. |
| Oral contraceptives | Decreases contraceptive effect. |
| Tetracycline | Decreases penicillin effect. |

**Interactions with other substances:**
- Taking ampicillin with food decreases effectiveness.

*See Glossary.

# Antacids

**Definition and description:** A group of products that neutralize stomach acid.

**Other names:** Antacids contain many substances. Substances commonly found in antacid products are calcium carbonate, aluminum hydroxide, aluminum carbonate, aluminum phosphate, aluminum aminoacetate, magnesium hydroxide, magnesium carbonate, magnesium trisilicate and sodium bicarbonate. See brand-name list, page 390, and Calcium, page 284, Magnesium, page 302, and Sodium, page 324.

 Dosage

**Safe dosage:**
- Follow instructions on the package.
- These products can be purchased without a prescription.

**Toxic dosage:**
- Frequent doses or prolonged use of sodium bicarbonate may cause sodium overload* and systemic alkalosis*.
- Taking sodium bicarbonate with milk may cause milk-alkali syndrome*, resulting in high calcium levels, kidney failure and systemic alkalosis*. Symptoms of milk-alkali syndrome* include nausea, vomiting, headache, confusion and loss of appetite. These symptoms have also been occasionally reported with calcium carbonate.
- Aluminum toxicity has been reported in persons with poor kidney function. Nervous-system damage occurs.
- High magnesium levels may develop in people using magnesium salts who have poor kidney function. Severe magnesium overdose can cause low blood pressure, lethargy, unsteadiness, changes in consciousness, nausea, vomiting, difficulty urinating, loss of consciousness and death.
- If you develop any of the above symptoms, discontinue use and contact your doctor.

 Possible benefits

**Benefits before pregnancy:**
- Relieves heartburn*.

**Benefits to mother:**
- See Benefits before pregnancy.

**Benefits to fetus:**
- None reported.

**Benefits during lactation:**
- None reported.

 Possible adverse effects

**Effects before pregnancy:**
- Sodium bicarbonate causes constipation, swelling, appetite loss and belching.
- Calcium carbonate causes constipation or diarrhea, high calcium blood levels and rebound acid secretion*.
- Aluminum causes constipation and lowers phosphate levels.
- Magnesium causes diarrhea and fluid and electrolyte loss. Kidney stones* may occur with use of trisilicate preparations.
- Discontinue use if you develop any adverse effects. If adverse effects are severe, notify your doctor.

**Effects on mother:**
- Pregnant women may develop swelling from excess sodium intake. Sodium bicarbonate is absorbed more than other antacids. Changes in pH may occur.
- Pregnant women may be at higher risk for milk-alkali syndrome* from sodium bicarbonate use or excessive calcium carbonate use because high calcium intake is encouraged during pregnancy.
- Pregnant women may have the same adverse effects as any other person.
- Discontinue use if you develop any adverse effects. If adverse effects persist, call your doctor.

### Effects on fetus:

- Sodium bicarbonate may produce alkalosis* in the fetus. It may also cause heart failure and swelling. Changes in fetal pH may occur.
- Magnesium trisilicate may damage the kidneys.

### Effects on newborn:

- Sodium bicarbonate is associated with bleeding in the brain of some newborns treated with high doses by injection.
- Adverse effects in newborns due to treatment of the mother are rare, in spite of frequent use of antacids during labor.

### Effects during lactation:

- Magnesium is found in breast milk.
- Lactating women may have the same adverse effects as any other person.

 **Additional information**

- Many antacids contain sodium as a manufacturing by-product. Ask your pharmacist for help in selecting one with a low-sodium content.
- High sodium intake has been implicated as a risk factor for high blood pressure and pre-eclampsia* or eclampsia*. Sodium bicarbonate has a very high sodium content.

 **Recommendations for use**

### Women considering pregnancy:

- Use as directed on the package.
- If symptoms are severe or persistent, call your doctor.

### Recommendations during pregnancy:

- See your doctor regularly.
- Ask your doctor for advice about management of heartburn*.
- Use antacids only after non-medication treatments fail and only if your doctor recommends use.
- Do not use sodium bicarbonate as an antacid during pregnancy.

### Recommendations during lactation:

- Use medication as directed on the package.
- Do not exceed the suggested dose.
- Use only when needed.
- Ask your doctor to recommend an antacid for use during lactation.

# Antacids, continued

 **Interactions**

**Interactions with medications, vitamins and minerals:**

| Interacts with | Combined effect |
| --- | --- |
| Aspirin | Decreases aspirin levels. |
| Beta-adrenergic blockers* | Decreases beta-adrenergic blocker absorption (with magnesium hydroxide). |
| Chloroquine | Decreases chloroquine absorption (with magnesium trisilicate). |
| Chlorpromazine | Decreases chlorpromazine absorption (with magnesium trisilicate). |
| Cimetidine | Decreases cimetidine absorption. |
| Corticosteroids | May decrease corticosteroid absorption. |
| Dicumerol | Increases dicumerol effect. |
| Diflunisal | Decreases diflunisal absorption. |
| Digoxin | Decreases digoxin effect. |
| Ephedrine | Increases ephedrine toxicity (with sodium bicarbonate). |
| Fluoride | Decreases fluoride effect (with aluminum and calcium antacids). |
| Indomethacin | Decreases indomethacin effect. |
| Iron preparations | Decreases iron absorption. |
| Isoniazid (INH) | Decreases isoniazid effect (with aluminum antacids). |
| Naproxen | Decreases naproxen absorption (except sodium bicarbonate). Increases naproxen absorption (with sodium bicarbonate). |
| Nitrofurantoin | Decreases nitrofurantoin absorption. |
| Pencillamine | Decreases pencillamine absorption. |
| Phenothiazines | Decreases phenothiazine absorption. |
| Phenytoin | May decrease phenytoin absorption. |
| Phosphorus | Decreases phosphorus absorption (with aluminum antacids). |
| Quinidine | Increases quinidine toxicity (with magnesium, calcium carbonate and magnesium-aluminum combinations). |
| Ranitidine | Decreases ranitidine absorption. |
| Sucralfate | Decreases sucralfate activity. |
| Tetracyclines | Decreases tetracycline effect. |

**Interactions with other substances:**
• None reported.

*See Glossary.

Note: This page purposely left blank.

# Anthraquinone laxatives

**Definition and description:** Acts as a laxative to relieve constipation.

**Other names:** Casanthranol, cascara sagrada, danthron, aloe, rhubarb, senna, aloin, fragula. Also see brand-name list, page 390.

 ## Dosage

**Safe dosage:**
- Usual adult dose varies with the agent. Follow instructions on the package.
- These products can be purchased without a prescription.

**Toxic dosage:**
- These medications are well-tolerated if used for short periods in recommended dosages.
- Laxative overuse can cause diarrhea, weak bones, decreased protein, liver disease, poor absorption of fats, colon problems and low blood levels of potassium, calcium and magnesium.

 ## Possible benefits

**Benefits before pregnancy:**
- Relieves constipation.

**Benefits to mother:**
- See *Benefits before pregnancy.*

**Benefits to fetus:**
- None reported.

**Benefits during lactation:**
- None reported.

 ## Possible adverse effects

**Effects before pregnancy:**
- Adverse effects are rare.
- Liver damage has been reported when danthron is used in combination with docusate.

**Effects on mother:**
- Pregnant women may have the same adverse effects as any other person.

**Effects on fetus:**
- Laxatives of this class have not been adequately studied as individual agents. Safety or risk has not been established.
- Some malformations have been reported after use of medications for stomach and intestinal complaints. These include central-nervous-system, genital, urinary-tract, eye and ear abnormalities. Risk of club foot* was also increased. Cascara sagrada and casanthranol were in this group of medications.

**Effects on newborn:**
- None reported. However, safety or risk has not been established.

**Effects during lactation:**
- These laxatives are found in breast milk. After use of senna, brown discoloration of milk has been reported.
- Diarrhea and colic* have been reported in infants whose mothers take anthraquinone laxatives.
- Lactating women may have the same adverse effects as any other person.

 ## Additional information

- Try non-medication therapies first. Your doctor or nurse can instruct you.
- Increasing fiber in your diet, exercise and adequate fluid intake are helpful. See Appendix 1, page 375, for fiber sources.

 ## Recommendations for use

**Women considering pregnancy:**
- Use as directed on the package.
- Overuse of laxatives can produce dependence on them.
- If you require a laxative for more than a few days, contact your doctor.

## Recommendations during pregnancy:

- Do not use these laxatives during pregnancy. Safety or risk has not been established.
- See your doctor regularly.
- Try non-medication therapies before using any laxative.
- Other laxatives are known to be safe during pregnancy. Ask your doctor for a recommendation.

## Recommendations during lactation:

- Do not use these laxatives while nursing. Your doctor can recommend an alternative.

 ## Interactions

### Interactions with medications, vitamins and minerals:

| Interacts with | Combined effect |
| --- | --- |
| **Docusate (with danthron only)** | Causes liver damage. |
| **Warfarin** | May increase or decrease warfarin effect. |

### Interactions with other substances:
- None reported.

*See Glossary.

MEDICATION

37

# Antibiabetic Agents (Oral)

**Definition and description:**Acts as an antidiabetic agent to lower blood sugar.

**Other names:**Acetohexamide, chlorpropamide, glipizide, glyburide, tolazamide, tolbutamide. Also see brand-name list, page 390.

 **Dosage**

### Safe dosage:
- Acetohexamide—250-1,500mg/day.
- Chlorpropamide—250mg/day.
- Glipizide—5-15mg/day.
- Glyburide—2.5-70mg/day.
- Tolazamide—100-250mg/day.
- Tolbutamide—0.5-2.0g/day.
- *Pregnant diabetic women should not use oral antidiabetic agents.*

### Toxic dosage:
- Exact toxic dose cannot be predicted.
- Overdose can produce serious low blood sugar, with loss of consciousness and death.
- Call your doctor, poison-control center of emergency room if you think you have taken an overdose.

 **Possible Benefits**

### Benefits before pregnancy:
- Maintains normal blood sugar in some (but not all) people who suffer from diabetes*.
- Oral antidiabetic agents must be used in combination with a diabetic diet. Your doctor or dietitian can prescribe a diet.

### Benefits to mother:
- Oral antidiabetic agents do not provide adequate blood-sugar control during pregnancy.
- *Most physicians do not recommend these medications during pregnancy. Insulin provides better diabetic control.*

### Benefits to fetus:
- Adequate blood-sugar control during pregnancy may decrease malformations, premature delivery, excessive size and low blood sugar in the newborn. *Insulin therapy is considered superior to oral antidiabetic agents.* See Insulin, page 146.

### Benefits during lactation:
- None reported.

 **Possible adverse effects**

### Effects before pregnancy:
- Adverse effects include low blood sugar, jaundice*, diarrhea, vomiting, loss of appetite, itching, rash and low blood-cell count.
- Fatal anemia* has occurred.
- Notify your doctor if you develop any adverse effects.

### Effects on mother:
- Pregnant women may have the same adverse effects as any other person.
- *Blood sugar is not well-controlled during pregnancy with oral-antidiabetic agents compared to insulin.* See Insulin, page 146.
- *Poor blood-sugar control is associated with complications of pregnancy.* See Insulin, page 146.

### Effects on fetus:
- These medications enter fetal circulation and alter the secretion of insulin in the fetus.
- Most evidence indicates the rate of malformations is not different than the rate of malformations in unexposed diabetic pregnancies.

### Effects on newborn:
- Low blood sugar persists for several days after delivery in infants exposed to these medications.

### Effects during lactation:
- Lactating women may have the same adverse effects as any other person.

**Additional information**

- *Diabetes mellitus\* may be diagnosed during pregnancy in women who have not been diabetic before. Many of these women will not be diabetic after pregnancy. During pregnancy these women may be treated with diet and/or insulin. Oral antidiabetic medications are not recommended.*
- Diabetes\* is usually harder to control during pregnancy.
- Insulin and diet are the treatments of choice for diabetes in pregnancy. See Insulin, page 146.

 **Recommendations for use**

### Women considering pregnancy:

- Notify your doctor if you plan to become pregnant. The possible risks to you and your baby must be considered on an individual basis.
- Pregnancy outcome is improved in diabetic women who maintain good blood-sugar control before and during pregnancy.
- Your doctor can recommend the best time to change to insulin.
- Follow your doctor's recommendations carefully.
- Follow diet instructions carefully.
- Monitor your blood sugar carefully.

### Recommendations during pregnancy:

- See your doctor as soon as you think you may be pregnant. He or she may want to change your medications.
- Insulin or diet is preferred. See Insulin, page 146.
- See your doctor regularly.
- Follow diet instructions carefully.
- Monitor your blood sugar carefully. Your doctor will recommend the best blood-sugar level for you.
- Even if you have never had diabetes mellitus\*, your doctor may recommend screening tests to make sure you have not become diabetic during pregnancy.
- If you continue this medication during pregnancy, it should be discontinued before delivery. Ask your doctor for recommendations.

### Recommendations during lactation:

- Avoid nursing while using this medication.

 **Interactions**

**Interactions with medications, vitamins and minerals:**

| Interacts with | Combined effect |
|---|---|
| **Clonidine** | Lowers blood sugar. |
| **Methyldopa (with tolbutamide only)** | Lowers blood sugar. |
| **Monoamine oxidase (MAO) inhibitors** | Lowers blood sugar. |
| **Propranolol** | Prolongs low blood sugar. Masks symptoms of low blood sugar. |
| **Rifampin** | Raises blood sugar. |
| **Sulfisoxazole** | Lowers blood sugar. |

**Interactions with other substances:**

- Use with alcohol may produce facial flushing, difficulty breathing, fast heart rate, low blood pressure, nausea and vomiting. Life-threatening symptoms have occurred rarely.
- Use of alcohol with oral antidiabetic agents decreases antidiabetic effectiveness.
- Large amounts of alcohol increase this medication's toxicity.
- Inappropriate diet decreases effectiveness of oral antidiabetic agents.

\*See Glossary.

# Aspirin

### Definition and description: Reduces pain, fever and inflammation. Relieves swelling, stiffness and joint pain of rheumatoid arthritis*, osteoarthritis* and similar diseases.

### Other names: Acetylsalicylic acid, ASA, salicylate. Also see brand-name list, page 390.

 ## Dosage

### Safe dosage:

- Usual adult dose—325-650mg every 4 to 6 hours for pain or fever.
- Higher doses are needed to control rheumatoid arthritis* and related disorders. Salicylate blood levels may be used to determine correct dose for arthritis* and other inflammatory conditions.
- Higher doses are used to treat premature labor. See *Benefits to fetus.*
- Aspirin can be purchased without a prescription. It is also found in products requiring a prescription.

### Toxic dosage:

- Dose ingested is inadequate to predict seriousness of toxicity. Salicylate blood levels are used to determine risk of serious complications.
- Excess use for a short period can produce nausea, stomach irritation, stomach bleeding and vomiting.
- Overdose produces serious heart and lung problems, seizures, loss of consciousness and possibly death.
- Chronic large doses in adults produce rapid breathing, loss of fluid, ringing in ears, confusion and acidosis*.
- Contact your doctor, poison-control center or emergency room if you think you have taken an overdose.

 ## Possible benefits

### Benefits before pregnancy:

- Relieves pain, fever or inflammation.
- Decreases joint pain and swelling of arthritis* or related conditions.

### Benefits to mother:

- Aspirin has been used to prevent pregnancy-induced hypertension* and pre-eclampsia* in some high-risk women. This use is *experimental. Do not* use this medication except as directed by your doctor.
- Also see *Benefits before pregnancy.*

### Benefits to fetus:

- Aspirin has been used to treat premature labor, usually in combination with other medications. This use is *experimental.* Do *not* use this medication except as directed by your doctor.

### Benefits during lactation:

- None reported.

 ## Possible adverse effects

### Effects before pregnancy:

- Adverse effects include nausea, vomiting, abdominal pain, heartburn*, indigestion, bruising, bleeding and ringing in ears.
- Serious adverse effects include drowsiness, jaundice*, hives*, rash, wheezing or vomiting blood.
- Notify your doctor of any new or unusual adverse effects.

### Effects on mother:

- Anemia*, serious bleeding during or after delivery, delayed onset of labor, long labor and Cesarean and forceps deliveries* are associated with aspirin use late in pregnancy.
- Pregnant women may have the same adverse effects as any other person.
- Call your doctor if you develop any new adverse effects or if adverse effects worsen during pregnancy.

### Effects on fetus:

- Occasional aspirin use in pregnancy has not been associated with increased stillbirths or birth defects.
- Regular use of aspirin has been associated with increased stillbirth, birth defects and growth retardation.
- Fetal death was reported after maternal overdose.

- Decreased intelligence and attention deficits have been reported in children whose mothers used aspirin during the first half of pregnancy.

### Effects on newborn:

- Exposure during the 10 days before delivery is associated with increased risk of serious bleeding during or shortly after delivery.
- Death in newborns is reported more frequently after daily exposure to aspirin throughout pregnancy.

### Effects during lactation:

- Small quantities are found in milk.
- An infant developed severe adverse effects possibly related to his mother's use of aspirin.
- Rash has been reported in nursing infants exposed to aspirin.
- It is unknown if the risk of Reye's syndrome* is increased in infants exposed to aspirin in breast milk.
- Lactating women may have the same adverse effects as any other person.

## Additional information

- Use of aspirin or similar medication may be necessary to control severe rheumatoid arthritis* or related disorders during pregnancy.
- Premature delivery is associated with a high infant-mortality rate. For each 2 weeks a fetus remains in the uterus between the 25th and 37th week of pregnancy, newborn mortality is cut in half.
- Premature delivery is associated with blindness, mental retardation and severe lung disease.
- Benefits to the baby from medication may outweigh the risks of using medication. Your doctor will select the safest medication for you and your baby if you need treatment for premature labor.

## Recommendations for use

### Women considering pregnancy:

- Use only recommended doses of this medication.

- Use this medication only when needed for pain and fever.
- Use this medication regularly as directed by your doctor for arthritis* and related disorders.
- If you use aspirin to control rheumatoid arthritis* or related disorders, notify your doctor if you plan to become pregnant. Possible risks to you and your baby must be considered on an individual basis.
- Your doctor can provide the best recommendation for you.

### Recommendations during pregnancy:

- See your doctor regularly.
- Use this medication only as directed by your doctor.
- Avoid unnecessary use during pregnancy.
- If you use aspirin to control rheumatoid arthritis* or related disorders, possible risks to you and your baby must be considered on an individual basis. Follow your doctor's recommendations carefully.
- Avoid use of this medication in the last 3 months of pregnancy, except as directed by your doctor.
- At the time of delivery, tell your doctor if you have taken aspirin any time in the 2 weeks before labor starts.
- Contact your doctor, poison-control center or emergency room immediately if you think you have taken a toxic dose. See *Toxic dosage.*

### Recommendations during lactation:

- Nursing is usually safe when aspirin is used in moderation.
- Notify your doctor or your baby's doctor if your baby is ill or develops a rash.
- Ask your baby's doctor for recommendations and precautions regarding Reye's syndrome*.
- Your baby's doctor can provide the best recommendation for you.

# Aspirin, continued

 **Interactions**

**Interactions with medications, vitamins and minerals:**

| Interacts with | Combined effect |
|---|---|
| **Ammonium chloride** | Possibly increases aspirin toxicity. |
| **Antacids** | Decreases aspirin levels. |
| **Ascorbic acid (vitamin C)** | Decreases ascorbic-acid levels. |
| **Captopril** | Decreases captopril effectiveness. |
| **Cimetidine** | Increases aspirin effect. |
| **Fenoprofen** | Decreases fenoprofen effect. |
| **Furosemide** | Decreases furosemide effectiveness. |
| **Heparin** | May increase risk of bleeding. |
| **Methotrexate** | Increases methotrexate toxicity. |
| **Oral antidiabetic agents** | Decreases blood sugar. |
| **Para-aminosalicylic acid (PAS)** | Increases toxicity of both. |
| **Phenytoin** | May decrease phenytoin effect. |
| **Probenecid** | Decreases probenecid effect. |
| **Steroids** | Decreases aspirin effect. |
| **Thiazides** | Decreases thiazides effectiveness. |
| **Warfarin** | Increases risk of bleeding. |

**Interactions with other substances:**

• Smoking may increase the possibility of having a baby with intrauterine growth retardation.
• Use with alcohol increases stomach irritation and blood loss. Use with alcohol may also decrease blood clotting.

*See Glossary.

Note: This page purposely left blank.

# Atropine

**Definition and description:** As an antispasmodic*, atropine may relieve irritable bowel, irritable bladder and irritable urethra. As a bronchodilator*, it relieves asthma*. As a decongestant, it dries nasal secretions. Atropine may not be effective as a nasal decongestant.

**Other names:** See brand-name list, page 390.

 ## Dosage

### Safe dosage:
- Usual adult dose in non-prescription medications—0.06 to 0.2mg.
- Higher doses may occasionally be prescribed by a doctor.
- This medication may be used by inhalation to treat asthma*.
- This medication can be purchased without a prescription. It is also found in products requiring a prescription.

### Toxic dosage:
- Exact toxic dose cannot be determined.
- Severe poisoning can occur. Symptoms include dry, hot skin, flushing, rapid heart rate, dilated pupils, slurred speech, restlessness, headache, staggering, hallucinations*, loss of consciousness and death.
- Contact your doctor, poison-control center or emergency room if you think you have taken an overdose.

 ## Possible benefits

### Benefits before pregnancy:
- Low doses found in non-prescription medications may decrease nasal secretions.
- May relieve bladder, bowel and urethra spasms.
- May relieve asthma* symptoms.

### Benefits to mother:
- See *Benefits before pregnancy.*

### Benefits to fetus:
- None reported.

### Benefits during lactation:
- None reported.

 ## Possible adverse effects

### Effects before pregnancy:
- Adverse effects include dry mouth, decreased sweating, increased heart rate, unusual heart rhythm, thirst, dilation of pupils, blurred vision, difficulty urinating and constipation.

### Effects on mother:
- Pregnant women may have the same adverse effects as any other person.
- Discontinue use and call your doctor if you develop any new adverse effects during pregnancy.

### Effects on fetus:
- One study found no increase in malformations after use of this medication during pregnancy.
- When used before anesthesia for Cesarean delivery, no adverse effects have been observed in the fetus.
- These results are inadequate to establish safety or risk in early pregnancy.

### Effects on newborn:
- None reported after use during Cesarean delivery.

### Effects during lactation:
- It is unknown if atropine enters breast milk.
- No adverse effects have been reported in nursing infants. However, safety or risk has not been established.
- May decrease breast-milk supply.
- Lactating women may have the same adverse effects as any other person.

 ## Additional information

- Atropine may not be effective as a decongestant in doses found in most non-prescription medications.

**Recommendations for use**

## Women considering pregnancy:

- Use medication as directed on the package.
- Do not exceed the suggested dose.
- Use only when needed for stuffy nose.
- If you use this medication for asthma* or as an antispasmodic, follow your doctor's instructions carefully.
- Notify your doctor if you plan to become pregnant.

## Recommendations during pregnancy:

- Safety or risk has not been established.
- See your doctor regularly.
- Avoid unnecessary use during pregnancy. Use only if directed by your doctor.
- This medication has not been proved effective for nasal stuffiness or irritable-bowel syndrome*, so risks outweigh benefits for these uses.

## Recommendations during lactation:

- Safety or risk has not been established.
- Close medical supervision is required if nursing is attempted.
- Your doctor or your baby's doctor can provide the best recommendation for you.

 **Interactions**

## Interactions with medications, vitamins and minerals:

*Significant medication interactions are unlikely to occur when using recommended doses for non-prescription products. However, these reactions may be significant when prescription-strength medications are used.*

| Interacts with | Combined effect |
|---|---|
| Acetaminophen | Delays acetaminophen effect. |
| Amantadine | Increases atropine effect. |
| Antidepressants | Increases antidepressant toxicity. |
| Antihistamines | Increases atropine effect. |
| Beta-adrenergic blockers* | Alters response to both. |
| Digoxin | Increases digoxin absorption. |
| Monoamine oxidase (MAO) inhibitors | Increases atropine activity. |
| Phenothiazines | Decreases phenothiazine absorption and effect. Increases intestinal pain. Causes heat sensitivity. |
| Potassium tablets | Increases intestinal pain. |

## Interactions with other substances:

- None reported.

*See Glossary.

45

# Belladonna

**Definition and description:** As an antispasmodic*, belladonna may relieve irritable bowel, irritable bladder and irritable urethra. As a decongestant, it dries nasal secretions. As an antidiarrheal, it decreases intestinal motility*.

**Other names:** See brand-name list, page 390.

 Dosage

## Safe dosage:
- Usual adult dose in non-prescription medications—0.06 to 0.2mg.
- Higher doses may occasionally be prescribed by a doctor.
- This medication can be purchased without a prescription. It is also found in products requiring a prescription.

## Toxic dosage:
- Exact toxic dose cannot be determined.
- Severe poisoning can occur. Symptoms include dry, hot skin, flushing, rapid heart rate, dilated pupils, slurred speech, restlessness, headache, staggering, hallucinations*, loss of consciousness and death.
- Contact your doctor, poison-control center or emergency room if you think you have taken an overdose.

 Possible benefits

## Benefits before pregnancy:
- Low doses found in non-prescription medications may decrease nasal secretions.
- May relieve bladder, bowel and urethra spasms.
- Decreases intestinal motility* associated with diarrhea.

## Benefits to mother:
- See *Benefits before pregnancy.*

## Benefits to fetus:
- None reported.

## Benefits during lactation:
- None reported.

 Possible adverse effects

## Effects before pregnancy:
- Adverse effects include dry mouth, decreased sweating, increased heart rate, unusual heart rhythm, thirst, dilation of pupils, blurred vision, difficulty urinating and constipation.

## Effects on mother:
- Pregnant women may have the same adverse effects as any other person.
- Discontinue use and call your doctor if you develop any adverse effects during pregnancy.

## Effects on fetus:
- An increased risk of malformations was found after exposure to this medication during the first 4 months of pregnancy. Malformations reported included lung, genital, eye and ear abnormalities and dislocated hip*.

## Effects on newborn:
- None reported after exposure during pregnancy.
- Infants treated with this medication may develop adverse effects.

## Effects during lactation:
- None reported in nursing infants.
- May decrease breast-milk supply.
- Lactating women may have the same adverse effects as any other person.

 Additional information

- Belladonna is a compound containing atropine (hyoscyamine), aminescopolamine (hyoscine), methylatropine nitrate, methscopolamine bromide and homoatropine methylbromide.
- It may not be effective in doses found in most non-prescription medications.
- Belladonna does not cure or shorten the course of an illness. It provides relief for symptoms, but otherwise it offers no benefit.

- Viral illnesses have been implicated as a cause of birth defects. It is unknown if colds or flu cause birth defects. Belladonna is often used to relieve symptoms of viral illnesses.
- This medication is often used in combination with other medications. Most studies did not study persons using it alone. It is difficult to determine if belladonna caused any malformations.

## Recommendations for use

### Women considering pregnancy:
- Use this medication as directed on the package.
- Do not exceed the suggested dose.
- Use only when needed for stuffy nose.
- Notify your doctor if you plan to become pregnant.

### Recommendations during pregnancy:
- Safety or risk has not been established.
- This medication has not been proved effective for nasal stuffiness or irritable bowel syndrome*, so risks outweigh benefits.
- See your doctor regularly.
- Avoid use during pregnancy. Use only if directed by your doctor.

### Recommendations during lactation:
- Safety or risk has not been established.
- Close medical supervision is required if nursing is attempted.
- Your doctor or your baby's doctor can provide the best recommendation for you.

## Interactions

### Interactions with medications, vitamins and minerals:
*Significant medication interactions are unlikely to occur when using recommended doses for non-prescription products. However, these interactions may be significant when prescription-strength medications are used.*

| Interacts with | Combined effect |
|---|---|
| Acetaminophen | Delays acetaminophen effect. |
| Amantadine | Increases belladonna effect. |
| Antihistamines | Increases belladonna effect. |
| Beta-adrenergic blockers* | Alters response to both. |
| Digoxin | Increases digoxin absorption. |
| Monoamine oxidase (MAO) inhibitors | Increases belladonna activity. |
| Phenothiazines | Decreases phenothiazine absorption and effect. Increases intestinal pain. Causes heat sensitivity. |
| Potassium tablets | Increases intestinal pain. |
| Tricyclic anti-depressants | Increases antidepressant toxicity. |

### Interactions with other substances:
- None reported.

*See Glossary.

# Brompheniramine

**Definition and description:** Acts as an antihistamine to relieve allergy symptoms, including sneezing, runny nose, itching and tearing.

**Other names:** Brompheniramine hydrochloride, brompheniramine maleate, Dimetane®, Histapp®, Rolabromophen®, Symptom 3®, Veltane®.

 ## Dosage

### Safe dosage:
- Usual adult dose—4mg every 4 to 6 hours, as needed for relief of symptoms.
- Long-acting products are available. Follow instructions on the package.

### Toxic dosage:
- Exact toxic dose cannot be predicted.
- Symptoms of overdose include sedation, dry mouth, large pupils, flushing and low blood pressure.
- Serious overdose may cause convulsions and death.
- Contact your doctor, poison-control center or emergency room if you think you have taken an overdose.

 ## Possible benefits

### Benefits before pregnancy:
- Relieves allergy symptoms.

### Benefits to mother:
- See *Benefits before pregnancy.*

### Benefits to fetus:
- None reported.

### Benefits during lactation:
- None reported.

 ## Possible adverse effects

### Effects before pregnancy:
- Adverse effects include drowsiness, rash, hives*, sweating, chills, dry mouth, headache, unusual heart rhythm, low blood pressure, low blood-cell count, confusion, ringing in ears, blurred vision, nausea, vomiting and difficulty urinating.
- Notify your doctor of any adverse effects.

### Effects on mother:
- Pregnant women may have the same adverse effects as any other person.
- Call your doctor if you develop any adverse effects.

### Effects on fetus:
- Other antihistamines as a group have not been shown to increase risk of malformations compared to unexposed pregnancies.
- Available evidence indicates an increased risk of malformations after use of this antihistamine during the first 4 months of pregnancy compared to unexposed pregnancies or pregnancies exposed to other antihistamines.

### Effects on newborn:
- None reported.

### Effects during lactation:
- An infant developed irritability and disturbed sleep patterns after exposure to brompheniramine and ephedrine. See Ephedrine, page 116.
- Lactating women may have the same adverse effects as any other person.

**Additional information**

- Brompheniramine does not cure colds, coughs or minor allergy complaints. It provides relief for symptoms. Occasionally, when allergic reactions are very serious, using antihistamines and other medications can be life-saving.
- Viral illnesses and fever have been implicated as a cause of birth defects. This medication is often used to relieve symptoms of viral illnesses. Contact your doctor if you have a fever.
- This medication is often used in combination with other medications. Most studies did not study persons using it alone. It is difficult to determine if brompheniramine caused any malformations.

 **Recommendations for use**

### Women considering pregnancy:
- Notify your doctor if you plan to become pregnant.
- Use only the recommended dose of this medication.
- Use brompheniramine only when needed.

### Recommendations during pregnancy:
- See your doctor regularly.
- Avoid brompheniramine during pregnancy.

### Recommendations during lactation:
- Nursing is usually safe while using antihistamines.
- Your doctor or your baby's doctor can provide the best recommendation for you.

 **Interactions**

### Interactions with medications, vitamins and minerals:

| Interacts with | Combined effect |
| --- | --- |
| Antianxiety agents | Increases drowsiness. |
| Anti-depressants | Increases drowsiness. |
| Other antihistamines | Increases drowsiness. |
| Tranquilizers | Increases drowsiness. |

### Interactions with other substances:
- Use with alcohol increases drowsiness and slows reaction time.

*See Glossary.

MEDICATION

# Bulk laxatives

**Definition and description:** Acts as a laxative to relieve constipation.

**Other names:** Methylcellulose, carboxymethyl cellulose, malt-soup extract, polycarbophyl, psyllium seeds. Also see brand-name list, page 390.

 ## Dosage

### Safe dosage:
- Usual adult dose varies with the agent. Follow instructions on the package.
- These medications can be purchased without a prescription.

### Toxic dosage:
- Bulk laxatives are well-tolerated if used for short periods in recommended dosages.
- Laxative overuse can cause diarrhea, weak bones, decreased protein, liver disease, poor absorption of fats, colon problems and low blood levels of potassium, calcium and magnesium.

 ## Possible benefits

### Benefits before pregnancy:
- Relieves constipation.

### Benefits to mother:
- See *Benefits before pregnancy*.

### Benefits to fetus:
- None reported.

### Benefits during lactation:
- None reported.

 ## Possible adverse effects

### Effects before pregnancy:
- Adverse effects are rare.

### Effects on mother:
- Pregnant women may have the same adverse effects as any other person.

### Effects on fetus:
- None reported.

### Effects on newborn:
- None reported.

### Effects during lactation:
- None reported in nursing infants.
- Lactating women may have the same adverse effects as any other person.

 ## Additional information

- Try non-medication therapies first. Your doctor or nurse can instruct you.
- Increasing fiber in your diet, exercise and adequate fluid intake are helpful. See Appendix 1, page 375, for fiber sources.

 ## Recommendations for use

### Women considering pregnancy:
- Use as directed on the package.
- Overuse of laxatives can produce dependence on them.
- If you require a laxative for more than a few days, contact your doctor.

### Recommendations during pregnancy:
- See your doctor regularly.
- Try non-medication therapies before using any laxative.
- Use these medications only as directed by your doctor.

### Recommendations during lactation:
- Nursing is usually safe while using these medications for short periods.
- Your doctor can provide the best recommendation for you.

 ## Interactions

### Interactions with medications, vitamins and minerals:

| Interacts with | Combined effect |
| --- | --- |
| Warfarin | May increase or decrease warfarin effect. |

### Interactions with other substances:
- None reported.

*See Glossary.

Note: This page purposely left blank.

# Carbamazepine

**Definition and description:** Acts as an anticonvulsant to prevent epileptic seizures.

**Other names:** Tegretol®.

 ## Dosage

### Safe dosage:
- Usual adult dose—200 to 1,800mg/day.
- Your doctor can use carbamazepine blood levels to determine correct dosage.

### Toxic dosage:
- Varies from person to person. Toxic effects include blood-cell damage.
- Call your doctor if you develop unusual bruising or bleeding, sore throat, fever, abdominal cramps, irregular menstruation, severe staggering or drowsiness.

 ## Possible benefits

### Benefits before pregnancy:
- Use of medication may prevent seizures. Seizures may result in serious injury from falls and accidents. Prolonged, frequent seizures or continuous epileptic seizures may also result in brain damage or death.

### Benefits to mother:
- See *Benefits before pregnancy.*

### Benefits to fetus:
- Use of medication may prevent seizures in the mother. Decreased oxygen supply due to maternal seizures may cause brain damage or death in the fetus.
- Injuries from the mother falling during a seizure may damage the fetus.

### Benefits during lactation:
- None reported.

 ## Possible adverse effects

### Effects before pregnancy:
- Women who are pregnant may have negative pregnancy tests while using carbamazepine. It may also affect home-pregnancy tests.
- Adverse effects include dizziness, drowsiness, confusion, headache, staggering, vision changes, unusual eye movements, diarrhea, skin rash, numbness, weakness, twitching, unusual bruising or bleeding, sore throat, sores in mouth, swollen lymph glands, chest pain and difficulty breathing.
- Notify your doctor of any new or unusual adverse effects.

### Effects on mother:
- Pregnant women may have same adverse effects as any other person.
- Call your doctor if you develop any new adverse effects or if adverse effects worsen during pregnancy.

### Effects on fetus:
- Malformations occur in 10% of children exposed to anticonvulsant medications before birth.
- Minor abnormalities of the hands, feet, face and head include wide nasal bridge, low-set ears, low-set forehead, malformations of eyes and ears, small or absent nails, finger-like thumbs, short fingers, skin folds in the corners of the eyes, single nasopharynx* and hip dislocation*.
- Serious adverse effects, such as malformations of heart, lungs and other breathing structures, small brain, oral clefts*, absent thyroid, absent gallbladder, meningomyelocele*, and slow mental and physical development have also been reported. Deaths due to serious malformations have been reported.
- Childhood cancers have been rarely reported in children who were exposed to carbamazepine before birth.
- Many of the children with malformations or cancers were also exposed to other anticonvulsants.

### Effects on newborn:
- Newborns may be sedated for a few days after birth.
- Infants may develop jitteriness, changes in sleep pattern and irritability for up to 4 weeks after birth.
- Poor sucking and vomiting have occurred up to 4 weeks after birth.

# Carbamazepine, continued

### Effects during lactation:
- Poor sucking has been reported in infants.
- Lactating women may have the same adverse effects as any other person.

 **Additional information**

- You have a 90% chance of having a normal child if you must take medication to control epilepsy*.
- Pregnancy may increase, decrease or have no effect on the frequency and severity of seizures.
- Very severe seizures have occurred when medication is discontinued without a doctor's supervision.
- Having epilepsy and taking anticonvulsant medications increase the risk of having a miscarriage, stillbirth or child with birth defects.

 **Recommendations for use**

### Women considering pregnancy:
- Notify your doctor if you plan to become pregnant. Possible risks to you and your baby must be considered on an individual basis.
- If you have been seizure-free for many years, your doctor may recommend slowly discontinuing this medication before pregnancy.
- If you have a severe seizure disorder, it is *absolutely necessary* to continue anticonvulsant medication throughout your pregnancy.
- Your doctor can provide the best recommendation for you. Do *not* stop taking this medication unless told to do so by your doctor.

### Recommendations during pregnancy:
- See your doctor regularly.
- Blood levels should be checked frequently during pregnancy and for a few weeks after delivery to balance adverse effects and effectiveness of medication.
- Your doctor may want to adjust medication dosage frequently during and after pregnancy. It is important to follow your doctor's instructions carefully.

- If seizures occur, contact your doctor immediately.
- At the time of delivery, tell your doctor you take carbamazepine.
- Get plenty of sleep during pregnancy.

### Recommendations during lactation:
- Nursing is usually safe when using this medication.
- Notify your baby's doctor immediately if your baby is sedated or sucks poorly.

 **Interactions**

### Interactions with medications, vitamins and minerals:

| Interacts with | Combined effect |
|---|---|
| Barbiturates | Alters carbamazepine effect. |
| Doxycycline | May decrease doxycycline effect. |
| Erythromycin | May increase carbamazepine toxicity. |
| Isoniazid (INH) | Increases toxicity of both. |
| Lithium | Increases lithium toxicity. |
| Monoamine oxidase (MAO) inhibitors | Increases monoamine oxidase inhibitor toxicity. |
| Oral contraceptives | Decreases oral contraceptive effectiveness. |
| Other anticonvulsant medications | Increases likelihood of birth defects when more than one medication is needed to control seizures. |
| Phenytoin | Alters phenytoin effect. |
| Theophylline | Increases theophylline toxicity. |
| Warfarin | Decreases warfarin effect. |

### Interactions with other substances:
- None reported.

*See Glossary.

# Castor oil

**Definition and description:** Acts as a laxative to relieve constipation.

**Other names:** Kellogg's Tasteless Castor Oil®, Emulsoil®.

##  Dosage

### Safe dosage:
- Usual adult dose—1 to 4 tablespoons/day.
- Castor oil can be purchased without a prescription.

### Toxic dosage:
- Castor oil is well-tolerated if used for short periods in recommended dosages.
- Laxative overuse can cause diarrhea, weak bones, decreased protein, liver disease, poor absorption of fats, colon problems, and low blood levels of potassium, calcium and magnesium.

##  Possible benefits

### Benefits before pregnancy:
- Relieves constipation.

### Benefits to mother:
- See *Benefits before pregnancy.*

### Benefits to fetus:
- None reported.

### Benefits during lactation:
- None reported.

##  Possible adverse effects

### Effects before pregnancy:
- Adverse effects are rare, but include diarrhea, nausea and vomiting.

### Effects on mother:
- Castor oil has been associated with premature labor.
- Pregnant women may have the same adverse effects as any other person.

### Effects on fetus:
- None reported. However, safety or risk has not been established.

### Effects on newborn:
- None reported. However, safety or risk has not been established.

### Effects during lactation:
- None reported in nursing infants.
- Lactating women may have the same adverse effects as any other person.

##  Additional information

- Try non-medication therapies first. Your doctor or nurse can instruct you.
- Increasing fiber in your diet, exercise and adequate fluid intake are helpful. See Appendix 1, page 375, for fiber sources.

**Recommendations for use**

### Women considering pregnancy:
- Use as directed on the package.
- Overuse of laxatives can produce dependence on them.
- If you require a laxative for more than a few days, contact your doctor.

### Recommendations during pregnancy:
- See your doctor regularly.
- Try non-medication therapies before using any laxative.
- Do not use castor oil during pregnancy.
- Other laxatives are safer during pregnancy. Ask your doctor or nurse for recommendations.

### Recommendations during lactation:
- Your doctor can provide the best recommendation for you.

 **Interactions**

**Interactions with medications, vitamins and minerals:**

| Interacts with | Combined effect |
| --- | --- |
| Isoniazid (INH) | Decreases isoniazid absorption. |
| Sulfonamides | May decrease sulfonamide absorption. |
| Warfarin | May increase or decrease warfarin effect. |

**Interactions with other substances:**
- None reported.

# Cefoxitin

**Definition and description:** Antibiotic of the cephalosporin* class. Treats susceptible bacterial infections.

**Other names:** Mefoxin®.

 ## Dosage

### Safe dosage:
- Usual adult dose—1 or 2g every 6 to 8 hours by injection. Smaller doses may be used in persons with some kidney diseases.
- Gonorrhea* can be treated with 2g of cefoxitin by injection as a single dose combined with 1g probenecid by mouth.

### Toxic dosage:
- Cephalosporin* antibiotics are well-tolerated.
- Exact toxic dose cannot be predicted.
- Life-threatening allergic reactions have occurred after use of cefoxitin. Contact your doctor or emergency room immediately if you have difficulty breathing or swelling of the face, mouth or throat. Hives* sometimes precede serious reactions.

 ## Possible benefits

### Benefits before pregnancy:
- Cures susceptible bacterial infections.

### Benefits to mother:
- Some bacterial infections may be very serious to the mother. This medication can cure susceptible infections.

### Benefits to fetus:
- Some bacterial infections in the mother may increase risk to the fetus. This medication can cure susceptible infections.

### Benefits during lactation:
- None reported.

 ## Possible adverse effects

### Effects before pregnancy:
- Adverse effects include pain and swelling at injection sites, rash, itching, fever, low blood pressure, diarrhea, vomiting, nausea, decreased blood-cell count, liver damage and kidney damage.
- Fatal allergic reactions have occurred rarely.
- Notify your doctor of any adverse effects.

### Effects on mother:
- Pregnant women may have the same adverse effects as any other person.
- Call your doctor if you develop any adverse effects.

### Effects on fetus:
- Cefoxitin enters fetal circulation throughout pregnancy.
- Experience with this medication in pregnancy is limited.
- Cephalosporin* antibiotics are usually considered safe for the fetus. See Cephalexin, page 60.

### Effects on newborn:
- None reported in infants exposed before birth.

### Effects during lactation:
- This medication is found in low levels in breast milk.
- Lactating women may have the same adverse effects as any other person.

 ## Additional information

- Some bacterial infections may be very serious to the mother or the baby. It is important to treat these infections.
- Risks from infection or medication must be considered on an individual basis. Your doctor can advise you.
- Levels of cefoxitin in the blood are lower in pregnant women than other women given the same dose. Your doctor will select the best dose for you.

## Recommendations for use

### Women considering pregnancy:
- Use this medication as directed by your doctor.
- Ask your doctor for advice if you use oral contraceptives while taking cefoxitin.

### Recommendations during pregnancy:
- Use cefoxitin as directed by your doctor.
- Notify your doctor of any adverse effects.
- Contact your doctor if symptoms continue.

### Recommendations during lactation:
- Your doctor can provide the best recommendation for you.

## Interactions

### Interactions with medications, vitamins and minerals:

| Interacts with | Combined effect |
|---|---|
| **Oral contraceptives** | Decreases contraceptive effect. |
| **Probenecid** | Increases cefoxitin effect. |

### Interactions with other substances:
- Cefoxitin produces false-positive results in blood-sugar tests, such as Clinitest®.

*See Glossary.

# Ceftriaxone

**Definition and description:** Antibiotic of the cephalosporin* class. Treats susceptible bacterial infections.

**Other names:** Rocephin®.

 ## Dosage

### Safe dosage:
- Usual adult dose—1 to 4g/day by injection.
- Gonorrhea* can be treated with 250mg by injection as a single dose.

### Toxic dosage:
- Cephalosporin* antibiotics are well-tolerated.
- Exact toxic dose cannot be predicted.
- Life-threatening allergic reactions have occurred after use of ceftriaxone. Contact your doctor or emergency room immediately if you have difficulty breathing or swelling of the face, mouth or throat. Hives* sometimes precede serious reactions.

 ## Possible benefits

### Benefits before pregnancy:
- Cures susceptible bacterial infections.

### Benefits to mother:
- Some bacterial infections may be very serious to the mother. This medication can cure susceptible infections.

### Benefits to fetus:
- Some bacterial infections in the mother may increase risk to the fetus. This medication can cure susceptible infections.

### Benefits during lactation:
- None reported.

 ## Possible adverse effects

### Effects before pregnancy:
- Adverse effects include pain at injection site, fever, rash, changes in blood-cell count, liver damage, kidney damage, headache, dizziness, sweating, flushing, bleeding and diarrhea.
- Severe allergic reactions have occurred rarely .
- Notify your doctor of any adverse effects.

### Effects on mother:
- Pregnant women may have the same adverse effects as any other person.
- Call your doctor if you develop any adverse effects.

### Effects on fetus:
- This medication enters fetal circulation throughout pregnancy.
- Experience with ceftriaxone in pregnancy is limited.
- Cephalosporin* antibiotics are usually considered safe for the fetus. See Cephalexin, page 60.

### Effects on newborn:
- None reported in infants exposed before birth.

### Effects during lactation:
- This medication is found in low levels in breast milk.
- Lactating women may have the same adverse effects as any other person.

 ## Additional information

- Some bacterial infections may be very serious to the mother or the baby. It is important to treat these infections.
- Risks from infection or medication must be considered on an individual basis. Your doctor can advise you.

**Recommendations for use**

### Women considering pregnancy:
- Use this medication as directed by your doctor.
- Notify your doctor of any adverse
- effects.

### Recommendations during pregnancy:
- Use this medication as directed by your doctor.
- Notify your doctor of any adverse effects.
- Risks from infection or medication must be considered on an individual basis. Your doctor can advise you.
- Notify your doctor if symptoms continue.

### Recommendations during lactation:
- Your doctor can provide the best recommendation for you.

 **Interactions**

### Interactions with medications, vitamins and minerals:
- None reported.

### Interactions with other substances:
- None reported. However, alcohol sensitivity has occurred with other cephalosporin medications.

*See Glossary.

MEDICATION

# Cephalexin

### Definition and description:
Antibiotic of the cephalosporin* class. Treats susceptible bacterial infections.

**Other names:** Keflex®.

 ## Dosage

### Safe dosage:
- Usual adult dose—250 to 500mg every 6 hours.
- Smaller or larger doses may be used for some infections.

### Toxic dosage:
- Cephalexin is well-tolerated. Adverse effects increase with increasing dose.
- Exact toxic dose cannot be predicted.
- Life-threatening allergic reactions have occurred after use of cephalexin. Contact your doctor or emergency room immediately if you have difficulty breathing or swelling of the face, mouth or throat. Hives* sometimes precede serious reactions.

 ## Possible benefits

### Benefits before pregnancy:
- Cures susceptible bacterial infections.

### Benefits to mother:
- Some bacterial infections may be very serious to the mother. This medication can cure susceptible infections.

### Benefits to fetus:
- Some bacterial infections in the mother may increase risk to the fetus. This medication can cure susceptible infections.

### Benefits during lactation:
- None reported.

 ## Possible adverse effects

### Effects before pregnancy:
- Adverse effects include nausea, vomiting, diarrhea, abdominal pain, jaundice*, liver damage, rash, hives*, dizziness, headache and decreased blood-cell count.

- Serious allergic reactions have been reported.
- Notify your doctor of any adverse effects.

### Effects on mother:
- Pregnant women may have the same adverse effects as any other person.
- Call your doctor if you develop any adverse effects.

### Effects on fetus:
- Cephalexin enters fetal blood and amniotic fluid.
- Cephalosporin* antibiotics are usually considered safe for the fetus.

### Effects on newborn:
- None reported in infants exposed before birth.
- Newborns treated with cephalexin may develop diarrhea.

### Effects during lactation:
- Cephalexin is found in low levels in breast milk.
- No adverse effects have been reported in infants exposed to this medication in breast milk. However, a similar medication has caused diarrhea and thrush*. See Ampicillin, page 30.
- Lactating women may have the same adverse effects as any other person.

 ## Additional information

- Some bacterial infections may be very serious to the mother or the baby. It is important to treat these infections.
- Risks from infection or medication must be considered on an individual basis. Your doctor can advise you.
- Levels of similar medication in the blood are lower in pregnant women than other women given the same dose. Your doctor will select the best dose for you. See Cefoxitin, page 56.

**Recommendations for use**

### Women considering pregnancy:
- Use this medication as directed by your doctor.
- Notify your doctor of any adverse effects.

### Recommendations during pregnancy:
- Use cephalexin as directed by your doctor.
- Notify your doctor of any adverse effects.
- Contact your doctor if symptoms continue.

### Recommendations during lactation:
- Nursing is usually safe while using this medication.
- Notify your doctor or your baby's doctor if you notice white patches in the baby's mouth or if your baby has diarrhea.
- Your doctor can provide the best recommendation for you.

 **Interactions**

### Interactions with medications, vitamins and minerals:
- None reported.

### Interactions with other substances:
- Taking cephalexin with food decreases effectiveness.

*See Glossary.

MEDICATION

# Cephradine

**Definition and description:** Antibiotic of the cephalosporin* class. Treats susceptible bacterial infections.

**Other names:** Anspor®, Eskacef®, Velocef®.

 ## Dosage

### Safe dosage:
- Usual adult dose—250 to 500mg every 6 hours.
- Smaller or larger doses may be used for some infections.

### Toxic dosage:
- Cephradine is well-tolerated. Adverse effects increase with increasing dose.
- Exact toxic dose cannot be predicted.
- Life-threatening allergic reactions have occurred after use of cephradine. Contact your doctor or emergency room immediately if you have difficulty breathing or swelling of the face, mouth or throat. Hives* sometimes precede serious reactions.

 ## Possible benefits

### Benefits before pregnancy:
- Cures susceptible bacterial infections.

### Benefits to mother:
- Some bacterial infections may be very serious to the mother. This medication can cure susceptible infections.

### Benefits to fetus:
- Some bacterial infections in the mother may increase risk to the fetus. This medication can cure susceptible infections.

### Benefits during lactation:
- None reported.

 ## Possible adverse effects

### Effects before pregnancy:
- Adverse effects include nausea, vomiting, diarrhea, swelling in the throat, abdominal pain, heartburn*, jaundice*, liver damage, kidney damage, rash, hives*, itching, dizziness, headache and decreased blood-cell count.
- Notify your doctor of any adverse effects.

### Effects on mother:
- Pregnant women may have the same adverse effects as any other person.
- Call your doctor if you develop any adverse effects.

### Effects on fetus:
- Cephradine enters fetal blood and amniotic fluid.
- Cephalosporin* antibiotics are usually considered safe for the fetus. See Cephalexin, page 60.

### Effects on newborn:
- None reported in infants exposed before birth.

### Effects during lactation:
- Cephradine is found in low levels in breast milk.
- No adverse effects have been reported in infants exposed to this medication in breast milk. However, similar medications have cause diarrhea and thrush*. See Ampicillin, page 30.
- Lactating women may have the same adverse effects as any other person.

**Additional information**

- Some bacterial infections may be very serious to the mother or the baby. It is important to treat these infections.
- Risks from infection or medication must be considered on an individual basis. Your doctor can advise you.
- Levels of similar medications in the blood are lower in pregnant women than other women given the same dose. Your doctor will select the best dose for you. See Cefoxitin, page 56.

 **Recommendations for use**

### Women considering pregnancy:
- Use this medication as directed by your doctor.
- Notify your doctor of any adverse effects.

### Recommendations during pregnancy:
- Use cephradine as directed by your doctor.
- Notify your doctor of any adverse effects.
- Contact your doctor if symptoms continue.

### Recommendations during lactation:
- Nursing is usually safe while using this medication.
- Notify your doctor or your baby's doctor if you notice white patches in the baby's mouth or if your baby has diarrhea.
- Your doctor can provide the best recommendation for you.

 **Interactions**

### Interactions with medications, vitamins and minerals:
- None reported.

### Interactions with other substances:
- Taking cephradine with food decreases effectiveness.

*See Glossary.

# Chlordiazepoxide

**Definition and description:** Acts as an antianxiety agent to relieve symptoms of anxiety. Also treats symptoms of acute alcohol withdrawal.

**Other names:** A-Poxide®, Brigen-G®, Libritabs®, Librium®, Menrium®.

 ## Dosage

### Safe dosage:
- Usual adult dose—15 to 100mg/day.
- Higher doses may be used to treat alcohol withdrawal.

### Toxic dosage:
- Exact toxic dose cannot be predicted.
- Symptoms of overdose include drowsiness, confusion and loss of consciousness.
- If you think you have taken an overdose, contact your doctor, poison-contol center or emergency room.

 ## Possible benefits

### Benefits before pregnancy:
- Relieves anxiety.
- Relieves symptoms of alcohol withdrawal.

### Benefits to mother:
- See *Benefits before pregnancy.*

### Benefits to fetus:
- None reported.

### Benefits during lactation:
- None reported.

 ## Possible adverse effects

### Effects before pregnancy:
- Adverse effects include drowsiness, staggering, tiredness, confusion, constipation, depression, changes in vision, headache, nausea, dizziness and slurred speech.

- Anxiety has worsened and hallucinations* have rarely occurred.
- Notify your doctor if you have any adverse effects.
- This medication is addicting.

### Effects on mother:
- Pregnant women may have the same adverse effects as any other person.
- Call your doctor if you develop any adverse effects.

### Effects on fetus:
- Malformations are noted in about 11% of exposures in the first 42 days of pregnancy. Unexposed pregnancies had a malformation rate of under 3%.
- There is controversy about the safety or risk of this medication.
- Some studies have demonstrated an increased risk of malformations and other abnormalities after use in early pregnancy. These include mental retardation, deafness, small brain, intestinal defects, spasticity*, heart defects and fetal death. However, other studies did not find an increased risk. Ask your doctor to provide specific information about the risk of this medication.

### Effects on newborn:
- Withdrawal has been reported in newborns exposed to chlordiazepoxide before birth.
- Infants exposed to this medication during labor have had poor muscle tone, low body temperature, poor feeding and unresponsiveness.

### Effects during lactation:
- Drowsiness has been reported in nursing infants.
- Lactating women may have the same adverse effects as any other person.

## Recommendations for use

### Women considering pregnancy:
- Notify your doctor if you plan to become pregnant.
- Discontinue use of this medication, if possible.
- Your doctor can advise you.

### Recommendations during pregnancy:
- See your doctor regularly.
- Avoid use of this medication during pregnancy.

### Recommendations during lactation:
- With medical supervision, nursing may be safe while using this medication.
- Your doctor or your baby's doctor can provide the best recommendation for you.
- Notify your doctor or your baby's doctor if your baby becomes drowsy.

 ## Interactions

### Interactions with medications, vitamins and minerals:

| Interacts with | Combined effect |
| --- | --- |
| Antacids (aluminum hydroxide) | Decreases chlordiazepoxide effect. |
| Anti-depressants | Increases sedation. |
| Cimetidine | Increases chlordiazepoxide effect. |
| Isoniazid (INH) | Increases chlordiazepoxide effect. |
| Lithium | Decreases body temperature. |
| Oral contraceptives | Decreases contraceptive effect. |
| Phenytoin | Increases phenytoin toxicity. |
| Valproic acid | Increases chlordiazepoxide effect. |

### Interactions with other substances:
- Use of alcohol with chlordiazepoxide increases drowsiness and slows reaction time.
- Food increases absorption of this medication.
- Smoking decreases chlordiazepoxide effectiveness.

*See Glossary.

# Chlorpheniramine

**Definition and description:** Acts as an antihistamine to relieve allergy symptoms, including sneezing, runny nose, itching and tearing.

**Other names:** See brand-name list, page 390.

 ## Dosage

### Safe dosage:
- Usual adult dose—4mg every 4 to 6 hours, as needed for relief of symptoms.
- Long-acting products are available. Follow instructions on the package.
- This medication can be purchased without a prescription. It is also found in products requiring a prescription.

### Toxic dosage:
- Exact toxic dose cannot be predicted.
- Symptoms of overdose include sedation, dry mouth, large pupils, flushing and low blood pressure.
- Serious overdose may cause convulsions and death.
- Contact your doctor, poison-control center or emergency room if you think you have taken an overdose.

 ## Possible benefits

### Benefits before pregnancy:
- Relieves allergy symptoms.

### Benefits to mother:
- See *Benefits before pregnancy.*

### Benefits to fetus:
- None reported.

### Benefits during lactation:
- None reported.

 ## Possible adverse effects

### Effects before pregnancy:
- Adverse effects include drowsiness, rash, hives*, sweating, chills, dry mouth, headache, unusual heart rhythm, low blood pressure, low blood-cell count, confusion, ringing in ears, blurred vision, nausea, vomiting and difficulty urinating.
- Notify your doctor of any adverse effects.

### Effects on mother:
- Pregnant women may have the same adverse effects as any other person.
- Call your doctor if you develop any adverse effects.

### Effects on fetus:
- Antihistamines as a group have not been shown to increase risk of malformations.
- Some evidence does not indicate an increased risk of total numbers of malformations after exposure to chlorpheniramine.

### Effects on newborn:
- None reported.

### Effects during lactation:
- Most antihistamines are found in breast milk.
- Lactating women may have the same adverse effects as any other person.

**Additional information**

- This medication does not cure colds, coughs or minor allergy complaints. It provides relief for symptoms. Occasionally, when allergic reactions are very serious, using antihistamines and other medications can be life-saving.
- Viral illnesses and fever have been implicated as a cause of birth defects. This medication is often used to relieve symptoms of viral illnesses. Contact your doctor if you have a fever.
- This medication is often used in combination with other medications. Most studies did not study persons using it alone. It is difficult to determine if chlorpheniramine caused any malformations.

 **Recommendations for use**

### Women considering pregnancy:

- Notify your doctor if you plan to become pregnant.
- Use only the recommended doses of this medication.
- Use this medication only when needed.

### Recommendations during pregnancy:

- Safety or risk has not been established.
- See your doctor regularly.
- Use this medication only as directed by your doctor.
- Do not use this medication during pregnancy unless instructed by your doctor.
- Avoid unnecessary use of this medication.

### Recommendations during lactation:

- Nursing is usually safe while using antihistamines.
- Your doctor or your baby's doctor can provide the best recommendation for you.

 **Interactions**

**Interactions with medications, vitamins and minerals:**

| Interacts with | Combined effect |
| --- | --- |
| Antianxiety agents | Increases drowsiness. |
| Anti-depressants | Increases drowsiness. |
| Other antihistamines | Increases drowsiness. |
| Phenytoin | May increase phenytoin levels. |
| Tranquilizers | Increases drowsiness. |

**Interactions with other substances:**

- Use with alcohol increases drowsiness and slows reaction time.

*See Glossary.

MEDICATION

# Chlorpromazine

**Definition and description:** Acts as a phenothiazine tranquilizer* to treat manifestations of psychiatric disorders. Also controls nausea and vomiting.

**Other names:** Chlorpromazine hydrochloride. See brand-name list, page 390.

 ## Dosage

### Safe dosage:
- Usual adult dose—10 to 2,000mg/day.
- For nausea and vomiting—10 to 25mg every 4 to 6 hours is usually effective.

### Toxic dosage:
- Exact toxic dose cannot be predicted.
- Symptoms of overdose include agitation, restlessness, convulsions, fever, dry mouth, bowel paralysis, loss of consciousness, low blood pressure and dangerous heart rhythm.
- Extrapyramidal symptoms* occur after overdose or occasionally after usual doses.
- Contact your doctor, poison-control center or emergency room if you think you have taken an overdose.

 ## Possible benefits

### Benefits before pregnancy:
- Controls psychiatric disorders.
- Controls nausea and vomiting.

### Benefits to mother:
- See *Benefits before pregnancy.*
- Chlorpromazine has been used to treat nausea and vomiting in all stages of pregnancy.

### Benefits to fetus:
- None reported.

### Benefits during lactation:
- None reported.

 ## Possible adverse effects

### Effects before pregnancy:
- Adverse effects include drowsiness, jaundice*, low blood-cell count, low blood pressure, unusual heart rhythm, seizures, rash, sensitivity to sunburn, dry mouth, nasal stuffiness, nausea, constipation, urinary retention, skin discoloration and eye damage. Tardive dyskinesia* occurs in some persons.
- Fatal anemia*, heart rhythm disturbances and allergic reactions have occurred.
- Abnormal milk production and absence of menstruation occur in some women after prolonged use. These symptoms are associated with decreased fertility.
- Notify your doctor of any new or unusual adverse effects.
- Impotence* and decreased sperm motility* have been reported in men.

### Effects on mother:
- Low blood pressure may occur when chlorpromazine is used during labor.
- Pregnant women may have the same adverse effects as any other person.
- Call your doctor if you develop any new adverse effects or if adverse effects worsen during pregnancy.

### Effects on fetus:
- Most evidence indicates the risk of birth defects is very low with phenothiazines. Malformations found in some studies include abnormalities of the hands, fingers, feet, toes, abdominal muscles, blood vessels, heart and small brain.

### Effects on newborn:
- Difficulty breathing has been reported infrequently in newborns of mothers who took high doses at the time of delivery.
- An infant exposed to very high doses during the last 10 days of pregnancy was lethargic and had poor muscle tone, decreased reflexes and jaundice*.
- Infants exposed to chlorpromazine have developed extrapyramidal symptoms*. Symptoms include excessive crying, abnormal motion, muscle rigidity, blood-pressure changes and delayed early learning. These symptoms may last for several months. They occur rarely.
- Intelligence at 4 years of age shown not to be affected in group of children exposed to phenothiazines before birth.

- Temporary paralysis of the bowel has been reported in a few infants.
- Phenothiazines do not adversely affect birth weight or infant mortality.
- Increased jaundice* was reported in premature infants exposed to phenothiazines.

### Effects during lactation:
- This medication enters breast milk in very low concentrations.
- An infant became lethargic after nursing. Breast-milk levels in the mother were higher than her blood levels.
- Children evaluated 16 months to 5 years after use of this medication during nursing were healthy.
- Lactating women may have the same adverse effects as any other person.

 ## Additional information

- Pregnancy may be complicated by development or recurrence of a serious mental disorder. Treatments other than medication should be tried first. If the risks of mental illness are considered serious, use of medication to treat the mother's illness is important.
- For nausea and vomiting, use medication *only* if nausea and vomiting interfere with eating or daily activities, and other treatments fail. Your doctor can prescribe other treatments. He or she should determine whether medication is necessary.
- Other treatments may include eating soda crackers or dry toast and drinking hot or cold liquids as soon as you get up in the morning.
- A severe form of nausea and vomiting of pregnancy is called *hyperemesis gravidarum*. This condition causes nutritional deficiencies, loss of electrolytes*, weight loss and starvation. It often requires hospitalization. Treatment with antiemetics* alone will not reverse hyperemesis gravidarum*.
- Your doctor will determine whether medication is necessary.

 ## Recommendations for use

### Women considering pregnancy:
- Use this medication as directed by your doctor.
- Do not exceed the dose recommended by your doctor.
- If you use chlorpromazine regularly, notify your doctor if you plan to become pregnant. Possible risks to you and your baby must be considered on an individual basis.
- Your doctor can provide the best recommendation for you.

### Recommendations during pregnancy:
- See your doctor regularly.
- Use chlorpromazine as directed by your doctor.
- Do not exceed the dose recommended by your doctor.
- If nausea and vomiting persist, contact your doctor. Do not increase the dose without your doctor's consent.
- Your doctor can advise you about ways to decrease nausea and vomiting without medication.
- If other treatments fail to reduce nausea and vomiting, contact your doctor *before* using any medication.
- If you use this medication regularly, follow your doctor's instructions carefully.
- Avoid use near the time of delivery, if possible.

### Recommendations during lactation:
- Nursing is usually safe while using this medication.
- Contact your doctor or your baby's doctor if your baby becomes drowsy or lethargic.

### Recommendations for newborn:
- If your baby develops extrapyramidal symptoms*, contact your doctor for treatment.

# Chlorpromazine, continued

 **Interactions**

**Interactions with medications, vitamins and minerals:**

| Interacts with | Combined effect |
| --- | --- |
| Amphetamines | Decreases effect of both. |
| Anticholinergic agents* | Decreases chlorpromazine effect. Increases anticholenergic effect. |
| Antacids | Decreases chlorpromazine absorption. |
| Cimetidine | May decrease chlorpromazine effect. |
| Guanethidine | Increases blood pressure. |
| Hydroxazine | May decrease chlorpromazine effect. |
| Insulin | Increases blood sugar. |
| Lithium | Decreases chlorpromazine effect. Increases delirium and seizures. |
| Merperidine | Increases toxicity of both. |
| Methyldopa | Increases blood pressure. |
| Narcotic analgesics | Increases narcotic toxicity. |
| Oral antidiabetic agents | Decreases antidiabetic effect. |
| Orphenadrine | Lowers blood sugar. |
| Phenobarbital | Decreases chlorpromazine effect. |
| Propranolol | Increases effect of both. |
| Tricyclic anti-depressants | Increases toxicity of both. |

**Interactions with other substances:**
- Use with alcohol increases drowsiness and slows reaction time.
- Smoking may decrease chlorpromazine effectiveness.

*See Glossary.

70

Note: This page purposely left blank.

# Cimetidine

**Definition and description:** Treats duodenal ulcer*, gastric ulcer* and reflux* of stomach contents into the esophagus.

**Other names:** Tagamet®.

 **Dosage**

**Safe dosage:**
• Usual adult dose—400mg twice/day, 800mg at bedtime or 300mg four times/day.
• Dose can vary from 300mg/day to 1,200mg/day.

**Toxic dosage:**
• Exact toxic dose cannot be predicted.

 **Possible benefits**

**Benefits before pregnancy:**
• Treats ulcer disease*.
• Treats symptoms of reflux*.

**Benefits to mother:**
• Cimetidine has been useful in decreasing gastric-acid secretion during labor and Cesarean delivery.
• Also see *Benefits before pregnancy.*

**Benefits to fetus:**
• None reported.

**Benefits during lactation:**
• None reported.

 **Possible adverse effects**

**Effects before pregnancy:**
• Adverse effects include dizziness, sleeplessness, confusion, agitation, depression, hallucinations*, abnormal heart rhythms, constipation, diarrhea, nausea, vomiting, liver damage, kidney damage, low blood-cell count, rash, allergic reactions and increased breast size.
• Notify your doctor if you develop any adverse effects.
• Impotence* and decreased sperm count have been reported in men.

**Effects on mother:**
• When used in labor, no change in duration of labor or contractions was noted.
• There may be an increase in the rate of Cesarean deliveries.
• Pregnant women may have the same adverse effects as any other person.

**Effects on fetus:**
• There is no experience with this medication in early pregnancy. Safety or risk has not been established in early pregnancy.
• A normal premature infant was delivered after the mother used this medication during her pregnancy, beginning in the 16th week.
• Cimetidine was not shown to affect the fetus adversely when used during labor.

**Effects on newborn:**
• A newborn developed liver damage after exposure to this medication before birth.
• Newborns have been treated with cimetidine without adverse effects.

**Effects during lactation:**
• This medication is found in very high concentrations in breast milk.
• Cimetidine increases prolactin secretion. Prolactin is necessary for milk production.
• Cimetidine may decrease stomach acid and cause central-nervous-system toxicity, such as excitation. It may interfere with metabolism of medications the baby takes.
• Lactating women may have the same adverse effects as any other person.

 **Recommendations for use**

**Women considering pregnancy:**
• There is no experience with this medication in early pregnancy.
• Safety or risk has not been established in early pregnancy.
• Use this medication as directed by your doctor.

- Notify your doctor if you plan to become pregnant. Risk to you and your baby must be considered on an individual basis.

## Recommendations during pregnancy:

- Safety or risk has not been established in early pregnancy.
- See your doctor regularly.
- Use this medication only as directed by your doctor.

## Recommendations during lactation:

- Avoid nursing while using cimetidine.
- Your doctor can provide the best recommendation for you.

 ## Interactions

### Interactions with medications, vitamins and minerals:

| Interacts with | Combined effect |
| --- | --- |
| Antacids | Decreases cimetidine effect. |
| Benzodiazepines | Increases benzodiazepine effect. |
| Beta-adrenergic blockers* | Increases beta-blocker effect. |
| Chlorpromazine | May decrease chlorpromazine effect. |
| Digoxin | Decreases digoxin effect. |
| Ketoconazole | May decrease ketoconazole effect. |
| Lidocaine | Decreases lidocaine effect. |
| Narcotic analgesics | Increases narcotic toxicity. |
| Nifedipine | Increases nifedipine effect. |
| Phenobarbital | May decrease cimetidine elimination. |
| Procainamide | Increases procainamide effect. |
| Quinidine | Increases quinidine effect. |
| Theophylline | Increases theophylline effect. |
| Tricyclic antidepressants | Increases tricyclic antidepressant toxicity. |
| Warfarin | Increases risk of bleeding. |

### Interactions with other substances:

- Use with alcohol increases drowsiness and slows reaction time.
- Cimetidine may decrease elimination of alcohol by the liver.

*See Glossary.

# Clemastine

**Definition and description:** Acts as an antihistamine to relieve allergy symptoms, including sneezing, runny nose, itching and tearing. Hives* and other skin reactions respond to high doses.

**Other names:** Tavist®.

 ## Dosage

### Safe dosage:
- Usual adult dose—1.34 to 2.68mg 2 to 3 times/day.
- Skin reactions require doses of 2.68mg.

### Toxic dosage:
- Exact toxic dose cannot be predicted.
- Symptoms of overdose include sedation, dry mouth, large pupils, flushing and low blood pressure.
- Serious overdose may cause convulsions and death.
- Contact your doctor, poison-control center or emergency room if you think you have taken an overdose.

 ## Possible benefits

### Benefits before pregnancy:
- Relieves allergy symptoms.

### Benefits to mother:
- See *Benefits before pregnancy.*

### Benefits to fetus:
- None reported.

### Benefits during lactation:
- None reported.

 ## Possible adverse effects

### Effects before pregnancy:
- Adverse effects include drowsiness, rash, hives*, sweating, chills, dry mouth, headache, unusual heart rhythm, low blood pressure, low blood-cell count, confusion, ringing in ears, blurred vision, nausea, vomiting and difficulty urinating.
- Severe allergic reactions have occurred.
- Notify your doctor of any adverse effects.

### Effects on mother:
- Safety or risk has not been established.
- Pregnant women may have the same adverse effects as any other person.
- Call your doctor if you develop any adverse effects.

### Effects on fetus:
- There is limited experience with this medication in pregnancy.
- Safety or risk has not been established.

### Effects on newborn:
- There is limited experience with clemastine in pregnancy.
- Safety or risk has not been established.

### Effects during lactation:
- An infant became drowsy, refused to feed and developed a stiff neck and high-pitched cry soon after the mother began use of clemastine. Symptoms disappear after discontinuing use.
- Lactating women may have the same adverse effects as any other person.

 ## Additional information

- This medication does not cure colds, coughs or minor allergy complaints. It provides relief for symptoms. Occasionally, when allergic reactions are very serious, using antihistamines and other medications can be life-saving.
- Viral illnesses and fever have been implicated as a cause of birth defects. This medication is often used to relieve symptoms of viral illnesses. Contact your doctor if you have a fever.
- This medication is often used in combination with other medications. Most studies did not study persons using it alone. It is difficult to determine if clemastine caused any malformations.

**Recommendations for use**

## Women considering pregnancy:
- Use only the recommended doses of this medication.
- Use this medication only when needed.
- Notify your doctor if you plan to become pregnant.

## Recommendations during pregnancy:
- Safety or risk has not been established.
- See your doctor regularly.
- Use this medication only as directed by your doctor.

## Recommendations during lactation:
- Do not use this medication if you breast-feed. Your doctor can recommend an alternative.

 **Interactions**

### Interactions with medications, vitamins and minerals:

| Interacts with | Combined effect |
| --- | --- |
| Antianxiety agents | Increases drowsiness. |
| Antidepressants | Increases drowsiness. |
| Other anti-histamines | Increases drowsiness. |
| Tranquilizers | Increases drowsiness. |

### Interactions with other substances:
- Use with alcohol increases drowsiness and slows reaction time.

*See Glossary.

# Clindamycin

**Definition and description:** Acts as an antibiotic to treat susceptible bacterial infections. Also used topically to treat acne.

**Other names:** Clindamycin hydrocholoride, clindamycin palmitate hydrochloride, clindamycin phosphate, Cleocin®, Cleocin T®.

 **Dosage**

### Safe dosage:
- Usual adult dose—300 to 600mg every 6 hours by mouth.
- Larger doses may be injected for severe infections.
- A topical solution may be used to treat acne.

### Toxic dosage:
- Exact toxic dose cannot be predicted.
- Severe colitis* from resistant bacteria may result in death. Notify your doctor if diarrhea develops.

 **Possible benefits**

### Benefits before pregnancy:
- Cures susceptible bacterial infections.
- Used on the skin to treat acne.

### Benefits to mother:
- See *Benefits before pregnancy.*
- Some bacterial infections may be very serious to the mother. This medication can cure susceptible infections.

### Benefits to fetus:
- Some bacterial infections in the mother may increase risk to the fetus. This medication can cure susceptible infections.

### Benefits during lactation:
- None reported.

 **Possible adverse effects**

### Effects before pregnancy:
- Adverse effects after ingestion or injection include nausea, vomiting, diarrhea, abdominal pain, rash, hives*, jaundice*, liver damage, decreased kidney function, decreased blood-cell count and joint pain. Fatal colitis* has been reported.
- Adverse effects after use on the skin
- include dry skin, abdominal pain, irritation, allergic reactions and infection of the hair follicles due to resistant bacteria.
- Topical use for acne results in absorption through the skin. Severe diarrhea and colitis* have been reported after topical use.
- Notify your doctor of any adverse effects.

### Effects on mother:
- Pregnant women may have the same adverse effects as any other person.
- Call your doctor if you develop any adverse effects.

### Effects on fetus:
- This medication reaches high concentrations in fetal blood and tissues after ingestion or injection by the mother.
- Safety or risk has not been established.

### Effects on newborn:
- None reported after exposure before birth.

### Effects during lactation:
- An infant developed bloody stools after exposure to clindamycin in breast milk. The mother was using clindamycin and another antibiotic.
- Lactating women may have the same adverse effects as any other person.

**Additional information**

- Some bacterial infections may be very serious to the mother or the baby. It is important to treat these infections.
- Risks from infection or medication must be considered on an individual basis. Your doctor can advise you.

 **Recommendations for use**

### Women considering pregnancy:
- Use this medication as directed by your doctor.
- Notify your doctor of any adverse effects, especially diarrhea.

### Recommendations during pregnancy:
- Use this medication as directed by your doctor.
- Notify your doctor of any adverse effects.
- Risks from infection or medication must be considered on an individual basis. Your doctor can advise you.

### Recommendations during lactation:
- With medical supervision, nursing is usually safe.

 **Interactions**

**Interactions with medications, vitamins and minerals:**

| Interacts with | Combined effect |
|---|---|
| Antidiarrhea medications | Increases risk of very severe colitis*. |

**Interactions with other substances:**
- None reported.

*See Glossary.

77

# Clonazepam

**Definition and description:** Acts as an anticonvulsant to prevent epileptic seizures.

**Other names:** Klonopin®.

 ## Dosage

**Safe dosage:**
- Usual adult dose—1.5 to 20mg/day.
- Your doctor can use clonazepam blood levels to determine correct dosage.

**Toxic dosage:**
- Varies from person to person.

 ## Possible benefits

**Benefits before pregnancy:**
- Use of medication may prevent seizures. Seizures may result in serious injury from falls and accidents. Prolonged, frequent seizures or continuous epileptic seizures may also result in brain damage or death.

**Benefits to mother:**
- See *Benefits before pregnancy.*

**Benefits to fetus:**
- Use of medication may prevent seizures in the mother. Decreased oxygen supply due to maternal seizures may cause brain damage or death in the fetus.
- Injuries from the mother falling during a seizure may damage the fetus.

**Benefits during lactation:**
- None reported.

 ## Possible adverse effects

**Effects before pregnancy:**
- Adverse effects include dizziness, drowsiness, insomnia*, headache, nightmares, skin rash, dry eyes, dry mouth, swollen lymph glands*, constipation, nausea, vomiting, abnormal heart rhythm, cold fingers and toes, and difficulty urinating.

- Notify your doctor of any new or unusual adverse effects.

**Effects on mother:**
- Pregnant women may have same adverse effects as any other persons.
- Call your doctor if you develop any new adverse effects or if adverse effects worsen during pregnancy.

**Effects on fetus:**
- None reported. Similar medications have been associated with malformations. See Diazepam, page 94.

**Effects on newborn:**
- Lethargy, sedation, weakness, irregular breathing and delays between breaths have occurred in newborns exposed to clonazepam before birth.

**Effects during lactation:**
- Irregular breathing and delays between breaths have been reported in babies exposed to this medication in breast milk.
- Lactating women may have the same adverse effects as any other person.

 ## Additional information

- You have a 90% chance of having a normal child if you must take medication to control epilepsy*.
- Pregnancy may increase, decrease or have no effect on the frequency and severity of seizures.
- Very severe seizures have occurred when medication is discontinued without a doctor's supervision.
- Having epilepsy and taking anticonvulsant medications increase the risk of having a miscarriage, stillbirth or child with birth defects.

**Recommendations for use**

### Women considering pregnancy:

- Notify your doctor if you plan to become pregnant. Possible risks to you and your baby must be considered on an individual basis.
- If you have been seizure-free for many years, your doctor may recommend slowly discontinuing this medication before pregnancy.
- If you have a severe seizure disorder, it is *absolutely necessary* to continue an anticonvulsant medication throughout your pregnancy.
- Your doctor may recommend changing medications.
- Your doctor can provide the best recommendation for you. Do *not* stop taking this medication unless told to do so by your doctor.

### Recommendations during pregnancy:

- See your doctor regularly.
- Your doctor may recommend changing medications.
- Blood levels should be checked frequently during pregnancy and for a few weeks after delivery to balance adverse effects and effectiveness of medication.
- Your doctor may want to adjust dosage of medication frequently during and after pregnancy. It is important to follow your doctor's instructions carefully.
- If seizures occur, contact your doctor immediately.
- At the time of delivery, tell your doctor you take clonazepam.
- Take only the vitamin supplements recommended by your doctor.
- Get plenty of sleep during your pregnancy.

### Recommendations during lactation:

- With medical supervision, nursing may be safe while using clonazepam. Your baby's doctor may want to check your baby's blood level of this medication.
- It may be necessary to stop nursing or to change medication if your baby's breathing becomes irregular or his blood level is high.
- Your doctor can provide the best recommendation for you. Follow your doctor's instructions carefully.
- Notify your baby's doctor immediately if the baby is sedated, has difficulty breathing or breathes irregularly.

 **Interactions**

### Interactions with medications, vitamins and minerals:

| Interacts with | Combined effect |
| --- | --- |
| Other anti-convulsant medications | Increases likelihood of birth defects when more than one medication is needed to control seizures. |

### Interactions with other substances:

- Alcohol consumption may increase risk of malformations.

*See Glossary.

Note: This page purposely left blank.

# Clotrimazole

**Definition and description:** Acts as an antifungal to treat susceptible fungal (yeast) infections.

**Other names:** Gyne-Lotrimin®, Lotrimin®, Mycelex®, Mycelex-G®.

 ## Dosage

**Safe dosage:**
- There are several preparations. Dose varies.
- This medication may be used on the skin or in the vagina.

**Toxic dosage:**
- Clotrimazole is well-tolerated.
- Exact toxic dose cannot be predicted.

 ## Possible benefits

**Benefits before pregnancy:**
- Cures susceptible fungal (yeast) infections.

**Benefits to mother:**
- Vaginal yeast infections are more common in pregnancy. These infections cause discomfort. Clotrimazole cures yeast infections.

**Benefits to fetus:**
- None reported.

**Benefits during lactation:**
- None reported.

 ## Possible adverse effects

**Effects before pregnancy:**
- Adverse effects include itching, burning, irritation and redness.
- Notify your doctor of any adverse effects.

**Effects on mother:**
- Pregnant women may have the same adverse effects as any other person.
- Call your doctor if you develop any adverse effects.

**Effects on fetus:**
- This medication has not been evaluated in early pregnancy.
- No malformations or other problems are reported when used after the 12th week of pregnancy.

**Effects on newborn:**
- None reported after exposure before birth.

**Effects during lactation:**
- None reported in nursing infants. Absorption through the skin or vagina is very low, so presence in milk is not expected.
- Lactating women may have the same adverse effects as any other person.

 ## Recommendations for use

**Women considering pregnancy:**
- Use clotrimazole as directed by your doctor.
- Notify your doctor of any adverse effects.

**Recommendations during pregnancy:**
- Use clotrimazole as directed by your doctor.
- Notify your doctor of any adverse effects.

**Recommendations during lactation:**
- Nursing is usually safe while using clotrimazole.
- Your doctor or your baby's doctor can provide the best recommendation for you.

 ## Interactions

**Interactions with medications, vitamins and minerals:**
- None reported.

**Interactions with other substances:**
- None reported.

# Codeine

**Definition and description:** Acts as a narcotic analgesic to relieve moderate to moderately severe pain. Also acts as an antitussive* to relieve cough.

**Other names:** Codeine phosphate, codeine polistirex, codeine sulfate. Also see brand-name list, page 390.

 **Dosage**

**Safe dosage:**
• Usual adult dose—10 to 120mg every 4 hours, as needed.

**Toxic dosage:**
• Exact toxic dose cannot be predicted.
• Symptoms of overdose include slow breathing, slow heartbeat, drowsiness or loss of consciousness.
• Death occurs after severe overdose.
• Call your doctor, poison-control center or emergency room if you think you have taken an overdose.

 **Possible benefits**

**Benefits before pregnancy:**
• Relieves cough.
• Relieves moderate to moderately severe pain.

**Benefits to mother:**
• See *Benefits before pregnancy.*

**Benefits to fetus:**
• None reported.

**Benefits during lactation:**
• None reported.

 **Possible adverse effects**

**Effects before pregnancy:**
• Adverse effects include depression, dizziness, drowsiness, hives*, rash, itching, flushing, blurred vision, constipation, abdominal pain, vomiting, difficulty urinating and fatigue.
• This medication is addicting.
• Notify your doctor of any adverse effects.

**Effects on mother:**
• Pregnant women may have the same adverse effects as any other person.
• Call your doctor if you develop any adverse effects.

**Effects on fetus:**
• Most evidence does not indicate an increase in birth defects after use of codeine.
• Growth retardation has been reported in babies of addicted mothers.

**Effects on newborn:**
• Infants exposed to codeine during labor may have difficulty breathing.
• Infants have rarely become addicted to codeine after prescribed use late in pregnancy.
• Infants of mothers addicted to narcotics are frequently addicted.
• Addicted infants experience withdrawal. Withdrawal symptoms include poor nursing, irritability, restlessness, continuous crying, sleeplessness, vomiting, diarrhea, nasal stuffiness, fever, tremors* and occasionally convulsions.

**Effects during lactation:**
• Codeine is found in very low concentrations in breast milk.
• Lactating women may have the same adverse effects as any other person.

 **Recommendations for use**

**Women considering pregnancy:**
• Notify your doctor if you plan to become pregnant.
• If you use this medication regularly, ask your doctor's advice about discontinuing use.
• Use only as directed by your doctor.

### Recommendations during pregnancy:
- See your doctor regularly.
- Avoid unnecessary use of codeine.

### Recommendations during lactation:
- Nursing is usually safe while using codeine.
- Avoid unnecessary use of this medication.
- Your doctor or your baby's doctor can provide the best recommendation for you.

 ## Interactions

**Interactions with medications, vitamins and minerals:**

| Interacts with | Combined effect |
|---|---|
| **Acetaminophen** | Increases analgesic effect. |
| **Antidepressants** | Increases drowsiness. |
| **Antihistamines** | Increases drowsiness. |
| **Aspirin** | Increases analgesic effect. |
| **Other narcotics** | Increases narcotic effect. |
| **Tranquilizers** | Increases drowsiness. |

**Interactions with other substances:**
- Use with alcohol increases drowsiness and slows reaction time.

*See Glossary.

MEDICATION

# Cromolyn

**Definition and description:** Acts as an antiasthmatic* to reduce reaction of airways to agents that may cause constriction. Cromolyn is preventive therapy. It is *not* intended to relieve acute asthma* attacks.

**Other names:** Sodium cromoglycate, Intal®, Nasalcrom®, Opticrom 4%®.

## Dosage

### Safe dosage:
- Usual adult dose—2 puffs 4 times a day, initially. Often it is possible to reduce the dose after a response is achieved.
- Cromolyn is used by inhalation. The usual administration system is a metered-dose inhaler*.
- Capsules are also available for use in a special device for inhalation.
- A solution is available for use in a nebulizer*.

### Toxic dosage:
- It is impossible to predict exact toxic dose. Less than 10% of the dose is absorbed from the lungs into the bloodstream.
- Use of capsules during an acute asthma* attack may worsen symptoms. Severe constriction of the airways has been reported.

## Possible benefits

### Benefits before pregnancy:
- Reduces reaction of airways to agents that may cause constriction.
- Prevents asthma* attacks.

### Benefits to mother:
- See *Benefits before pregnancy.*

### Benefits to fetus:
- Severe asthma* may have detrimental effects on the fetus. This medication relieves the symptoms of asthma* and improves oxygen exchange in the mother.

### Benefits during lactation:
- None reported.

## Possible adverse effects

### Effects before pregnancy:
- With the metered-dose inhaler*, adverse effects include throat irritation, bad taste, coughing, wheezing* and nausea.
- After use of capsules and solution, severe constriction of the airways has been reported. Coughing, swelling of the throat, nasal congestion and wheezing* have also occurred.
- Other adverse reactions include dizziness, discomfort on urination, frequent urination, joint swelling, tearing, nausea, headache, rash, hives*, muscle damage and severe allergic reaction.
- Notify your doctor of any new or unusual adverse effects.

### Effects on mother:
- Pregnant women may have the same adverse effects as any other person.
- Call your doctor if you develop any new adverse effects or if adverse effects worsen during pregnancy.

### Effects on fetus:
- Malformations have not been reported in a group of infants exposed to cromolyn. However, this does not establish safety or risk in early pregnancy.
- Ask your doctor to provide specific information about this medication.

### Effects on newborn:
- None reported.

### Effects during lactation:
- None reported.

## Additional information

- Pregnancy may affect asthma*. About 50% of pregnant asthmatic women have no change in symptoms during pregnancy, 30% improve and 20% worsen.

• Premature delivery, low birth weight, stillbirth, newborn deaths and maternal deaths are more likely to occur in women with asthma*. Treatment of asthma* improves outcome.

 ## Recommendations for use

### Women considering pregnancy:

• Notify your doctor if you plan to become pregnant. Possible risks to you and your baby must be considered on an individual basis.
• Use this medication as directed by your doctor.
• If you have frequent asthma* attacks, it is important to work with your doctor to control your asthma* *before* pregnancy.
• Your doctor can provide the best recommendation for you. Do not change your medications unless your doctor tells you to do so.

### Recommendations during pregnancy:

• See your doctor regularly.
• Avoid anything that worsens your asthma* symptoms.
• Use this medication as directed by your doctor.

### Recommendations during lactation:

• Due to low levels in your blood and poor absorption after oral use, adverse effects to your baby are not expected.
• Your doctor can provide the best recommendation for you.

 ## Interactions

### Interactions with medications, vitamins and minerals:

| Interacts with | Combined effect |
| --- | --- |
| Corticosteroids | May decrease need for corticosteroids. |

### Interactions with other substances:

• None reported.

*See Glossary.

# Cyclizine

**Definition and description:** Antihistamine that acts as an antiemetic* to control nausea, vomiting and dizziness of motion sickness.

**Other names:** Marzine®, Valoid®.

 ## Dosage

### Safe dosage:
- Usual adult dose—50mg every 4 to 6 hours, to a maximum of 200mg a day.
- This medication can be purchased without a prescription.

### Toxic dosage:
- Exact toxic dose cannot be predicted.
- Serious toxicity has occurred with antihistamine overdose. Contact your doctor, poison-control center or emergency room if you think you have taken an overdose.

 ## Possible benefits

### Benefits before pregnancy:
- Treats nausea and vomiting.

### Benefits to mother:
- May relieve nausea and vomiting.
- Effectiveness of non-prescription antiemetics* has not been proved for nausea and vomiting in pregnancy.

### Benefits to fetus:
- None reported.

### Benefits during lactation:
- None reported.

 ## Possible adverse effects

### Effects before pregnancy:
- Adverse effects include drowsiness, dry mouth, rash, hives*, nervousness, sleeplessness, loss of appetite, nausea, vomiting, diarrhea, constipation, ringing in ears, changes in heart rhythm, difficulty urinating, hallucinations* and blurred vision.
- Notify your doctor of any adverse effects.

### Effects on mother:
- Pregnant women may have the same adverse effects as any other person.
- Call your doctor if you develop any adverse effects.

### Effects on fetus:
- Cyclizine has not been shown to increase malformation rates.
- Antihistamines as a group were not found to increase risk of malformations compared to unexposed pregnancies.

### Effects on newborn:
- None reported.

### Effects during lactation:
- None reported in nursing infants.
- Lactating women may have the same adverse effect as any other person.

 ## Additional information

- In 1966, the FDA* required cyclizine to carry warnings against use by pregnant women. The warning was based on animal studies that demonstrated increased fetal death and malformations. Since then, the warning has been removed, based on evaluation of use by pregnant women. Risk from this medication is low. See *Effects on fetus*.
- Use medication *only* if nausea and vomiting interfere with eating or daily activities, and other treatments fail. Your doctor can prescribe other treatments. He or she should determine whether medication is necessary.
- Other treatments may include eating soda crackers or dry toast and drinking hot or cold liquids as soon as you get up in the morning.
- A severe form of nausea and vomiting of pregnancy is called *hyperemesis gravidarum*. This condition causes nutritional deficiencies, loss of electrolytes*, weight loss and starvation. It often requires hospitalization. Treatment with antiemetics* alone will not reverse hyperemesis gravidarum*.

**Recommendations for use**

### Women considering pregnancy:
- Use cyclizine as directed on the package.
- Use this medication only as needed.
- Notify your doctor if you plan to become pregnant. Before pregnancy, your doctor can advise you about ways to decrease nausea and vomiting without medication.

### Recommendations during pregnancy:
- If you have severe vomiting, contact your doctor as soon as possible.
- See your doctor regularly.
- Your doctor can advise you about ways to decrease nausea and vomiting without medication.
- If other treatments fail to reduce nausea and vomiting, contact your doctor *before* using any medication.
- Use this medication only as directed by your doctor.

### Recommendations during lactation:
- Nursing is usually safe while using antihistamines.
- Your doctor or your baby's doctor can provide the best recommendation for you.

 **Interactions**

### Interactions with medications, vitamins and minerals:

| Interacts with | Combined effect |
| --- | --- |
| Antianxiety agents | Increases drowsiness. |
| Antidepressants | Increases drowsiness. |
| Other antihistamines | Increases drowsiness. |
| Tranquilizers | Increases drowsiness. |

### Interactions with other substances:
- Use with alcohol increases drowsiness and slows reaction time.

*See Glossary.

MEDICATION

# Cyproheptadine

**Definition and description:** Acts as an antihistamine and antiserotonin* to relieve allergy symptoms, including sneezing, runny nose, itching, tearing, hives* and other skin reactions. May be used with epinephrine for severe, life-threatening allergic reactions.

**Other names:** Periactin®.

 **Dosage**

**Safe dosage:**
• Usual adult dose—4mg 3 times/day.

**Toxic dosage:**
• Exact toxic dose cannot be predicted.
• Symptoms of overdose include sedation, dry mouth, large pupils, flushing and low blood pressure.
• Serious overdose may cause convulsions and death.
• Contact your doctor, poison-control center or emergency room if you think you have taken an overdose.

 **Possible benefits**

**Benefits before pregnancy:**
• Relieves allergy symptoms.

**Benefits to mother:**
• See *Benefits before pregnancy.*

**Benefits to fetus:**
• None reported.

**Benefits during lactation:**
• None reported.

 **Possible adverse effects**

**Effects before pregnancy:**
• Adverse effects include drowsiness, dizziness, confusion, restlessness, irritability, tingling in extremities, hallucinations*, faintness, rash, hives*, sensitivity to sunburn, vertigo*, blurred vision, ringing in ears, low blood pressure, unusual heart rhythm, low blood-cell count, dry mouth, vomiting, diarrhea, jaundice*, changes in urination, chills and headache.

**Effects on mother:**
• Pregnant women may have the same adverse effects as any other person.
• Call your doctor if you develop any adverse effects.

**Effects on fetus:**
• When cyproheptadine has been used to prevent recurring miscarriages, no malformations were noted.
• A person treated with this medication for Cushing's disease* delivered a normal infant. The medication was discontinued after 3 months of pregnancy. This evidence is insufficient to establish safety or risk in early pregnancy.

**Effects on newborn:**
• None reported.

**Effects during lactation:**
• Lactating women may have the same adverse effects as any other person.

 **Additional information**

• Cyproheptadine does not cure colds, coughs or minor allergy complaints. It provides relief for symptoms. Occasionally, when allergic reactions are very serious, using antihistamines and other medications can be life-saving.
• Viral illnesses and fever have been implicated as a cause of birth defects. This medication is often used to relieve symptoms of viral illnesses. Contact your doctor if you have a fever.

**Recommendations for use**

### Women considering pregnancy:
- Notify your doctor if you plan to become pregnant.
- Use only the recommended doses of cyproheptadine.
- Use this medication only when needed.

### Recommendations during pregnancy:
- Safety or risk has not been established.
- See your doctor regularly.
- Use cyproheptadine only as directed by your doctor.
- Avoid unnecessary use of this medication.

### Recommendations during lactation:
- Avoid use during lactation.

 **Interactions**

### Interactions with medications, vitamins and minerals:

| Interacts with | Combined effect |
| --- | --- |
| **Antianxiety agents** | Increases drowsiness. |
| **Antidepressants** | Increases drowsiness. |
| **Other anti-histamines** | Increases drowsiness. |
| **Tranquilizers** | Increases drowsiness. |

### Interactions with other substances:
- Use with alcohol increases drowsiness and slows reaction time.

*See Glossary.

# Desipramine

**Definition and description:** Acts as an antidepressant to relieve symptoms of depression.

**Other names:** Norpramin®, Pertofrane®.

 ## Dosage

**Safe dosage:**
- Usual adult dose—100 to 300mg/day.

**Toxic dosage:**
- Exact toxic dose cannot be predicted.
- Overdose has produced serious, life-threatening toxicity.
- Symptoms include confusion, hallucinations*, drowsiness, decreased or increased body temperature, muscle rigidity, dangerous heart rhythm, dilated pupils, low blood pressure, seizures and loss of consciousness.
- Death may occur after severe overdose.
- Contact your doctor, poison-control center or emergency room if you think you have taken an overdose.

 ## Possible benefits

**Benefits before pregnancy:**
- Controls symptoms of depression.

**Benefits to mother:**
- See *Benefits before pregnancy.*

**Benefits to fetus:**
- None reported.

**Benefits during lactation:**
- None reported.

 ## Possible adverse effects

**Effects before pregnancy:**
- Adverse reactions include low blood pressure or (less often) high blood pressure, rapid heart rate, unusual heart rhythm, altered mental state, tingling, staggering, ringing in the ears, seizures, dry mouth, blurred vision, constipation, difficulty urinating, rash, hives*, sensitivity to sunburn, low blood-cell count, nausea, vomiting, diarrhea, jaundice*, dizziness, headache and drowsiness.
- Notify your doctor of any new or unusual adverse effects.

**Effects on mother:**
- Pregnant women may have the same adverse effects as any other person.
- Call your doctor if you develop any new adverse effects or if adverse effects worsen during pregnancy.

**Effects on fetus:**
- No malformations have been reported with use of this medication. However, experience is limited with desipramine.
- Safety or risk has not been established in early pregnancy.

**Effects on newborn:**
- Use of this medication produced withdrawal symptoms in newborns, including weight loss, sweating, fast heart rate and decreased oxygen in the blood.
- Inability to urinate was reported in one infant.

**Effects during lactation:**
- Desipramine is found in breast milk.
- Lactating women may have the same adverse effects as any other person.

 ## Additional information

- Pregnancy may be complicated by development or recurrence of a serious mental disorder. Treatments other than medication should be tried first. If the risks of mental illness are considered serious, use of medications to treat the mother's illness is important.
- Depression during pregnancy may threaten you or your fetus if you are suicidal, unable to eat or if you have impaired judgment.
- Your doctor will determine if medication is necessary.

# Desipramine, continued

 ## Recommendations for use

### Women considering pregnancy:
- Use this medication as directed by your doctor.
- Do not exceed the dose or frequency recommended by your doctor.
- Notify your doctor if you plan to become pregnant. Possible risks to you and your baby must be considered on an individual basis.
- Your doctor can provide the best recommendation for you.

### Recommendations during pregnancy:
- See your doctor regularly.
- Use this medication as directed by your doctor.
- Do not exceed the dose recommended by your doctor.
- Avoid use near the time of delivery, if possible.

### Recommendations during lactation:
- Nursing is usually safe while using desipramine.
- Your doctor or your baby's doctor can provide the best recommendation for you.

 ## Interactions

### Interactions with medications, vitamins and minerals:

| Interacts with | Combined effect |
| --- | --- |
| Amphetamines | Increases amphetamine toxicity. |
| Anticholinergics* | Increases toxicity of both. |
| Barbiturates | Decreases antidepressant effect. |
| Cimetidine | Increases antidepressant toxicity. |
| Clonidine | Increases blood pressure. |
| Debrisoquin | Increases blood pressure. |
| Epinephrine | Increases blood pressure. |
| Guanethidine | Increases blood pressure. |
| Methyldopa | Increases blood pressure. |
| Monoamine oxidase (MAO) inhibitors | Causes fever and seizures. |
| Phenothiazines | Increases toxicity. |
| Phenylephrine (intravenous*) | Increases blood pressure. |
| Phenytoin | Increases phenytoin toxicity. |

### Interactions with other substances:
- Use with alcohol increases drowsiness and slows reaction time.
- Smoking may decrease desipramine effectiveness.

*See Glossary.

91

# Dextromethorphan

**Definition and description:** Acts as an antitussive* to relieve cough.

**Other names:** See brand-name list, page 390.

 ## Dosage

### Safe dosage:
- Usual adult dose—10 to 20mg every 4 hours or 30mg every 6 to 8 hours, as needed.
- This medication can be purchased without a prescription. It is also found in products requiring a prescription.

### Toxic dosage:
- Large doses in adults have produced intoxication and bizarre behavior.
- Children have developed an unusual gait and change of consciousness after receiving more than the recommended dose.

 ## Possible benefits

### Benefits before pregnancy:
- Relieves cough.

### Benefits to mother:
- See *Benefits before pregnancy.*

### Benefits to fetus:
- None reported.

### Benefits during lactation:
- None reported.

 ## Possible adverse effects

### Effects before pregnancy:
- Adverse effects include drowsiness, nausea and vomiting.

### Effects on mother:
- Pregnant women may have the same adverse effects as any other person.
- Discontinue use, and call your doctor if you develop any adverse effects during pregnancy.

### Effects on fetus:
- Safety or risk has not been established.
- Cough mixtures as a group are associated with an increased risk of eye and ear abnormalities.
- Antitussives* as a group are associated with an increased risk of malformations of the central nervous system, heart, blood vessels, muscles, bones, intestinal tract, stomach, genitals, eyes and ears and tumors* after exposure during the first 4 months of pregnancy.

### Effects on newborn:
- None reported.

### Effects during lactation:
- Lactating women may have the same adverse effects as any other person.

 ## Additional information

- Dextromethorphan does not cure or shorten the course of an illness. It provides relief for symptoms, but otherwise it offers no benefit.
- Viral illnesses and fever have been implicated as a cause of birth defects. Dextromethorphan is often used to relieve symptoms of viral illnesses. Contact your doctor if you have a fever.
- This medication is often used in combination with other medications. Most studies did not study persons using it alone. It is difficult to determine if dextromethorphan caused any malformations.

**Recommendations for use**

### Women considering pregnancy:
- Use medication as directed on the package.
- Do not exceed the suggested dose.
- Use only when needed.

### Recommendations during pregnancy:
- Safety or risk has not been established.
- See your doctor regularly.
- Avoid unnecessary use during pregnancy. Use only if directed by your doctor.

### Recommendations during lactation:
- Safety or risk has not been established.
- Your doctor or your baby's doctor can provide the best recommendation for you.

 **Interactions**

### Interactions with medications, vitamins, minerals

| Interacts with | Combined effect |
|---|---|
| **Phenelzine (an MAO inhibitor)** | May cause very high blood pressure, leading to death. |

### Interactions with other substances:
- None reported.

*See Glossary.

MEDICATION

# Diazepam

**Definition and description:** Acts as an antianxiety agent to relieve symptoms of anxiety. As an anticonvulsant, diazepam (administered by injection) can treat prolonged, life-threatening seizures. May be used by mouth in combination with other medications to control seizures. As an antispasmodic*, it relieves muscle spasm. Also treats symptoms of acute alcohol withdrawal. Diazepam is converted to oxazepam in the liver.

**Other names:** Valcaps®, Valium®, Valrelease®, T-Quil®.

 Dosage

## Safe dosage:
- Usual adult dose by mouth—4 to 40mg/day for anxiety, muscle spasm or alcohol withdrawal.
- Injectable doses for seizures or alcohol withdrawal may be higher.

## Toxic dosage:
- Exact toxic dose cannot be predicted.
- Symptoms of overdose include drowsiness, confusion and loss of consciousness.
- If you think you have taken an overdose, contact your doctor, poison-control center or emergency room.

 Possible benefits

## Benefits before pregnancy:
- Relieves anxiety, symptoms of alcohol withdrawal, muscle spasm or seizures. Prolonged, frequent seizures or continuous epileptic seizures may result in brain damage or death.

## Benefits to mother:
- See *Benefits before pregnancy.*

## Benefits to fetus:
- Use of medication may prevent seizures in the mother. Decreased oxygen supply due to maternal seizures may cause brain damage or death in the fetus.

## Benefits during lactation:
- None reported.

 Possible adverse effects

## Effects before pregnancy:
- Adverse effects include drowsiness, staggering, tiredness, confusion, constipation, depression, changes in vision, headache, nausea, dizziness and slurred speach.
- In rare cases, anxiety has worsened and hallucinations* have occurred.
- This medication is addicting.
- Notify your doctor if you have any adverse effects.

## Effects on mother:
- Pregnant women may have the same adverse effects as any other person.
- Call your doctor if you develop any adverse effects.

## Effects on fetus:
- There is controversy about the safety or risk of this medication.
- In most studies, no increased risk of malformations were reported after use of diazepam. However, cleft lip*, cleft palate*, hernias* and heart, blood-vessle, stomach, limb and facial malformations have been reported after diazepam use in some studies.
- Ask your doctor to provide specific information about the risk of this medication.

## Effects on newborn:
- This medication may reach higher levels in the fetus than in the mother. Newborns do not eliminate this medication as rapidly as adults.
- Infants have experienced sucking problems, lethargy, poor muscle tone and withdrawal after exposure to diazepam during pregnancy.
- Use of diazepam in labor is associated with poor temperature control, sedation and poor responsiveness in the newborn.

## Effects during lactation:

- Diazepam is found in breast milk. Occasionally breast-milk levels are higher than the mother's blood level.
- One infant had low blood levels of this medication after exposure to diazepam in breast milk.
- Jaundice* has been reported in the first few weeks of life after exposure to diazepam in breast milk.
- Lethargy and drowsiness have also been reported.
- Lactating women may have the same adverse effects as any other person.

 **Additional information**

- Diazepam is converted in the liver to several compounds. Many of these compounds produce the same effects as diazepam. One of these is oxazepam. See Oxazepam, page 194.

 **Recommendations for use**

### Women considering pregnancy:

- Notify your doctor if you plan to become pregnant.
- Discontinue use of this medication, if possible.
- Your doctor can advise you.

### Recommendations during pregnancy:

- See your doctor regularly.
- Avoid use of this medication during pregnancy, if possible.

### Recommendations during lactation:

- Do not nurse while using this medication if you take doses of 10mg or more. Small doses may be safe with medical supervision.
- Notify your baby's doctor if your baby is drowsy.
- Your doctor or your baby's doctor can provide the best recommendation for you.

 **Interactions**

### Interactions with medications, vitamins and minerals:

| Interacts with | Combined effect |
| --- | --- |
| Antidepressants | Increases drowsiness. |
| Cimetidine | Increases diazepam effect. |
| Digoxin | Increases digoxin effect. |
| Isoniazid (INH) | Increases diazepam effect. |
| Lithium | May decrease body temperature. |
| Oral contraceptives | Decreases contraceptive effect. |
| Phenytoin | Increases phenytoin toxicity. |
| Rifampin | Decreases diazepam effect. |
| Valproic acid | Increases diazepam effect. |

### Interactions with other substances:

- Use with alcohol increases drowsiness and slows reaction time.
- Food increases absorption of this medication.
- Smoking decreases diazepam effectiveness.

*See Glossary.

MEDICATION

# Dicloxacillin

**Definition and description:** Antibiotic of the penicillin class. Treats susceptible bacterial infections.

**Other names:** Dicloxacillin sodium, Dycill®, Dynapen®, Pathocil®, Veracillin®.

 ## Dosage

**Safe dosage:**
• Usual adult dose—125 to 250mg every 6 hours.

**Toxic dosage:**
• Exact toxic dose cannot be predicted.
• Kidney or liver damage, changes in reflexes and seizures occur very rarely after intravenous* use.
• Life-threatening allergic reactions have occurred after use of dicloxacillin. Contact your doctor or emergency room immediately if you have difficulty breathing or swelling of the face, mouth or throat. Hives* sometimes precede serious reactions.

 ## Possible benefits

**Benefits before pregnancy:**
• Cures susceptible bacterial infections.

**Benefits to mother:**
• Some bacterial infections may be very serious to the mother. This medication can cure susceptible infections.

**Benefits to fetus:**
• Some bacterial infections in the mother may increase risk to the fetus. This medication can cure susceptible infections.

**Benefits during lactation:**
• None reported.

 ## Possible adverse effects

**Effects before pregnancy:**
• Adverse effects include nausea, vomiting, diarrhea, flatulence, rash, hives*, itching, fever and changes in blood-cell count.

• Fatal allergic reactions have rarely occurred.
• Notify your doctor of any adverse effects.

**Effects on mother:**
• Pregnant women may have the same adverse effects as any other person.
• Call your doctor if you develop any adverse effects.

**Effects on fetus:**
• Penicillin antibiotics are usually considered safe for the fetus.

**Effects on newborn:**
• None reported in infants exposed before birth.

**Effects during lactation:**
• None reported in nursing infants.
• Other penicillins have caused thrush* and diarrhea. See Ampicillin, page 30.
• Lactating women may have the same adverse effects as any other person.

 ## Additional information

• Some doctors believe exposure to penicillins during breast-feeding may be associated with allergy to penicillins. There is no supporting evidence in humans.
• Some bacterial infections may be very serious to the mother or the baby. It is important to treat these infections.
• Risks from infection or medication must be considered on an individual basis. Your doctor can advise you.

 ## Recommendations for use

**Women considering pregnancy:**
• Use this medication as directed by your doctor.
• Notify your doctor of any adverse effects.

## Recommendations during pregnancy:
- Use this medication as directed by your doctor.
- Notify your doctor of any adverse effects.
- Contact your doctor if symptoms continue.

## Recommendations during lactation:
- Nursing is usually safe while using this medication.
- Notify your doctor or your baby's doctor if you notice white patches in the baby's mouth or if your baby has diarrhea.

 ## Interactions

### Interactions with medications, vitamins and minerals:

| Interacts with | Combined effect |
| --- | --- |
| Methotrexate | Increases methotrexate toxicity. |
| Tetracycline | Decreases dicloxacillin effectiveness. |

### Interactions with other substances:
- Taking dicloxacillin with food decreases effectiveness.

*See Glossary.

MEDICATION

# Diflunisal

**Definition and description:** Relieves swelling, stiffness and pain of rheumatoid arthritis* or osteoarthritis*. Relieves mild to moderate pain.

**Other names:** Dolobid®.

 **Dosage**

**Safe dosage:**
- Usual adult dose—500 to 1,500mg/day.

**Toxic dosage:**
- Exact toxic dose cannot be predicted.
- Mild overdose symptoms include low blood pressure, rapid heart rate and loss of consciousness in adults.
- Severe overdose has produced ringing in ears, rapid breathing, rapid heart rate, heart failure and death.

 **Possible benefits**

**Benefits before pregnancy:**
- Relieves swelling, stiffness and joint pain of rheumatoid arthritis* or osteoarthritis*.
- Relieves mild to moderate pain.

**Benefits to mother:**
- See *Benefits before pregnancy.*

**Benefits to fetus:**
- None reported.

**Benefits during lactation:**
- None reported.

 **Possible adverse effects**

**Effects before pregnancy:**
- Adverse effects include dizziness, headache, nervousness, depression, confusion, rash, ringing in ears, nausea, heartburn*, abdominal pain, swelling, decreased blood-cell count, kidney damage and liver damage.
- Notify your doctor if you develop any adverse effects.

**Effects on mother:**
- Pregnant women may have the same adverse effects as any other person.
- Call your doctor if you develop any new adverse effects or if adverse effects worsen during pregnancy.
- Anemia*, excessive bleeding during and after labor, and prolonged or delayed labor have been reported with similar medications. Experience with this medication in pregnancy is limited. See Aspirin, page 40.

**Effects on fetus:**
- Serious adverse effects have been reported after exposure to similar medications. Experience with this medication in pregnancy is limited. See Aspirin, page 40.

**Effects on newborn:**
- Serious adverse effects have been reported after use of similar medications. Experience with this medication in pregnancy is limited. See Indomethacin, page 142, and Aspirin, page 40.

**Effects during lactation:**
- Diflunisal is found in low concentrations in breast milk.
- Lactating women may have the same adverse effects as any other person.

 **Additional information**

- Use of this or similar medications may be necessary to control severe rheumatoid arthritis* or related disorders during pregnancy.

**Recommendations for use**

### Women considering pregnancy:

- Use diflunisal only when needed for mild to moderate pain.
- Use this medication regularly as directed by your doctor for arthritis* or related disorders.
- If you use diflunisal regularly, notify your doctor if you plan to become pregnant. Possible risks to you and your baby must be considered on an individual basis.
- Your doctor can provide the best recommendation for you.

### Recommendations during pregnancy:

- Avoid unnecessary use of diflunisal for mild to moderate pain in pregnancy.
- See your doctor regularly.
- If you use diflunisal to control rheumatoid arthritis* or related disorders, possible risks to you and your baby must be considered on an individual basis. Follow your doctor's recommendations carefully.
- Avoid use of this medication near your expected delivery date, except as directed by your doctor.
- At the time of delivery, tell your doctor you take diflunisal.

### Recommendations during lactation:

- Safety or risk has not been established.
- Your doctor or your baby's doctor can provide the best recommendation for you.

 **Interactions**

### Interactions with medications, vitamins and minerals:

| Interacts with | Combined effect |
|---|---|
| **Acetaminophen** | Increases acetaminophen levels. |
| **Antacids** | Decreases diflunisal effect. |
| **Thiazides** | Decreases uric-acid levels. |
| **Warfarin** | Increases risk of bleeding. |

### Interactions with other substances:

- None reported.

*See Glossary.

# Dimenhydrinate

### Definition and description:
Antihistamine that acts as an antiemetic*
to control nausea, vomiting and dizziness
of motion sickness.

**Other names:** See brand-name list,
page 390.

 ## Dosage

### Safe dosage:
- Usual adult dose—50 to 100mg every 4
  hours, to a maximum of 400mg/day.
- This medication can be purchased without a prescription.

### Toxic dosage:
- Exact toxic dose cannot be predicted.
- Serious toxicity has occurred with anti-
  histamine overdose.

 ## Possible benefits

### Benefits before pregnancy:
- Treats nausea and vomiting associated
  with motion sickness.

### Benefits to mother:
- May relieve nausea and vomiting.
- Effectiveness of non-prescription
  antiemetics* has not been proved for
  nausea and vomiting in pregnancy.

### Benefits to fetus:
- None reported.

### Benefits during lactation:
- None reported.

 ## Possible adverse effects

### Effects before pregnancy:
- Adverse effects include drowsiness,
  dizzines, dry mouth, blurred vision, difficulty urinating, headache, loss of
  appetite, nervousness, rash, fast heart
  rate, nausea and vomiting.
- Discontinue use if you develop any
  adverse effects.

### Effects on mother:
- This medication may relax or stimulate
  the uterus, depending on your stage of
  pregnancy.
- Pregnant women may have the same
  adverse effects as any other person.
- Call your doctor if you develop any
  adverse effects.

### Effects on fetus:
- No increase in total number of
  malformations was found in a group of
  exposed pregnancies. The number of
  exposures is too small to establish
  safety or risk. However, heart defects,
  lung defects and hernias* have
  occurred with greater frequency.

### Effects on newborn:
- None reported. A similar medication
  produced withrawal in a newborn. See
  Diphenhydramine, page 104.

### Effects during lactation:
- This medication enters breast milk.
- Lactating women may have the same
  adverse effect as any other person.

 ## Additional information

- Use medication *only* if nausea and vomiting interfere with eating or daily
  activities, and other treatments fail. Your
  doctor can prescribe other treatments.
  He or she should determine whether
  medication is necessary.
- Other treatments may include eating
  soda crackers or dry toast and drinking
  hot or cold liquids as soon as you get
  up in the morning.
- A severe form of nausea and vomiting
  of pregnancy is called *hyperemesis
  gravidarum\**. This condition causes
  nutritional deficiencies, loss of
  electrolytes*, weight loss and starvation. It often requires hospitalization.
  Treatment with antiemetics* alone will
  not reverse hyperemesis gravidarum*.

**Recommendations for use**

### Women considering pregnancy:
- Use this medication as directed on the package.
- Use dimenhydrinate only as needed.
- Notify your doctor if you plan to become pregnant. Before pregnancy, your doctor can advise you about ways to decrease nausea and vomiting without medication.

### Recommendations during pregnancy:
- If you have severe vomiting, contact your doctor as soon as possible.
- See your doctor regularly.
- Your doctor can advise you about ways to decrease nausea and vomiting without medication.
- If other treatments fail to reduce nausea and vomiting, contact your doctor *before* using any medication.
- Use this medication only as directed by your doctor.

### Recommendations during lactation:
- Nursing is usually safe while using antihistamines.
- Your doctor or your baby's doctor can provide the best recommendation for you.

 **Interactions**

### Interactions with medications, vitamins and minerals:

| Interacts with | Combined effect |
| --- | --- |
| **Amino-glycosides** | Masks damage to inner-ear structures (responsible for hearing and balance). |
| **Antianxiety agents** | Increases drowsiness. |
| **Antidepressants** | Increases drowsiness. |
| **Antihistamines** | Increases drowsiness. |
| **Tranquilizers** | Increases drowsiness. |

### Interactions with other substances:
- Use with alcohol increases drowsiness and slows reaction time.

*See Glossary.

MEDICATION

# Dimethylmethane laxatives

**Definition and description:** Acts as a laxative to relieve constipation.

**Other names:** Bisacodyl and phenolphthalein. Also see brand-name list, page 390.

 **Dosage**

### Safe dosage:
- Dose varies with the agent. Follow instructions on the package.
- These medications can be purchased without a prescription.

### Toxic dosage:
- These medications are well-tolerated if used for short periods in recommended dosages.
- Laxative overuse can cause diarrhea, weak bones, decreased protein, liver disease, poor absorption of fats, colon problems and low blood levels of potassium, calcium and magnesium.

 **Possible benefits**

### Benefits before pregnancy:
- Relieves constipation.

### Benefits to mother:
- See *Benefits before pregnancy.*

### Benefits to fetus:
- None reported.

### Benefits during lactation:
- None reported.

 **Possible adverse effects**

### Effects before pregnancy:
- Adverse effects of bisacodyl include low blood-calcium levels, muscle paralysis, alkalosis* or acidosis* and malabsorption*.
- Adverse effects of phenolphthalein include diarrhea, low blood-calcium levels, weak bones, colic*, heart problems, lung problems and shock after large doses. Skin rash and sensitivity to sunburn have also been reported. Discontinue use, and notify your doctor if you develop any skin reactions.
- Notify your doctor if you develop any adverse effects.

### Effects on mother:
- Pregnant women may have the same adverse effects as any other person.
- Call your doctor if you develop any adverse effects.

### Effects on fetus:
- Bisacodyl has not been evaluated. Safety or risk has not been established.
- Phenolphthalein alone was not associated with an increased risk of malformations. However, some malformations have been reported after use of medications for stomach and intestinal complaints. These include central-nervous-system, genital, urinary-tract, eye and ear abnormalities. Risk of club foot* was also increased. Phenolphthalein was one of this group.

### Effects on newborn:
- Safety or risk has not been established.

### Effects during lactation:
- Bisacodyl is found in breast milk.
- Phenolphthalein has caused adverse effects in nursing infants.
- Lactating women may have the same adverse effects as any other person.

 **Additional information**

- Try non-medication therapies before using any laxative. Your doctor or nurse can instruct you.
- Increasing fiber in your diet, exercise and adequate fluid intake are helpful. See Appendix 1, page 375, for fiber sources.

**Recommendations for use**

## Women considering pregnancy:
- Use only as directed on the package.
- Overuse of laxatives can produce dependence on them.
- If you require a laxative for more than a few days, contact your doctor.

## Recommendations during pregnancy:
- See your doctor regularly.
- Try non-medication therapies before using any laxative.
- Do not use bisacodyl and phenolphthalein during pregnancy.
- Other laxatives are safer during pregnancy. Ask your doctor or nurse for recommendations.

## Recommendations during lactation:
- Your doctor can suggest an alternative. Avoid use of bisacodyl and phenolphthalein while nursing.

 **Interactions**

**Interactions with medications, vitamins and minerals:**

| Interacts with | Combined effect |
| --- | --- |
| **Docusate** | Possible phenophthalein toxicity. |
| **Sulfonamides** | May decrease sulfonamide absorption. |
| **Warfarin** | May increase or decrease warfarin effect. |

**Interactions with other substances:**
- None reported.

*See Glossary.

MEDICATION

# Diphenhydramine

**Definition and description:** Acts as an antihistamine to relieve allergy symptoms, including sneezing, runny nose, itching, tearing, hives* and other skin reactions. May be used in addition to epinephrine for severe, life-threatening allergic reactions. Also relieves or prevents motion sickness.

**Other names:** Diphenhydramine citrate, diphenhydramine hydrochloride. Also see brand-name list, page 390.

## Dosage

### Safe dosage:
- Usual adult dose—25 to 50mg every 4 to 6 hours.
- This medication can be purchased without a prescription. It is also found in products requiring a prescription.

### Toxic dosage:
- Exact toxic dose cannot be predicted.
- Symptoms of overdose include drowsiness, dry mouth, large pupils, flushing and low blood pressure.
- Serious overdose may cause convulsions and death.
- Contact your doctor, poison-control center or emergency room if you think you have taken an overdose.

## Possible benefits

### Benefits before pregnancy:
- Relieves allergy symptoms.

### Benefits to mother:
- See *Benefits before pregnancy.*

### Benefits to fetus:
- None reported.

### Benefits during lactation:
- None reported.

## Possible adverse effects

### Effects before pregnancy:
- Adverse effects include drowsiness, sedation, dizziness, confusion, restlessness, blurred vision, ringing in ears, nausea, vomiting, diarrhea, constipation, changes in urination, decreased blood-cell count, unusual heart rhythm, low blood pressure, hives*, rash and dry mouth.
- Severe allergic reactions have occurred.
- Notify your doctor of any adverse effects.

### Effects on mother:
- Pregnant women may have the same adverse effects as any other person.
- Call your doctor if you develop any adverse effects.

### Effects on fetus:
- Most evidence does not indicate an increase in malformations after exposure to diphenhydramine. Evaluations of use in the first 13 weeks of pregnancy do not indicate an increase in malformations. However, one evaluation of 595 pregnancies reported club foot*, hernia* and genital, urinary, eye and ear malformations. Total numbers of malformations were not increased.
- There is controversy about diphenhydramine's role in club foot. Ask your doctor to advise you.
- Antihistamines as a group have not been shown to increase risk of malformations compared to unexposed pregnancies.
- Fetal death occurred after one mother used diphenhydramine and temazepam. Animal studies done after this death confirmed increased fetal death rates when these medications are used together. Based on this information, combination of these medications should be avoided during pregnancy.

### Effects on newborn:
- Withdrawal symptoms were reported in an infant after exposure to diphenhydramine before birth.

### Effects during lactation:
- This medication is found in breast milk.
- No adverse effects are reported in nursing infants.
- Lactating women may have the same adverse effects as any other person.

## Additional information

- Diphenhydramine does not cure colds, coughs or minor allergy complaints. It provides relief for symptoms. Occasionally, when allergic reactions are very serious, using antihistamines and other medications can be life-saving.
- Viral illnesses and fever have been implicated as a cause of birth defects. This medication is often used to relieve symptoms of viral illnesses. Contact your doctor if you have a fever.
- This medication is often used in combination with other medications. Most studies did not study persons using it alone. It is difficult to determine if diphenhydramine caused any malformations.
- Do not take diphenhydramine and temazepam together during pregnancy. See *Effects on fetus.*

## Recommendations for use

### Women considering pregnancy:
- Use only the recommended doses of diphenhydramine.
- Use this medication only when needed.
- Notify your doctor if you plan to become pregnant.

### Recommendations during pregnancy:
- See your doctor regularly.
- Use diphenhydramine only as directed by your doctor.
- Avoid unnecessary use of this medication.

### Recommendations during lactation:
- Nursing is usually safe while using this medication.
- Your doctor or your baby's doctor can provide the best recommendation for you.

## Interactions

### Interactions with medications, vitamins and minerals:

| Interacts with | Combined effect |
| --- | --- |
| Antianxiety agents | Increases drowsiness. |
| Antidepressants | Increases drowsiness. |
| Other anti-histamines | Increases drowsiness. |
| Para-aminosalicylic acid (PAS) | Decreases paraaminosalicylic-acid absorption. |
| Temazepam | Possibly increases incidence of fetal death. |
| Tranquilizers | Increases drowsiness. |

### Interactions with other substances:
- Use with alcohol increases drowsiness and slows reaction time.

*See Glossary.

# Divalporex

**Definition and description:** Acts as an anticonvulsant to prevent epileptic seizures. Divalporex is converted into valproate (valproic acid) in the body.

**Other names:** Depakote®.

 ## Dosage

### Safe dosage:
- Usual adult dose—500 to 1,250mg/day.
- Dosage requirements may change during and after pregnancy. Your doctor can use valproate blood levels to determine correct dose. *See Additional information.*

### Toxic dosage:
- Exact toxic dose cannot be predicted.
- Toxic effects include liver and blood-cell damage.
- Call your doctor if you develop unusual bruising or bleeding, sore throat, fever, abdominal cramps, irregular menstruation or jaundice*.

 ## Possible benefits

### Benefits before pregnancy:
- Use of medication may prevent seizures. Seizures may result in serious injury from falls and accidents. Prolonged, frequent seizures or continuous epileptic seizures may also result in brain damage or death.

### Benefits to mother:
- See *Benefits before pregnancy.*

### Benefits to fetus:
- Use of medication may prevent seizures in the mother. Decreased oxygen supply due to maternal seizures may cause brain damage or death in the fetus.
- Injuries from the mother falling during a seizure may damage the fetus.

### Benefits during lactation:
- None reported.

 ## Possible adverse effects

### Effects before pregnancy:
- Adverse effects include drowsiness, weakness, depression, lack of coordination, unsteady gait, headache, vision changes, nausea, vomiting and skin rash.
- Notify your doctor of any new or unusual adverse effects.

### Effects on mother:
- Pregnant women may have same adverse effects as any other person.
- Call your doctor if you develop any new adverse effects or if adverse effects worsen during pregnancy.

### Effects on fetus:
- Serious malformations of the brain and spinal cord, including small brain, absent brain, meningocele* and spina bifida*, are reported more frequently in children of women who use valproate compared to other anticonvulsant medications. Deaths due to serious malformations have been reported. See *Additional information* and Valproic acid, page 276.
- Malformations of the skeleton, skull and face, including cleft lip*, cleft palate*, high forehead, flat nasal bridge, small nose, widely spaced eyes, hip dislocation*, absence of ribs, absence of radius* and abnormal development of sternum*, have also been reported after use of valproic acid.
- Malformations of the digestive tract, kidneys, genital tract, liver, abdominal wall, heart and blood vessels have been reported.
- Fetal distress during labor may require Cesarean delivery.
- Growth retardation has been reported.

### Effects on newborn:
- Liver damage has been reported in infants exposed to a similar medication in combination with other anticonvulsant medications. Effect of this medication may increase during the first week of life. See *Additional information* and Valproic Acid, page 276.

- High maternal doses of similar medication may be associated with poor breathing, poor muscle tone and lethargy in the newborn period. See *Additional information* and Valproic Acid, page 276.
- Slow mental and physical development have been reported.

### Effects during lactation:

- Valproic acid is found in low concentrations in breast milk. See *Additional information*.
- Lactating women may have the same adverse effects as any other person.

 **Additional information**

- Divalporex is converted in the body to valproate. Valproate is the active form of valproic acid. See Valproic Acid, page 276.
- You have a 90% chance of having a normal child if you must take medication to control epilepsy.*
- Pregnancy may increase, decrease or have no effect on the frequency and severity of seizures.
- Very severe seizures have occurred when medication is discontinued without a doctor's supervision.
- Having epilepsy and taking anticonvulsant medications increase the risk of having a miscarriage, stillbirth or child with birth defects.

 **Recommendations for use**

### Women considering pregnancy:

- Notify your doctor if you plan to become pregnant. Possible risks to you and your baby must be considered on an individual basis.
- If you have been seizure-free for many years, your doctor may recommend slowly discontinuing this medication before pregnancy.

- If you have a severe seizure disorder, it is *absolutely necessary* to continue anticonvulsant medication throughout your pregnancy.
- Your doctor may recommend changing your medication.
- Your doctor can provide the best recommendation for you. Do *not* stop taking this medication unless told to do so by your doctor.

### Recommendations during pregnancy:

- See your doctor regularly.
- Blood levels should be checked often during pregnancy and for a few weeks after delivery to balance adverse effects and effectiveness of medication.
- Your doctor may want to adjust dosage of medication frequently during and after pregnancy. It is important to follow your doctor's instructions carefully.
- Your doctor may recommend blood screening, sonography*, amniocentesis* or other tests to diagnose spina bifida* or similar birth defects before your baby is born.
- If seizures occur, contact your doctor immediately.
- At the time of delivery, tell your doctor you take divalporex.
- Take only the vitamin supplements recommended by your doctor.
- Get plenty of sleep during your pregnancy.

### Recommendations during lactation:

- Nursing is usually safe when using this medication.
- Notify your baby's doctor if you notice anything unusual, especially bruising, bleeding or jaundice*.

# Divalporex, continued

 **Interactions**

**Interactions with medications, vitamins and minerals:**

| Interacts with | Combined effect |
|---|---|
| **Diazepam** | Increases diazepam effect. |
| **Other anti-convulsant medications** | Increases likelihood of birth defects when more than one medication is needed to control seizures. |
| **Phenobarbital** | Alters phenobarbital effect. |
| **Phenytoin** | Alters effect of both. |
| **Zinc** | May decrease zinc levels. |

**Interactions with other substances:**
• None reported.

*See Glossary.

Note: This page purposely left blank.

# Docusate

**Definition and description:** Acts as a stool softener to relieve constipation.

**Other names:** Docusate sodium, docusate calcium, docusate potassium. Also see brand-name list, page 390.

 ## Dosage

### Safe dosage:
- Usual adult dose—50 to 250mg/day.
- This medication can be purchased without a prescription. It is also found in products requiring a prescription, including some prenatal vitamins.

### Toxic dosage:
- Docusate is well-tolerated if used for short periods in recommended dosages.
- Laxative overuse can cause diarrhea, weak bones, decreased protein, liver disease, poor absorption of fats, colon problems and low blood levels of potassium, calcium and magnesium.

 ## Possible benefits

### Benefits before pregnancy:
- Relieves constipation.

### Benefits to mother:
- See *Benefits before pregnancy.*

### Benefits to fetus:
- None reported.

### Benefits during lactation:
- None reported.

 ## Possible adverse effects

### Effects before pregnancy:
- Adverse effects are rare.
- Liver damage has been reported when docusate was used in combination with danthron or mineral oil. See Anthraquinone laxatives (for danthron), page 36, and Mineral oil, page 182.

### Effects on mother:
- Pregnant women may have the same adverse effects as any other person.

### Effects on fetus:
- Docusate alone was not associated with an increased risk of any malformations. Most doctors consider it safe during pregnancy.
- Some malformations have been reported after use of medication for stomach and intestinal complaints. These include central-nervous-system, genital, urinary-tract, eye and ear abnormalities. Risk of club foot* was also increased. Docusate was one of the medications in this group of medications.

### Effects on newborn:
- Most evidence does not indicate an increased risk of adverse effects.

### Effects during lactation:
- None reported in nursing infants.
- Lactating women may have the same adverse effects as any other person.

 ## Additional information

- Try non-medication therapies first. Your doctor or nurse can instruct you.
- Increasing fiber in your diet, exercise and adequate fluid intake are helpful. See Appendix 1, page 375, for fiber sources.

 ## Recommendations for use

### Women considering pregnancy:
- Use as directed on the package.
- Overuse of laxatives can produce dependence on them.
- If you require a laxative for more than a few days, contact your doctor.

### Recommendations during pregnancy:
- See your doctor regularly.
- Try non-medication therapies before using any laxative.
- Use this medication only as directed by your doctor.

### Recommendations during lactation:
- Nursing is usually safe while using this medication for short periods.
- Your doctor can provide the best recommendation for you.

 ## Interactions

### Interactions with medications, vitamins and minerals:

| Interacts with | Combined effect |
| --- | --- |
| **Danthron** | Increases incidence of liver damage. |
| **Digoxin** | Increases digoxin toxicity. |
| **Mineral oil** | Increases liver damage. |
| **Phenophthalein** | May increase phenophthalein toxicity. |
| **Quinidine** | May increase liver damage. |

### Interactions with other substances:
- None reported.

*See Glossary.

# Doxepin

**Definition and description:** Acts as an antidepressant to relieve symptoms of depression.

**Other names:** Adapin®, Sinequan®.

 ## Dosage

### Safe dosage:
- Usual adult dose—75 to 150mg/day.

### Toxic dosage:
- Exact toxic dose cannot be predicted.
- Overdose has produced serious, life-threatening toxicity.
- Symptoms include confusion, hallucinations*, drowsiness, decreased or increased body temperature, muscle rigidity, dangerous heart rhythm, dilated pupils, low blood pressure and loss of consciousness.
- Contact your doctor, poison-control center or emergency room if you think you have taken an overdose.

 ## Possible benefits

### Benefits before pregnancy:
- Controls symptoms of depression.

### Benefits to mother:
- See *Benefits before pregnancy*.

### Benefits to fetus:
- None reported.

### Benefits during lactation:
- None reported.

 ## Possible adverse effects

### Effects before pregnancy:
- Adverse reactions include low blood pressure or (less often) high blood pressure, rapid heart rate, unusual heart rhythm, altered mental state, tingling, staggering, ringing in ears, seizures, dry mouth, blurred vision, constipation, difficulty urinating, rash, hives*, sensitivity to sunburn, low blood-cell count, nausea, vomiting, diarrhea, jaundice*, dizziness, headache and drowsiness.

- Notify your doctor of any new or unusual adverse effects.

### Effects on mother:
- Pregnant women may have the same adverse effects as any other person.
- Call your doctor if you develop any new adverse effects or if adverse effects worsen during pregnancy.

### Effects on fetus:
- No malformations have been reported after use of this medication. However, experience is limited with doxepin.
- Safety or risk in early pregnancy has not been established.

### Effects on newborn:
- Use of doxepin in combination with chlorpromazine late in pregnancy temporarily paralyzed the bowel of one newborn.

### Effects during lactation:
- Doxepin is found in breast milk.
- Lactating women may have the same adverse effects as any other person.

 ## Additional information

- Pregnancy may be complicated by development or recurrence of a serious mental disorder. Treatments other than medication should be tried first. If the risks of mental illness are considered serious, use of medications to treat the mother's illness is important.
- Depression during pregnancy may threaten you or your fetus if you are suicidal, unable to eat or if you have impaired judgment.
- Your doctor will determine if medication is necessary.

 ## Recommendations for use

### Women considering pregnancy:
- Use this medication as directed by your doctor.
- Do not exceed the dose recommended by your doctor.

- Notify your doctor if you plan to become pregnant. Possible risks to you and your baby must be considered on an individual basis.
- Your doctor can provide the best recommendation for you.

## Recommendations during pregnancy:
- See your doctor regularly.
- Use this medication as directed by your doctor.
- Do not exceed the dose recommended by your doctor.
- Avoid use near the time of delivery, if possible.

## Recommendations during lactation:
- Your doctor or your baby's doctor can provide the best recommendation for you.

 Interactions

**Interactions with medications, vitamins and minerals:**

| Interacts with | Combined effect |
| --- | --- |
| **Amphetamines** | Increases amphetamine toxicity. |
| **Anti-cholinergics*** | Increases toxicity of both. |
| **Barbiturates** | Decreases antidepressant effect. |
| **Cimetidine** | Increases antidepressant toxicity. |
| **Clonidine** | Increases blood pressure. |
| **Debrisoquin** | Increases blood pressure. |
| **Epinephrine** | Increases blood pressure. |
| **Guanethidine** | Increases blood pressure. |
| **Methyldopa** | Increases blood pressure. |
| **Monoamine oxidase (MAO) inhibitors** | Causes fever and seizures. |
| **Phenothiazines** | Increases toxicity of both. |
| **Phenylephrine (intravenous*)** | Increases blood pressure. |
| **Phenytoin** | Increases phenytoin toxicity. |
| **Propoxyphene** | Increases doxepin toxicity. |

**Interactions with other substances:**
- Use with alcohol increases drowsiness and slows reaction time.
- Smoking may decrease doxepin effectiveness.

*See Glossary.

MEDICATION

# Doxycycline

**Definition and description:** Acts as an antibiotic to treat susceptible bacterial infections.

**Other names:** Doxycycline calcium, doxycycline hyclate, doxycycline mono-hydrate, Vibra-Tabs®, Vibramycin®, Vivox®.

 **Dosage**

**Safe dosage:**
• Usual adult dose—100 to 200mg/day.

**Toxic dosage:**
• Adverse effects increase with doses larger than the recommended dose.
• Do *not* exceed the dose recommended by your physician.
• Exact toxic dose cannot be predicted.

 **Possible benefits**

**Benefits before pregnancy:**
• Cures susceptible bacterial infections.

**Benefits to mother:**
• See *Benefits before pregnancy.*

**Benefits to fetus:**
• None reported.

**Benefits during lactation:**
• None reported.

 **Possible adverse effects**

**Effects before pregnancy:**
• Adverse effects include loss of appetite, nausea, vomiting, diarrhea, swelling in the throat, liver damage, rash, hives*, kidney damage, decreased blood-cell counts, sensitivity to sunburn and ulcers* in the esophagus.
• Serious allergic reactions have rarely occurred.
• Notify your doctor of any adverse effects.

**Effects on mother:**
• Pregnant women are more likely to develop severe liver damage than other persons. Kidney damage and pancreatitis* are associated with liver toxicity. Maternal deaths have occurred. Premature delivery and stillbirths are reported in affected women.
• Pregnant women may have the same adverse effects as any other person.
• Call your doctor if you develop any adverse effects.

**Effects on fetus:**
• Children exposed during the last half of pregnancy have developed permanent staining of forming primary and permanent teeth. Up to 50% of all exposed children may be affected by similar medications. See Tetracycline, page 256.
• Abnormal development of tooth enamel has been reported.
• Malformations of limbs have been reported after exposure to similar medications. See Tetracycline, page 256.

**Effects on newborn:**
• Staining of developing primary and permanent teeth is reported in children exposed in the last half of pregnancy. This effect is also noted after administration of this medication to newborns or older children up to 8 years of age.
• Similar medications have been shown to inhibit bone growth in premature infants. See Tetracycline, page 256.
• Similar medications have also caused bulging fontanel*. See Tetracycline, page 256.

**Effects during lactation:**
• Doxycycline is found in moderate levels in breast milk.
• Lactating women may have the same adverse effects as any other person.

## Recommendations for use

### Women considering pregnancy:
- Notify your doctor if you plan to become pregnant.
- If you use this medication on a regular basis, ask your doctor for advice about the risks of this medication to you or your baby. Your doctor can provide the best recommendation for you.
- Avoid unnecessary exposure to doxycycline in early pregnancy.

### Recommendations during pregnancy:
- Avoid use of this medication during pregnancy.
- Your doctor or your baby's doctor can provide the best recommendation for you.

### Recommendations during lactation:
- Nursing is usually safe while using doxycycline.
- Risk of tooth discoloration must be considered.
- Your baby's doctor can provide the best recommendation for you.

 ## Interactions

**Interactions with medications, vitamins and minerals:**

| Interacts with | Combined effect |
| --- | --- |
| Antacids | Decreases doxycycline absorption. |
| Carbamazepine | Decreases doxycycline effect. |
| Phenobarbital | Decreases doxycycline effect. |
| Phenytoin | Decreases doxycycline effect. |

**Interactions with other substances:**
- None reported.

*See Glossary.

# Ephedrine

**Definition and description:** Acts as a decongestant to decrease nasal secretions. Acts as a bronchodilator* to treat asthma*, chronic bronchitis* and emphysema*.

**Other names:** See brand-name list, page 390.

 Dosage

### Safe dosage:
- Usual adult dose—12.5 to 25mg every 4 hours, as needed.
- Nasal spray or drops can be used as directed on the package. Rebound congestion* is common.
- This medication can be purchased without a prescription.

### Toxic dosage:
- Exact toxic dose cannot be predicted.
- Symptoms of overdose include anxiety, confusion, delirium*, tremors* and increased heart rate.

 Possible benefits

### Benefits before pregnancy:
- Decreases nasal congestion from allergies and colds.
- Relieves symptoms of asthma*, chronic bronchitis* and emphysema*.

### Benefits to mother:
- See *Benefits before pregnancy.*

### Benefits to fetus:
- None reported.

### Benefits during lactation:
- None reported.

 Possible adverse effects

### Effects before pregnancy:
- Adverse effects include drowsiness, excitation, tenseness, headache, dizziness, unusual heart rhythm and tremor*.

### Effects on mother:
- Pregnant women may have the same adverse effects as any other person.
- Call your doctor if you develop any adverse effects during pregnancy.

### Effects on fetus:
- Safety or risk has not been established.
- When used in large doses, fetal heart rate increases.

### Effects on newborn:
- Safety or risk has not been established.
- When given to mothers during Cesarean delivery, no adverse effects were noted in newborns.

### Effects during lactation:
- One infant developed irritability, high-pitched crying and altered sleep patterns after exposure to ephedrine in combination with brompheniramine. Symptoms disappeared when these medications were discontinued.
- Lactating women may have the same adverse effects as any other person.

 Recommendations for use

### Women considering pregnancy:
- Use medication as directed on the package.
- Do not exceed the suggested dose.
- Use only when needed.

### Recommendations during pregnancy:
- Safety or risk has not been established.
- See your doctor regularly.
- Avoid unnecessary use during pregnancy. Use only as directed by your doctor.

### Recommendations during lactation:
- Safety or risk has not been established.
- Your doctor or your baby's doctor can provide the best recommendation for you.

## Interactions

**Interactions with medications, vitamins and minerals:**

| Interacts with | Combined effect |
| --- | --- |
| Acetazolamide | Increases ephedrine toxicity. |
| Ammonium chloride | May decrease ephedrine effect. |
| Dexamethasone | Decreases dexamethasone effect. |
| Digoxin | Causes abnormal heart rhythm. |
| Guanethidine | Increases blood pressure. |
| High-blood-pressure medications | Increases blood pressure. |
| Indomethacin | Causes very high blood pressure. |
| Methyldopa | Decreases ephedrine effect. |
| Monoamine oxidase (MAO) inhibitor | Causes very high blood pressure, leading to death. |
| Reserpine | Decreases ephedrine effect. |
| Sodium bicarbonate | Causes ephedrine toxicity. |
| Theophylline | Increases sleeplessness and nervousness. |

**Interactions with other substances:**
• None reported.

*See Glossary.

# Epinephrine

**Definition and description:** Relieves potentially fatal allergic reactions (anaphylaxis*). Also relieves symptoms of asthma*.

**Other names:** Epinephrine bitartrate, racemic epinephrine. Also see brand-names list, page 390.

 ## Dosage

**Safe dosage:**
- Epinephrine can be taken by injection or inhalation.
- Dose is determined by route of administration.
- Epinephrine should not be used more often than every 4 hours.
- Epinephrine inhalers are available for purchase without a prescription. This medication is also found in products that require a prescription.

**Toxic dosage:**
- Toxic dose is influenced by the person's condition, size and age.
- Exact toxic dose cannot be predicted.
- Deaths have occurred from excessive use by inhalation. See *Effects before pregnancy.*

 ## Possible benefits

**Benefits before pregnancy:**
- Relieves symptoms of asthma* and life-threatening allergic reactions (anaphylaxis*).

**Benefits to mother:**
- See *Benefits before pregnancy.*

**Benefits to fetus:**
- Severe asthma* may have detrimental effects on the fetus. Epinephrine relieves asthma* symptoms and improves oxygen exchange in the mother.

**Benefits during lactation:**
- None reported.

 ## Possible adverse effects

**Effects before pregnancy:**
- Adverse effects include nervousness, tremor, headache, increased heart rate, unusual heart rhythm, drowsiness, nausea, vomiting, sweating and muscle cramps.
- Notify your doctor of any adverse effects.
- Deaths have been reported from overuse of inhaled epinephrine.

**Effects on mother:**
- Pregnant women may have the same adverse effects as any other person.
- Call your doctor if you develop any new or unusual adverse effects.

**Effects on fetus:**
- Safety or risk in early pregnancy has not been established.
- One study demonstrated an increase in malformations after exposure to epinephrine before the 16th week of pregnancy.

**Effects on newborn:**
- None reported.

**Effects during lactation:**
- None reported. It is unknown if epinephrine enters breast milk.
- Lactating women may have the same adverse effects as any other person.

 ## Additional information

- Pregnancy may affect asthma*. About 50% of pregnant asthmatic women have no change in symptoms during pregnancy, 30% improve and 20% worsen. If symptoms worsen during one pregnancy, they are more likely to worsen in other pregnancies.
- Premature delivery, low birth weight, stillbirth, newborn deaths and maternal deaths are more likely to occur in women with asthma*. Treatment of asthma* improves outcome.

## Recommendations for use

### Women considering pregnancy:

- Notify your doctor if you plan to become pregnant. Risks to you and your baby must be considered on an individual basis.
- Do not exceed the recommended dose.
- If you use a non-prescription product, follow instructions on the package carefully.
- If you use a non-prescription product, such as decongestants or asthma inhalers, tell your doctor you use this medication.
- If you have frequent asthma* attacks, it is important to work with your doctor to control your asthma* *before* pregnancy.
- Notify your doctor if symptoms worsen while using epinephrine.
- Your doctor can provide the best recommendation for you. Do *not* change your medications unless your doctor tells you to do so.

### Recommendations during pregnancy:

- See your doctor regularly.
- Do not exceed the dose recommended by your doctor.
- Notify your doctor if symptoms worsen while using this medication.
- If your asthma* improves, your doctor may decrease your medications.
- If your asthma* worsens, your doctor may increase your medications. Do not adjust your dose without medical supervision.
- Avoid exposure to anything that worsens your asthma*.
- If you use a non-prescription product, tell your doctor you use this medication.

### Recommendations during lactation:

- Your doctor or your baby's doctor can provide the best recommendation for you.

 ## Interactions

### Interactions with medications, vitamins and minerals:

| Interacts with | Combined effect |
| --- | --- |
| Antihypertensive medications | Decreases antihypertensive effect. |
| Beta-adrenergic blockers* | Increases blood pressure. |
| Digoxin | Causes abnormal heart rate. |
| Monoamine oxidase (MAO) inhibitors | Increases blood pressure. |
| Oral antidiabetic agents | Increases blood sugar. |
| Tricyclic anti-depressants | Increases blood pressure (intravenous* epinephrine only). |

### Interactions with other substances:

- None reported.

*See Glossary.

MEDICATION

119

# Erythromycin

**Definition and description:** Acts as an antibiotic to treat susceptible bacterial infections.

**Other names:** Erythromycin estolate, Ilosone®, erythromycin ethlysuccinate, E.E.S.®, E-Mycin E®, EryPed®, Pediamycin®, Wyamycin®, erythromycin gluceptate, Ilotycin®, erythromycin lactobionate, Erythrocin Lactobionate®, erythromycin stearate, Erythrocin Stearate Filmtab®, Ethril®, SK-Erythromycin®.

 ## Dosage

**Safe dosage:**
- Erythromycin, erythromycin estolate, erythromycin stearate: Usual adult dose—250 to 500mg every 6 hours by mouth. Dose varies with condition treated. Smaller or larger doses may be used for some infections.
- Erythromycin ethylsuccinate: Usual adult dose—400 to 800mg every 6 hours by mouth. Dose varies with condition treated. Smaller or larger doses may be used for some infections.
- Erythromycin gluceptate: Up to 4g/day by injection.
- Erythromycin lactobionate: Up to 4g/day by injection.

**Toxic dosage:**
- Adverse effects increase with increasing dose.
- Exact toxic dose cannot be predicted.

 ## Possible benefits

**Benefits before pregnancy:**
- Cures susceptible bacterial infections.

**Benefits to mother:**
- Some bacterial infections may be very serious to the mother. Erythromycin can cure susceptible infections.
- Used in pregnancy for infections usually treated by more-toxic medications.

**Benefits to fetus:**
- Some bacterial infections in the mother may increase risk to the fetus. Erythromycin can cure susceptible infections.

**Benefits during lactation:**
- None reported.

 ## Possible adverse effects

**Effects before pregnancy:**
- Adverse effects include abdominal cramps, nausea, vomiting, diarrhea, hives*, rash and hearing changes.
- Serious allergic reactions have rarely occurred.
- Liver damage is reported more frequently after use of *erythromycin estolate* compared to other forms of erythromycin.
- Notify your doctor of any adverse effects.

**Effects on mother:**
- Liver damage is reported in pregnant women treated with *erythromycin estolate*.
- Pregnant women may have the same adverse effects as any other person.
- Call your doctor if you develop any adverse effects.

**Effects on fetus:**
- Erythromycin is considered safe for the fetus.

**Effects on newborn:**
- None reported in infants exposed before birth.

**Effects during lactation:**
- Erythromycin is found in high levels in breast milk.
- Lactating women may have the same adverse effects as any other person.

 ## Additional information

- Some bacterial infections may be very serious to the mother or the baby. It is important to treat these infections.

- Risks from infection or medication must be considered on an individual basis. Your doctor can advise you.
- Blood levels of erythromycin are lower in pregnant women than other women given the same dose. Your doctor will select the best dose for you.

## Recommendations for use

**Women considering pregnancy:**
- Use this medication as directed by your doctor.
- Notify your doctor of any adverse effects.

### Recommendations during pregnancy:
- Avoid erythromycin estolate.
- Use other forms of erythromycin as directed by your doctor.
- Notify your doctor of any adverse effects.
- Contact your doctor if symptoms continue.

### Recommendations during lactation:
- Nursing is usually safe when using this medication.
- Lactating women may have the same adverse effects as any other person.

## Interactions

**Interactions with medications, vitamins and minerals:**

| Interacts with | Combined effect |
| --- | --- |
| Aminophylline | Increases aminophylline toxicity. |
| Carbamazepine | Increases carbamazepine effect. |
| Digoxin | May increase digoxin effect. |
| Penicillins | Decreases penicillin effect. |
| Riboflavin | Decreases riboflavin absorption. |
| Theophylline | Increases theophylline toxicity. |
| Warfarin | Increases warfarin effect. |

**Interactions with other substances:**
- Taking erythromycin with food decreases the effectiveness of some preparations. Ask your doctor or pharmacist for advice.

*See Glossary.

MEDICATION

# Ethambutol

**Definition and description:** Acts as an antibacterial to treat susceptible tuberculosis* bacteria.

**Other names:** Myambutol®.

 ## Dosage

### Safe dosage:
- Usual adult dose—15 to 25mg/kg of body weight/day.

### Toxic dosage:
- Exact toxic dose cannot be predicted.

 ## Possible benefits

### Benefits before pregnancy:
- Used in combination with other medications to treat active tuberculosis*.

### Benefits to mother:
- Some bacterial infections may be very serious to the mother. Ethambutol can treat susceptible infections.

### Benefits to fetus:
- Some bacterial infections in the mother may increase risk to the fetus. Ethambutol can treat susceptible infections.

### Benefits during lactation:
- None reported.

 ## Possible adverse effects

### Effects before pregnancy:
- Adverse effects include decreased vision, itching, joint pain, skin changes, loss of appetite, nausea, vomiting, abdominal pain, fever, headache, dizziness, confusion, hallucinations*, numbness, tingling, gout* and liver damage.
- Decreased vision is usually reversible but rarely may persist.
- Notify your doctor of any adverse effects.

### Effects on mother:
- Pregnant women may have the same adverse effects as any other person.
- Call your doctor if you develop any adverse effects.

### Effects on fetus:
- Ethambutol is used in combination with isoniazid (INH) or other medications. There is no information regarding its use alone.
- Available evidence has not indicated an increase in birth defects when ethambutol is used in combination with isoniazid (INH). See Isoniazid, page 150.
- Safety or risk has not been established, especially in early pregnancy.

### Effects on newborn:
- None reported.

### Effects during lactation:
- It is unknown if ethambutol enters breast milk.
- Lactating women may have the same adverse effects as any other person.

 ## Additional information

- Tuberculosis* can be a very serious infection in mothers and newborns. It is necessary to treat pregnant women with recent positive skin tests. Your doctor will determine which medication and how many medications are needed for you.
- In some cases, it will also be necessary to treat newborns of women with tuberculosis*. Your doctor or your baby's doctor can advise you.
- Some bacterial infections may be very serious to the mother or the baby. It is important to treat these infections.
- Risks from infection or medication must be considered on an individual basis. Your doctor can advise you.
- Elimination of ethambutol is faster in pregnant women than other women given the same dose. Your doctor will select the best dose for you.

**Recommendations for use**

### Women considering pregnancy:

- Notify your doctor if you plan to become pregnant. Possible risks to you and your baby must be considered on an individual basis.
- Your doctor can provide the best recommendation for you.

### Recommendations during pregnancy:

- See your doctor regularly.
- Risks from infection or medication must be considered on an individual basis. Your doctor can advise you.
- Use this medication as directed by your doctor.
- Notify your doctor of any adverse effects.

### Recommendations during lactation:

- Your baby's doctor can provide the best recommendation for you.

 **Interactions**

### Interactions with medications, vitamins and minerals:

- None reported.

### Interactions with other substances:

- None reported.

*See Glossary.

# Ethosuximide

**Definition and description:** Acts as an anticonvulsant to prevent petit mal epileptic seizures*.

**Other names:** Emeside®, Simatin®, Zarontin®.

 ## Dosage

### Safe dosage:
- Usual adult dose—500 to 2,000mg/day.
- Your doctor can use blood levels to determine correct dosage.

### Toxic dosage:
- Exact toxic dose cannot be predicted.
- Toxic effects include blood-cell damage. Call your doctor if you develop fever, sore throat, swollen lymph glands*, unusual bruising or bleeding.

 ## Possible benefits

### Benefits before pregnancy:
- Use of medication may prevent seizures. Seizures may result in serious injury from falls and accidents.

### Benefits to mother:
- See *Benefits before pregnancy.*

### Benefits to fetus:
- Use of medication may prevent seizures in the mother. Injuries from the mother falling during a seizure may damage the fetus.

### Benefits during lactation:
- None reported.

 ## Possible adverse effects

### Effects before pregnancy:
- Adverse effects include dizziness, drowsiness, headache, rash, nausea, vomiting, diarrhea and stomach cramps.
- Notify your doctor of any new or unusual adverse effects.

### Effects on mother:
- Pregnant women may have same adverse effects as any other person.
- Call your doctor if you develop any new adverse effects or if adverse effects worsen during pregnancy.

### Effects on fetus:
- The association between birth defects and ethosuximide is unclear because ethosuximide is frequently used with other medications to control seizures.
- Malformations reported when this medication is used alone include heart defects, cleft lip*, cleft palate*, head, face and eye abnormalities, short neck, altered palm crease in the hand, accessory nipple* and hydrocephalus*.
- Ask your doctor to review the evidence with you.

### Effects on newborn:
- Serious bleeding during the first day after birth can frequently be prevented by specific vitamin therapy. In some cases, a Cesarean delivery may be necessary to avoid trauma to the newborn.

### Effects during lactation:
- Ethosuximide is found in breast milk in amounts similar to the mother's blood level.
- Lactating women may have the same adverse effects as any other person.

 ## Additional information

- You have a 90% chance of having a normal child if you must take medication to control epilepsy*.
- Pregnancy may increase, decrease or have no effect on the frequency and severity of seizures.
- Very severe seizures have occurred when medication is discontinued without a doctor's supervision.
- Having epilepsy and taking anticonvulsant medications increase the risk of having a miscarriage, stillbirth or child with birth defects.

## Recommendations for use

### Women considering pregnancy:

- Notify your doctor if you plan to become pregnant. Possible risks to you and your baby must be considered on an individual basis.
- If you have been seizure-free for many years, your doctor may recommend slowly discontinuing this medication before pregnancy.
- If you have frequent seizures, it may be necessary to continue anticonvulsant medication throughout your pregnancy.
- Your doctor can provide the best recommendation for you. Do not stop taking this medication unless told to do so by your doctor.

### Recommendations during pregnancy:

- See your doctor regularly.
- Blood levels should be checked frequently during pregnancy and for a few weeks after delivery to balance adverse effects and effectiveness of medication.
- Your doctor may want to adjust dosage of medication frequently during and after pregnancy. It is important to follow your doctor's instructions carefully.
- If seizures occur, contact your doctor immediately.
- At the time of delivery, tell your doctor you take ethosuximide.
- Get plenty of sleep during your pregnancy.

### Recommendations during lactation:

- Nursing is considered safe when using this medication.

 ## Interactions

### Interactions with medications, vitamins and minerals:

| Interacts with | Combined effect |
| --- | --- |
| Oral contraceptives | Decreases effectiveness of oral contraceptives. |
| Other anticonvulsant medications | Increases likelihood of birth defects when more than one medication is needed to control seizures. |
| Pyridoxine | Decreases levels of pyridoxine. |

### Interactions with other substances:

- None reported.

*See Glossary.

# Fenoprofen

**Definition and description:** Relieves swelling, stiffness and pain of rheumatoid arthritis* or osteoarthritis*. Relieves mild to moderate pain.

**Other names:** Nalfon®, Nalfon 200®.

 ## Dosage

**Safe dosage:**
• Usual adult dose—900 to 3,200mg/day.

**Toxic dosage:**
• Exact toxic dose cannot be predicted.

 ## Possible benefits

**Benefits before pregnancy:**
• Relieves swelling, stiffness and joint pain of rheumatoid arthritis* or osteoarthritis*.
• Relieves mild to moderate pain.

**Benefits to mother:**
• See *Benefits before pregnancy*.

**Benefits to fetus:**
• None reported.

**Benefits during lactation:**
• None reported.

 ## Possible adverse effects

**Effects before pregnancy:**
• Adverse effects include dizziness, headache, drowsiness, tremor*, itching, rash, ringing in ears, nausea, heartburn*, abdominal pain, constipation, vomiting, bruising, bleeding, fast heartbeat, swelling, fatigue, anemia*, kidney damage, liver damage and vision changes.
• Notify your doctor if you develop any adverse effects.

**Effects on mother:**
• Pregnant women may have the same adverse effects as any other person.
• Call your doctor if you develop any new adverse effects or if adverse effects worsen during pregnancy.

• Anemia*, excessive bleeding during and after labor, and prolonged or delayed labor have been reported with similar medications. Experience with this medication in pregnancy is limited. See Aspirin, page 40.

**Effects on fetus:**
• Serious adverse effects have been reported after exposure to similar medications. Experience with this medication in pregnancy is limited. See Indomethacin, page 142, and Aspirin, page 40.

**Effects on newborn:**
• Serious adverse effects have been reported after use of similar medications. Experience with this medication in pregnancy is limited. See Indomethacin, page 142, and Aspirin, page 40.

**Effects during lactation:**
• Fenoprofen is found in very low concentrations in breast milk.
• Lactating women may have the same adverse effects as any other person.

 ## Additional information

• Use of fenoprofen or similar medications may be necessary to control severe rheumatoid arthritis* or related disorders during pregnancy.

 ## Recommendations for use

**Women considering pregnancy:**
• Use only the recommended doses of fenoprofen.
• Use fenoprofen only when needed for mild to moderate pain.
• Use this medication regularly as directed by your doctor for arthritis* and related disorders.
• If you use fenoprofen regularly, notify your doctor if you plan to become pregnant. Possible risks to you and your baby must be considered on an individual basis.
• Your doctor can provide the best recommendation for you.

## Recommendations during pregnancy:
- See your doctor regularly.
- Avoid unnecessary use of fenoprofen for mild to moderate pain during pregnancy.
- If you use this medication to control rheumatoid arthritis* or related disorders, possible risks to you and your baby must be considered on an individual basis. Follow your doctor's recommendations carefully.
- Avoid use of fenoprofen near your expected delivery date, except as directed by your doctor.
- At the time of delivery, tell your doctor you take fenoprofen.

## Recommendations during lactation:
- Your doctor or your baby's doctor can provide the best recommendation for you.

 ## Interactions

### Interactions with medications, vitamins and minerals:

| Interacts with | Combined effect |
|---|---|
| **Phenobarbital** | Decreases fenoprofen effectiveness. |
| **Warfarin** | Increases risk of bleeding. |

### Interactions with other substances:
- None reported.

*See Glossary.

# Fluphenazine

**Definition and description:** Acts as a phenothiazine tranquilizer* to treat manifestations of psychiatric disorders.

**Other names:** Fluphenazine hydrochloride, fluphenazine decanoate, Permitil®, Prolixin®.

 ## Dosage

### Safe dosage:
• Usual adult dose—2.5 to 20mg/day.
• A long-acting injectable form is also available.

### Toxic dosage:
• Exact toxic dose cannot be predicted.
• Symptoms of overdose include agitation, restlessness, convulsions, fever, dry mouth, bowel paralysis, loss of consciousness, low blood pressure and dangerous heart rhythm.
• Extrapyramidal symptoms* occur after overdose or occasionally after usual doses.
• Contact your doctor, poison-control center or emergency room if you think you have take an overdose.

 ## Possible benefits

### Benefits before pregnancy:
• Controls psychiatric disorders.

### Benefits to mother:
• See *Benefits before pregnancy.*

### Benefits to fetus:
• None reported.

### Benefits during lactation:
• None reported.

 ## Possible adverse effects

### Effects before pregnancy:
• Adverse effects include drowsiness, jaundice*, low blood-cell count, changes in blood pressure, unusual heart rhythm, seizures, rash, sensitivity to sunburn, dry mouth, nasal stuffiness, nausea, constipation, urinary retention, skin discoloration and eye damage. Tardive dyskinesia* occurs in some persons.
• Fatal anemia*, heart-rhythm disturbances and allergic reactions have occurred.
• Abnormal milk production and absence of menstruation occur in some women after prolonged use. These symptoms are associated with decreased fertility.
• False-positive pregnancy tests have been reported.
• Notify your doctor of any new or unusual adverse effects.
• Impotence* has been reported in men.

### Effects on mother:
• Pregnant women may have the same adverse effects as any other person.
• Call your doctor if you develop any new adverse effects or if adverse effects worsen during pregnancy.

### Effects on fetus:
• Most evidence indicates risk of birth defects is very low with phenothiazine medications.

### Effects on newborn:
• Extrapyramidal symptoms* have been reported several weeks after birth. Symptoms include excessive crying, abnormal motion, muscle rigidity, blood-pressure changes and delayed early learning.
• Intelligence at 4 years of age was not shown to be affected in a group of children exposed to phenothiazines before birth.
• Phenothiazines do not adversely affect birth weight or infant mortality.
• Increased jaundice* has been reported in premature infants exposed to phenothiazines.

### Effects during lactation:
• Effects of fluphenazine on nursing infants is unknown.
• Other phenothiazines do not have serious adverse effects on nursing infants.
• Lactating women may have the same adverse effects as any other person.

**Additional information**

- Pregnancy may be complicated by development or recurrence of a serious mental disorder. Treatments other than medication should be tried first. If the risks of mental illness are considered serious, use of medications to treat the mother's illness is important.
- Your doctor will determine whether medication is necessary.

 **Recommendations for use**

**Women considering pregnancy:**

- Use fluphenazine as directed by your doctor.
- Do not exceed the dose or frequency recommended by your doctor.
- Notify your doctor if you plan to become pregnant. Possible risks to you and your baby must be considered on an individual basis.
- Your doctor can provide the best recommendation for you.

**Recommendations during pregnancy:**

- See your doctor regularly.
- Use this medication as directed by your doctor.
- Do not exceed the dose recommended by your doctor.
- Avoid use near the time of delivery, if possible.

**Recommendations during lactation:**

- Your doctor or your baby's doctor can provide the best recommendation for you.

**Recommendations for newborn:**

- If your baby develops extrapyramidal symptoms*, contact your doctor or the baby's doctor for treatment.

 **Interactions**

**Interactions with medications, vitamins and minerals:**

| Interacts with | Combined effect |
| --- | --- |
| **Antacids** | Decreases fluphenazine absorption. |
| **Guanethidine** | Increases blood pressure. |
| **Insulin** | Increases blood sugar. |
| **Lithium** | Decreases fluphenazine effect and fluphenazine levels. |
| **Methyldopa** | Increases blood pressure. |
| **Orphenadrine** | Lowers blood sugar. |
| **Phenobarbital** | Decreases fluphenazine effect. |
| **Propranolol** | Increases effect of both. |

**Interactions with other substances:**

- Use with alcohol increases drowsiness and slows reaction time.

*See Glossary.

MEDICATION

# Guaifenesin

**Definition and description:** As an expectorant, guaifenesin may promote removal of secretions from airways. Increasing fluid intake to 6 to 8 glasses of water a day may be as effective.

**Other names:** Glyceryl guaiacolate. Also see brand-name list, page 390.

 ## Dosage

### Safe dosage:
- Usual adult dose—200 to 400mg every 4 hours, as needed.
- This medication can be purchased without a prescription. It is also found in products requiring a prescription.

### Toxic dosage:
- Toxicity is rare.

 ## Possible benefits

### Benefits before pregnancy:
- May help remove secretions from the airways.
- Used to decrease thickness of cervical mucus in some types of infertility. Use only as directed by your doctor.

### Benefits to mother:
- See *Benefits before pregnancy.*

### Benefits to fetus:
- None reported.

### Benefits during lactation:
- None reported.

 ## Possible adverse effects

### Effects before pregnancy:
- Adverse effects include nausea and vomiting.

### Effects on mother:
- Pregnant women may have the same adverse effects as any other person.
- Discontinue use and call your doctor if you develop any new adverse effects during pregnancy.

### Effects on fetus:
- Some studies have found an increase in malformations after the use of guaifenesin in early pregnancy.
- Cough mixtures and expectorants, as separate groups, are each associated with an increased risk of eye and ear abnormalities.

### Effects on newborn:
- One infant was born with fetal alcohol syndrome* after exposure to high doses of a cough syrup containing guaifenesin and other medications with alcohol. Withdrawal symptoms were reported. These effects were likely due to alcohol, not guaifenesin. See Alcohol, page 346.

### Effects during lactation:
- None reported. However, safety or risk has not been established.
- Lactating women may have the same adverse effects as any other person.

 ## Additional information

- Guaifenesin does not cure or shorten the course of an illness. It provides relief for symptoms, but otherwise it offers no benefit.
- Viral illnesses and fever have been implicated as a cause of birth defects. This medication is often used to relieve symptoms of viral illnesses. Contact your doctor if you have a fever.
- This medication is often used in combination with other medications. Most studies did not study persons using it alone. It is difficult to determine if guaifenesin caused any malformations.

**Recommendations for use**

### Women considering pregnancy:

- Use medication as directed on the package to treat a cough.
- Do not exceed the suggested dose.
- This medication works better with adequate fluid intake.
- Drink 6 to 8 large glasses of water each day.
- When used to treat infertility, use only as directed by your doctor.
- Use only when needed.
- Adequate fluid intake may make this medication unnecessary.

### Recommendations during pregnancy:

- Safety or risk has not been established.
- See your doctor regularly.
- Adequate fluid intake may make this medication unnecessary.
- Drink 6 to 8 large glasses of water each day.
- Avoid use during pregnancy. Use only if directed by your doctor.

### Recommendations during lactation:

- Safety or risk has not been established.
- Your doctor or your baby's doctor can provide the best recommendations for you.

 **Interactions**

### Interactions with medications, vitamins and minerals:

- None reported.

### Interactions with other substances:

- None reported.

*See Glossary.

MEDICATION

# Haloperidol

**Definition and description:** Acts as a tranquilizer to treat manifestations of psychiatric disorders.

**Other names:** Haloperidol decanoate, Haldol®.

 ## Dosage

### Safe dosage:
- Usual adult dose—1 to 15mg/day.
- Doses as high as 100mg/day may be used.

### Toxic dosage:
- Exact toxic dose cannot be predicted.
- Extrapyramidal symptoms* occur after overdose or occasionally after usual doses. Overdose produces low blood pressure, shock, drowsiness and loss of consiousness.
- Contact your doctor, poison-control center or emergency room if you think you have taken an overdose.

 ## Possible benefits

### Benefits before pregnancy:
- Controls psychiatric disorders.

### Benefits to mother:
- May be used to control nausea and vomiting in pregnancy. This is not an FDA*-approved use.
- Also see *Benefits before pregnancy*.

### Benefits to fetus:
- None reported.

### Benefits during lactation:
- None reported.

 ## Possible adverse effects

### Effects before pregnancy:
- Adverse effects include drowsiness, jaundice*, low blood-cell count, blood-pressure changes, fast heart rate, seizures, rash, sensitivity to sunburn, nausea, constipation and urinary retention. Tardive dyskinesia* occurs in some persons.

- Fatal anemia*, heart-rhythm disturbances, heat intolerance and allergic reactions have occurred.
- Abnormal milk production and absence of menstruation occur in some women after prolonged use. These symptoms are associated with decreased fertility.
- Notify your doctor of any new or unusual adverse effects.
- Impotence* has been reported in men.

### Effects on mother:
- Pregnant women may have the same adverse effects as any other person.
- Call your doctor if you develop any new adverse effects or if adverse effects worsen during pregnancy.

### Effects on fetus:
- Although risk appears low, there is inadequate data to establish safety or risk in early pregnancy. However, limb malformations have been reported occasionally.

### Effects on newborn:
- This medication has not produced adverse effects in newborns after use in labor.
- There is limited experience with infants exposed to long-term use before birth. Safety or risk has not been established.

### Effects during lactation:
- Haloperidol is found in high concentrations in breast milk.
- Lactating women may have the same adverse effects as any other person.

 ## Additional information

- Pregnancy may be complicated by development or recurrence of a serious mental disorder. Treatments other than medication should be tried first. If the risks of mental illness are considered serious, use of medications to treat the mother's illness is important.
- Use medication *only* if nausea and vomiting interfere with eating or daily activities, and other treatments fail. Your doctor can prescribe other treatments. He or she should determine whether medication is necessary.

- Other treatments may include eating soda crackers or dry toast and drinking hot or cold liquids as soon as you get up in the morning.
- A severe form of nausea and vomiting of pregnancy is called *hyperemesis gravidarum\**. This condition causes nutritional deficiencies, loss of electrolytes\*, weight loss and starvation. It often requires hospitalization. Treatment with antiemetics\* alone will not reverse hyperemesis gravidarum\*.
- Your doctor will determine whether medication is necessary.

 **Recommendations for use**

### Women considering pregnancy:
- Use this medication as directed by your doctor.
- Do not exceed the dose recommended by your doctor.
- Notify your doctor if you plan to become pregnant. Possible risks to you and your baby must be considered on an individual basis.
- Your doctor can provide the best recommendation for you.

### Recommendations during pregnancy:
- See your doctor regularly.
- Use haloperidol as directed by your doctor.
- Do not exceed the dose recommended by your doctor.
- If you have severe vomiting, contact your doctor as soon as possible.
- Your doctor can advise you about ways to decrease nausea and vomiting without medication.
- If other treatments fail to reduce nausea and vomiting, contact your doctor *before* using any medication.

### Recommendations during lactation:
- With medical supervision, nursing may be safe while using this medication.
- Contact your doctor or your baby's doctor if your baby becomes drowsy or lethargic.

 **Interactions**

**Interactions with medications, vitamins and minerals:**

| Interacts with | Combined effect |
|---|---|
| Guanethidine | Increases blood pressure. |
| Lithium | Increases central-nervous-system adverse effects. |
| Methyldopa | Increases haloperidol toxicity. |
| Phenobarbital | Decreases haloperidol effect. |
| Phenytoin | Decreases haloperidol effect. |
| Propranolol | Increases effect of both. |

**Interactions with other substances:**
- Use with alcohol increases drowsiness and slows reaction time.

\*See Glossary.

# Heparin

**Definition and description:** Acts at an anticoagulant to prevent blood clotting.

**Other names:** See brand-name list, page 390.

 ## Dosage

### Safe dosage:
- Dose is adjusted for each individual.
- Blood tests are used to determine the correct dose.

### Toxic dosage:
- Exact toxic dose cannot be determined.

 ## Possible benefits

### Benefits before pregnancy:
- Treats deep-vein thrombosis* and pulmonary embolism*.
- Prevents expansion of blood clot.

### Benefits to mother:
- See *Benefits before pregnancy.*

### Benefits to fetus:
- None reported.

### Benefits during lactation:
- None reported.

 ## Possible adverse effects

### Effects before pregnancy:
- Adverse effects include bleeding, changes in platelet function, pain or bruising at injection site, chills, fever, hives*, headache, nausea, vomiting, serious allergic reactions, itching and burning.
- Changes in platelet count may be associated with myocardial infarction*, stroke* and pulmonary embolism*.
- Long-term use of heparin is associated with osteoporosis*.

### Effects on mother:
- Pregnant women may have the same adverse effects as any other person.
- Miscarriage has been associated with use of heparin.

### Effects on fetus:
- Heparin does not enter fetal circulation. No malformations have been reported.
- Premature delivery is associated with use of this medication.

### Effects on newborn:
- Stillbirths are associated with use of heparin.

### Effects during lactation:
- Heparin is not active after oral use. No adverse effects are expected in nursing infants.
- Lactating women may have the same adverse effects as any other person.

 ## Additional information

- Deep-vein thrombosis* and pulmonary embolism* may be fatal. Use of anticoagulants is necessary to treat these disorders. In some cases, it is necessary to continue therapy for several months. Your doctor can recommend the safest option for you.
- Artificial heart valves also require use of anticoagulants throughout pregnancy.
- Heparin is usually considered safer in pregnancy than warfarin. Your doctor will advise you.

 ## Recommendations for use

### Women considering pregnancy:
- Notify your doctor if you plan to become pregnant. Risks to you and your baby must be considered on an individual basis.
- Your doctor may discontinue this medication or change to a different medication.
- Your doctor can provide the best recommendation for you.
- Do not stop taking this medication unless told to do so by your doctor.

## Recommendations during pregnancy:

- Contact your doctor as soon as you think you are pregnant.
- Follow your doctor's instructions carefully.

## Recommendations during lactation:

- Nursing is safe while using this medication.

 ## Interactions

### Interactions with medications, vitamins and minerals:

| Interacts with | Combined effect |
|---|---|
| **Antihistamines** | Decreases heparin effect. |
| **Aspirin** | Increases risk of bleeding. |
| **Digoxin** | Decreases heparin effect. |
| **Tetracycline** | Decreases heparin effect. |

### Interactions with other substances:

- Smoking decreases heparin effect.

*See Glossary.

# Hydrocodone

**Definition and description:** Acts as an antitussive* to relieve cough. It also acts as a narcotic analgesic to relieve pain.

**Other names:** Hydrocodone bitartrate, hydrocodone resin complex. Also see brand-name list, page 390.

##  Dosage

### Safe dosage:
- Usual adult dose—5mg every 4 to 6 hours.

### Toxic dosage:
- Exact toxic dose cannot be predicted.
- Symptoms of overdose include slow breathing, slow heartbeat, drowsiness or loss of consciousness.
- Death occurs after severe overdose.
- Call your doctor, poison-control center or emergency room if you think you have taken an overdose.

##  Possible benefits

### Benefits before pregnancy:
- Relieves cough.
- Relieves pain.

### Benefits to mother:
- See *Benefits before pregnancy*.

### Benefits to fetus:
- None reported.

### Benefits during lactation:
- None reported.

##  Possible adverse effects

### Effects before pregnancy:
- Adverse effects include depression, dizziness, drowsiness, hives*, rash, itching, flushing, blurred vision, constipation, abdominal pain, vomiting, difficulty urinating and fatigue.
- This medication is addicting.
- Notify your doctor of any adverse effects.

### Effects on mother:
- Pregnant women may have the same adverse effects as any other person.
- Call your doctor if you develop any adverse effects.

### Effects on fetus:
- Similar medications have been associated with growth retardation. See Codeine, page 82.

### Effects on newborn:
- Withdrawal has occurred after use of similar medications. See Codeine, page 82, and Methadone, page 174.

### Effects during lactation:
- Experience in nursing women is limited.
- Lactating women may have the same adverse effects as any other person.

**Recommendations for use**

### Women considering pregnancy:
- Notify your doctor if you plan to become pregnant.
- If you use hydrocodone regularly, ask your doctor's advice about discontinuing use.
- Use only as directed by your doctor.

### Recommendations during pregnancy:
- See your doctor regularly.
- Avoid unnecessary use of hydrocodone.
- Use only as directed by your doctor.

### Recommendations during lactation:
- Your doctor can provide the best recommendation for you.

 **Interactions**

**Interactions with medications, vitamins and minerals:**

| Interacts with | Combined effect |
| --- | --- |
| Acetaminophen | Increases analgesic effect. |
| Antidepressants | Increases drowsiness. |
| Antihistamines | Increases drowsiness. |
| Aspirin | Increases analgesic effect. |
| Other narcotics | Increases narcotic effect. |
| Tranquilizers | Increases drowsiness. |

**Interactions with other substances:**
- Use with alcohol increases drowsiness and slows reaction time.

*See Glossary.

# Ibuprofen

**Definition and description:** Relieves swelling, stiffness and pain of rheumatoid arthritis* or osteoarthritis*. Relieves mild to moderate pain. Relieves menstrual discomfort.

**Other names:** See brand-name list, page 390.

 **Dosage**

### Safe dosage:
• Usual adult dose—1.2 to 3.2g/day.
• Ibuprofen may be purchased without a prescription. It is also found in products requiring a prescription.

### Toxic dosage:
• Exact toxic dose cannot be predicted.
• Symptoms of toxicity have occurred in about 20% of acute ingestions.
• Chronic use has produced toxicity in some people.

 **Possible benefits**

### Benefits before pregnancy:
• Relieves swelling, stiffness and joint pain of rheumatoid arthritis* or osteoarthritis*.
• Relieves mild to moderate pain.
• Relieves menstrual discomfort.

### Benefits to mother:
• See *Benefits before pregnancy,* except for menstrual discomfort.

### Benefits to fetus:
• None reported.

### Benefits during lactation:
• See *Benefits before pregnancy.*

 **Possible adverse effects**

### Effects before pregnancy:
• Adverse effects include dizziness, headache, drowsiness, depression, rash, ringing in ears, nausea, heartburn*, abdominal pain, bruising,

bleeding, swelling, fatigue, weakness, anemia*, kidney damage, liver damage and vision changes.
• Notify your doctor if you develop any adverse effects.

### Effects on mother:
• Pregnant women may have the same adverse effects as any other person.
• Call your doctor if you develop any new adverse effects or if adverse effects worsen during pregnancy.
• Anemia*, excessive bleeding during and after labor, and prolonged or delayed labor have been reported with similar medications. Experience with ibuprofen in pregnancy is limited. See Aspirin, page 40.

### Effects on fetus:
• Experience with ibuprofen in pregnancy is limited. Miscarriage and fetal death have been reported after use of this medication.
• Absence of the brain, seizure disorder, cerebral palsy*, abnormal eyes, facial clefts* and skin discoloration have been reported in children of mothers who took ibuprofen during pregnancy.
• Serious adverse effects have been reported after exposure to similar medications. See Aspirin, page 40, and Indomethacin, page 142.

### Effects on newborn:
• Transient kidney malfunction has been reported.
• Serious problems have been reported after use of similar medications. Experience with ibuprofen in pregnancy is limited. See Aspirin, page 40, and Indomethacin, page 142.

### Effects during lactation:
• This medication is found in very low concentrations in breast milk.
• Lactating women may have the same adverse effects as any other person.

**Additional information**

• Use of this or similar medications may be necessary to control severe rheumatoid arthritis* or related disorders during pregnancy.

 **Recommendations for use**

### Women considering pregnancy:

• Use only the recommended doses of ibuprofen.
• Use this medication only when needed for minor pain and menstrual discomfort.
• Use this medication regularly as directed by your doctor for arthritis* and related disorders.
• If you use ibuprofen regularly to control arthritis* and related disorders, notify your doctor if you plan to become pregnant. Possible risks to you and your baby must be considered on an individual basis.
• Your doctor can provide the best recommendation for you.

### Recommendations during pregnancy:

• See your doctor regularly.
• Avoid unnecessary use of ibuprofen for mild to moderate pain in pregnancy.
• If you use this medication to control rheumatoid arthritis* or related disorders, possible risks to you and your baby must be considered on an individual basis. Follow your doctor's recommendations carefully.
• Avoid use of this medication near your expected delivery date, except as directed by your doctor.
• At the time of delivery, tell your doctor you take ibuprofen.

### Recommendations during lactation:

• Nursing is usually safe when using this medication.

 **Interactions**

**Interactions with medications, vitamins and minerals:**

| Interacts with | Combined effect |
| --- | --- |
| **Aspirin** | Decreases effectiveness of both. |
| **Digoxin** | Increases digoxin effect. |
| **Furosemide** | Decreases furosemide effectiveness. |

**Interactions with other substances:**
• None reported.

*See Glossary.

MEDICATION

# Imipramine

**Definition and description:** Acts as an antidepressant to relieve symptoms of depression. Imipramine is converted to desipramine in the liver.

**Other names:** Imipramine hydrochloride, imipramine pamoate, Presamine®, Tanimine®, Tofranil®.

 **Dosage**

**Safe dosage:**
• Usual adult dose—75 to 200mg/day.

**Toxic dosage:**
• Exact toxic dose cannot be predicted.
• Overdose has produced serious, life-threatening toxicity.
• Symptoms include confusion, hallucinations*, drowsiness, decreased or increased body temperature, muscle rigidity, dangerous heart rhythm, dilated pupils, low blood pressure and loss of consciousness.
• Death may occur after severe overdose.
• Contact your doctor, poison-control center or emergency room if you think you have taken an overdose.

 **Possible benefits**

**Benefits before pregnancy:**
• Controls symptoms of depression.

**Benefits to mother:**
• See Benefits before pregnancy.

**Benefits to fetus:**
• None reported.

**Benefits during lactation:**
• None reported.

 **Possible adverse effects**

**Effects before pregnancy:**
• Adverse reactions include low blood pressure or (less often) high blood pressure, rapid heart rate, unusual heart rhythm, altered mental state, tingling, staggering, ringing in the ears, seizures, dry mouth, blurred vision, constipation, difficulty urinating, rash, hives*, sensitivity to sunburn, low blood-cell count, nausea, vomiting, diarrhea, jaundice*, dizziness, headache and drowsiness.
• Notify your doctor of any new or unusual adverse effects.

**Effects on mother:**
• Pregnant women may have the same adverse effects as any other person.
• Call your doctor if you develop any new adverse effects or if adverse effects worsen during pregnancy.

**Effects on fetus:**
• Most evidence indicates imipramine does not increase risk of malformations. However, some controversy exists regarding limb defects.
• Ask your doctor to review the evidence with you.

**Effects on newborn:**
• Use of this medication late in pregnancy produced withdrawal symptoms in newborns, including irritability, rapid heart rate, sweating and seizures.
• Inability to urinate was reported in one infant after use of a similar medication. See Nortriptyline, page 188.

**Effects during lactation:**
• Imipramine and desipramine are found in breast milk after use of imipramine. See Additional information.
• Lactating women may have the same adverse effects as any other person.

 **Additional information**

• Imipramine is converted to desipramine in the liver. Both imipramine and desipramine are active antidepressants.
• Pregnancy may be complicated by development or recurrence of a serious mental disorder. Treatments other than medication should be tried first. If the risks of mental illness are considered serious, use of medications to treat the mother's illness is important.
• Depression during pregnancy may threaten you or your fetus if you are suicidal, unable to eat or if you have impaired judgment.

- Your doctor will determine if medication is necessary.

##  Recommendations for use

### Women considering pregnancy:
- Use imipramine as directed by your doctor.
- Do not exceed the dose or frequency recommended by your doctor.
- Notify your doctor if you plan to become pregnant. Possible risks to you and your baby must be considered on an individual basis.
- Your doctor can provide the best recommendation for you.

### Recommendations during pregnancy:
- See your doctor regularly.
- Use this medication as directed by your doctor.
- Do not exceed the dose recommended by your doctor.
- Avoid use near the time of delivery, if possible.

### Recommendations during lactation:
- Nursing is usually safe while using imipramine.
- Your doctor or your baby's doctor can provide the best recommendation for you.

##  Interactions

### Interactions with medications, vitamins and minerals:

| Interacts with | Combined effect |
| --- | --- |
| Amphetamines | Increases amphetamine toxicity. |
| Anti-cholinergics* | Increases toxicity of both. |
| Barbiturates | Decreases antidepressant effect. |
| Cimetidine | Increases antidepressant toxicity. |
| Clonidine | Increases blood pressure. |
| Debrisoquin | Increases blood pressure. |
| Epinephrine | Increases blood pressure. |
| Guanethidine | Increases blood pressure. |
| Methyldopa | Increases blood pressure. |
| Monoamine oxidase (MAO) inhibitors | Causes fever and seizures. |
| Phenothiazines | Increases toxicity. |
| Phenylephrine (intravenous*) | Increases blood pressure. |
| Phenytoin | Increases phenytoin toxicity. |

### Interactions with other substances:
- Use with alcohol increases drowsiness and slows reaction time.
- Smoking may decrease imipramine effectiveness.

*See Glossary.

141

# Indomethacin

**Definition and description:** Relieves swelling, stiffness and pain of rheumatoid arthritis*, ankylosing spondylitis*, osteoarthritis*, bursitis*, tendonitis* and gout*.

**Other names:** See brand-name list, page 390.

## Dosage

**Safe dosage:**
- Usual adult dose—75 to 200mg/day.
- Doses up to 350mg/day have been used to treat premature labor. See *Benefits to fetus*.

**Toxic dosage:**
- Exact toxic dose cannot be predicted.
- Bleeding, convulsions and severe confusion are symptoms of serious toxicity.
- Contact your doctor or emergency room immediately if you experience any toxic effects.

## Possible benefits

**Benefits before pregnancy:**
- Relieves swelling, stiffness and joint pain of rheumatoid arthritis* and related disorders.

**Benefits to mother:**
- See *Benefits before pregnancy*.

**Benefits to fetus:**
- Indomethacin has been used alone or in combination with other medications to treat premature labor. This use is experimental. Neonatal outcome has been good in some studies. In other studies, serious adverse effects to the fetus were reported. Risks and benefits should be evaluated on an individual basis. See *Possible adverse effects*, *Additional information* and *Recommendations during pregnancy*.
- Other medications are preferred to treat premature labor. See Ritodrine, page 238, and Terbutaline, page 252.

**Benefits during lactation:**
- None reported.

## Possible adverse effects

**Effects before pregnancy:**
- Adverse effects include dizziness, headache, drowsiness, depression, rash, ringing in ears, nausea, heartburn*, abdominal pain, swelling, fatigue, weakness, kidney damage, liver damage and vision changes.
- Notify your doctor if you develop any adverse effects.

**Effects on mother:**
- Anemia* and excessive bleeding during and after labor are more common in pregnant women who use indomethacin.
- Pregnant women may have the same adverse effects as any other person.
- Call your doctor if you develop any new adverse effects or if adverse effects worsen during pregnancy.

**Effects on fetus:**
- Bleeding in the brain, premature closure of the ductus arteriosus* and fetal death have been reported.
- Fetal kidney failure has been reported. Decreased production of amniotic fluid* and Potter's face are associated with fetal kidney failure.

**Effects on newborn:**
- Most studies evaluating the use of indomethacin in premature labor do not indicate an increase in premature closure of the ductus arteriosus*, persistent fetal circulation*, respiratory distress syndrome*, low levels of calcium and sugar in the blood, infection or newborn deaths. However, premature closure of the ductus arteriosus*, persistent fetal circulation*, respiratory distress, heart failure and hydrops fetalis* are reported in many individuals.
- Complications resulting from use of this medication occur more frequently after the 35th week of pregnancy.
- Intestinal perforation* has been reported rarely in newborns treated with indomethacin or exposed to the medication before birth.

## Effects during lactation

- Seizures in one infant may have been caused by indomethacin use by the mother.
- Lactating women may have the same adverse effects as any other person.

 **Additional information**

- Use of indomethacin or similar medications may be necessary to control severe rheumatoid arthritis* or related disorders during pregnancy.
- Premature delivery is associated with high infant-mortality rates. For each 2 weeks a fetus remains in the uterus between the 25th and 37th week of pregnancy, newborn mortality is cut in half.
- Premature delivery is associated with blindness, mental retardation and severe lung disease.
- Benefits to the baby from medication may outweigh the risks of using medication. Other medications are preferred. See Ritodrine, page 238, and Terbutaline, page 252. Your doctor will select the safest medication for you and your baby if you need treatment for premature labor.

 **Recommendations for use**

### Women considering pregnancy:

- Use this medication regularly as directed by your doctor for arthritis* and related disorders.
- If you use indomethacin to control arthritis* or related disorders, notify your doctor if you plan to become pregnant. Possible risks to you and your baby must be considered on an individual basis.
- Your doctor can provide the best recommendation for you.

### Recommendations during pregnancy:

- See your doctor regularly.
- If you use this medication to control rheumatoid arthritis* or related disorders, possible risks to you and your baby must be considered on an individual basis. Follow your doctor's recommendations carefully.
- If you require medication to treat premature labor, your doctor will choose the best medication for you and your baby. Possible risks to you and your baby must be considered on an individual basis. Follow your doctor's recommendations carefully.
- Avoid use of this medication near your expected delivery date, except as directed by your doctor.
- At the time of delivery, tell your doctor you take indomethacin.

### Recommendations during lactation:

- With medical supervision, nursing is usually safe while using indomethacin.
- Your doctor or your baby's doctor can provide the best recommendation for you.

# Indomethacin, continued

 **Interactions**

**Interactions with medications, vitamins and minerals:**

| Interacts with | Combined effect |
| --- | --- |
| Captopril | Decreases captopril effectiveness. |
| Diflunisal | Increases risk of bleeding. |
| Furosemide | Decreases furosemide effectiveness. |
| Hydralazine | Decreases hydralazine effectiveness. |
| Lithium | Increases lithium toxicity. |
| Methotrexate | Increases methotrexate toxicity. |
| Prazosin | Decreases prazosin effectiveness. |
| Propranolol and similar agents | Decreases propranolol effectiveness. |
| Steroids | Increases risk of bleeding. |
| Thiazides | Decreases thiazide effectiveness. |
| Triamterene | Decreases triamterene effectiveness. |
| Warfarin | Increases risk of bleeding. |

**Interactions with other substances:**
• Use with alcohol increases stomach irritation. It may also increase drowsiness and slow reaction time.

*See Glossary.

144

Note: This page purposely left blank.

# Insulin

**Definition and description:** Acts as a hormone to lower blood sugar.

**Other names:** See brand-name list, page 390.

 ## Dosage

### Safe dosage:
- Correct dose must be determined for each individual.

### Toxic dosage:
- Exact toxic dose cannot be predicted.
- Overdose can cause severe low blood sugar, with loss of consciousness and death.
- Call your doctor, poison-control center or emergency room if you think you have taken an overdose.

 ## Possible benefits

### Benefits before pregnancy:
- Maintains normal blood sugar in diabetic persons.

### Benefits to mother:
- Adequate blood-sugar control may decrease risk of pre-eclampsia* or eclampsia*, premature labor, Cesarean delivery, excessive production of amniotic fluid* and kidney infection.
- Insulin is the medication of choice for diabetic women who need a medication to control their diabetes during pregnancy.
- See *Benefits before pregnancy.*

### Benefits to fetus:
- Adequate blood-sugar control during pregnancy may decrease malformations, premature delivery, excessive size and low blood sugar in the newborn. Insulin therapy is considered superior to oral antidiabetic agents.

### Benefits during lactation:
- None reported.

 ## Possible adverse effects

### Effects before pregnancy:
- Adverse effects include low blood sugar, sweating, fast heart rate, dizziness, confusion, redness, swelling, itching at injection site and allergic reactions.
- Notify your doctor if you develop any adverse reactions.

### Effects on mother:
- Pregnant women may have the same adverse reactions as any other person.
- Call your doctor if you develop any new adverse reactions during pregnancy.

### Effects on fetus:
- Most evidence indicates the rate of malformations is not different than the rate of malformations in unexposed *diabetic* pregnancies. See *Additional information.*

### Effects on newborn:
- Problems arising in the newborn are related to the mother's disease, not the use of insulin.
- See *Additional information.*

### Effects during lactation:
- Insulin does not enter breast milk.
- Lactating women may have the same adverse effects as any other person.

 ## Additional information

- Diabetes* is usually harder to control during pregnancy.
- Most investigators have found a small but significant increase in malformations in children of diabetic mothers. Malformations reported include defects of the skeleton, stomach, intestines, heart, genital system, urinary system, palate, ears, nose and eyes. Neural-tube defects* have also been reported in children of diabetics.
- Malformations are more frequent in infants of women who have poor blood-sugar control during the early weeks of pregnancy.

- Good blood-sugar control before conception and early in pregnancy has been shown to decrease the risk of malformations and improve intelligence of children.
- Higher fetal-death and infant-death rates have been reported in diabetic pregnancies.
- Newborns of diabetic mothers develop low blood sugar, low blood levels of calcium and magnesium, and breathing problems more often than newborns of non-diabetic mothers. Good blood-sugar control late in pregnancy and during delivery decreases these complications.
- Pregnant diabetic women are at higher risk of some complications of pregnancy, such as pre-eclampsia* or eclampsia*, premature labor, Cesarean delivery, excessive production of amniotic fluid* and kidney infection. Good blood-sugar control may decrease these complications.
- Diabetes mellitus* may be diagnosed during pregnancy in women who have not been diabetic before. Many of these women will not be diabetic after pregnancy. During pregnancy these women may be treated with diet and/or insulin.
- Insulin is superior to oral antidiabetic agents. Oral antidiabetic medications are not recommended during pregnancy.

## Recommendations for use

### Women considering pregnancy:
- Notify your doctor if you plan to become pregnant. The possible risks to you and your baby must be considered on an individual basis.

- Pregnancy outcome is improved in diabetic women who maintain good blood-sugar control before and during pregnancy.
- Follow your doctor's recommendations carefully.
- Follow diet instructions carefully.
- Monitor your blood sugar carefully.

### Recommendations during pregnancy:
- See your doctor as soon as you think you may be pregnant. He or she may want to adjust your dose.
- See your doctor regularly.
- Follow diet instructions carefully.
- Monitor your blood sugar carefully. Your doctor will recommend the best blood-sugar level for you.
- Even if you have never had diabetes mellitus*, your doctor may recommend screening tests to make sure you have not become diabetic during pregnancy.

### Recommendations during lactation:
- Nursing is safe while using insulin.

## Interactions

### Interactions with medications, vitamins and minerals:

| Interacts with | Combined effect |
| --- | --- |
| **Propranolol** | Prolongs low blood sugar. Masks symptoms of low blood sugar. |

### Interactions with other substances:
- Inappropriate diet increases blood sugar.
- Large amounts of alcohol may decrease blood sugar.

*See Glossary.

# Isoetharine

**Definition and description:** Acts as a bronchodilator* to treat asthma*, chronic bronchitis* and emphysema*.

**Other names:** Bronkosol®.

 ## Dosage

### Safe dosage:
- Usual adult dose—1 or 2 puffs every 4 hours.

### Toxic dosage:
- Toxic dose is influenced by person's condition, size and age.
- Exact toxic dose cannot be predicted.
- Deaths have occurred from excessive use by inhalation.

 ## Possible benefits

### Benefits before pregnancy:
- Relieves symptoms of asthma*, chronic bronchitis* and emphysema*.

### Benefits to mother:
- See *Benefits before pregnancy.*

### Benefits to fetus:
- Severe asthma* may have detrimental effects on the fetus. Isoetharine relieves asthma* symptoms and improves oxygen exchange in the mother.

### Benefits during lactation:
- None reported.

 ## Possible adverse effects

### Effects before pregnancy:
- Adverse effects include tremor, headache, increased heart rate, unusual heart rhythm, insomnia* or drowsiness, nausea, vomiting, sweating and muscle cramps.
- Chest pain (angina*), hypertension* and nervousness have been reported.
- Notify your doctor of any adverse effects.
- Inhalation of isoetharine has rarely worsened asthma* symptoms.
- Deaths have been reported from overuse of inhaled isoetharine.

### Effects on mother:
- Pregnant women may have the same adverse effects as any other person.
- Call your doctor if you develop any new or unusual adverse effects.

### Effects on fetus:
- Hernias*, club foot* and minor malformations have been found to be more frequent after exposure to some bronchodilators. See Isoproterenol, page 152.

### Effects on newborn:
- Similar medications cause low blood sugar. See Terbutaline, page 252.

### Effects during lactation:
- None reported. It is unknown if isoetharine enters breast milk.
- Lactating women may have the same adverse effects as any other person.

 ## Additional information

- Pregnancy may affect asthma*. About 50% of pregnant asthmatic women have no change in symptoms during pregnancy, 30% improve and 20% worsen. If symptoms worsen during one pregnancy, they are more likely to worsen in other pregnancies.
- Premature delivery, low birth weight, stillbirth, newborn deaths and maternal deaths are more likely to occur in women with asthma*. Treatment of asthma* improves outcome.
- Premature delivery is associated with a high infant-mortality rate. For each 2 weeks a fetus remains in the uterus between the 25th and 37th week of pregnancy, newborn mortality is cut in half.
- Premature delivery is associated with blindness, mental retardation and severe lung disease.

**Recommendations for use**

### Women considering pregnancy:
- Notify your doctor if you plan to become pregnant. Risks to you and your baby must be considered on an individual basis.
- Do not exceed the dose recommended by your doctor.
- Notify your doctor if symptoms worsen while using isoetharine.
- If you have frequent asthma* attacks, it is important to work with your doctor to control your asthma* *before* pregnancy.
- Your doctor can provide the best recommendation for you. Do *not* change your medications unless your doctor tells you to do so.

### Recommendations during pregnancy:
- See your doctor regularly.
- Do not exceed the dose recommended by your doctor.
- Notify your doctor if symptoms worsen while using isoetharine.
- If your asthma* improves, your doctor may decrease your medications.
- If your asthma* worsens, your doctor may increase your medications. Do not adjust your dose without medical supervision.
- Avoid exposure to anything that worsens your asthma*.

### Recommendations during lactation:
- Your doctor can provide the best recommendation for you.

 **Interactions**

**Interactions with medications, vitamins and minerals:**

| Interacts with | Combined effect |
| --- | --- |
| Adrenergic stimulants* | Increases heart rate. |
| Beta-adrenergic blockers* | Decreases isoetharine effectiveness. |

**Interactions with other substances:**
- None reported.

*See Glossary.

MEDICATION

# Isoniazid

**Definition and description:** Acts as an antibiotic to treat susceptible tuberculosis* bacteria.

**Other names:** INH. Also see brand-name list, page 390.

 ## Dosage

### Safe dosage:
- Usual adult dose—300mg/day.

### Toxic dosage:
- Exact toxic dose cannot be predicted.
- Severe liver damage has rarely been fatal.

 ## Possible benefits

### Benefits before pregnancy:
- Prevents active tuberculosis* in women at risk.
- Isoniazid (INH) is used in combination with other medications to treat active tuberculosis*.

### Benefits to mother:
- Some bacterial infections may be very serious to the mother. This medication can treat susceptible infections. Also see *Benefits before pregnancy*.

### Benefits to fetus:
- Some bacterial infections in the mother may increase risk to the fetus. This medication can treat susceptible infections.

### Benefits during lactation:
- None reported.

 ## Possible adverse effects

### Effects before pregnancy:
- Adverse effects include nausea, vomiting, decreased blood-cell count, fever, rash, swollen lymph glands*, tingling in the hands and feet, convulsions, memory loss, high blood sugar, rheumatic syndrome*, systemic lupus erythematosus syndrome* and encephalopathy*.

- Pyridoxine deficiency occurs in some women who take this medication. See Pyridoxine, page 318.
- Notify your doctor of any adverse effects.

### Effects on mother:
- Pregnant women may have the same adverse effects as any other person.
- Call your doctor if you develop any adverse effects.

### Effects on fetus:
- Most evidence indicates no increase in the risk of malformations. However, some controversy exists. Ask your doctor to review the evidence with you.

### Effects on newborn:
- Convulsions have been reported in infants exposed to high doses before birth.
- Serious bleeding after birth can be prevented by specific vitamin therapy.

### Effects during lactation:
- Isoniazid (INH) is found in high concentrations in breast milk.
- Lactating women may have the same adverse effects as any other person.

 ## Additional information

- Tuberculosis* can be a very serious infection in mothers and newborns. It is necessary to treat pregnant women with recent positive skin tests. Your doctor will determine which medication and how many medications are needed for you.
- In some cases, it will also be necessary to treat newborns of women with tuberculosis*. Your doctor or your baby's doctor can advise you.
- Some bacterial infections may be very serious to the mother or the baby. It is important to treat these infections.
- Risks from infection or medication must be considered on an individual basis. Your doctor can advise you.

## Recommendations for use

### Women considering pregnancy:
- Notify your doctor if you plan to become pregnant. Possible risks to you and your baby must be considered on an individual basis.
- Your doctor can provide the best recommendation for you.
- Take the vitamin supplements recommended by your doctor.
- Avoid alcohol while using this medication.

### Recommendations during pregnancy:
- Risks from infection or medication must be considered on an individual basis. Your doctor can advise you.
- Use this medication as directed by your doctor.
- Notify your doctor of any adverse effects.
- Take the vitamin supplements recommended by your doctor.
- Avoid alcohol while using this medication.

### Recommendations during lactation:
- With medical supervision, nursing is safe while using isoniazid (INH).
- The amount of medication absorbed may be decreased if you avoid nursing for 1 or 2 hours after taking isoniazid (INH).
- Your doctor or your baby's doctor may recommend vitamin supplements for your baby.
- Your baby's doctor can provide the best recommendation for you.

 ## Interactions

### Interactions with medications, vitamins and minerals:

| Interacts with | Combined effect |
| --- | --- |
| Antacids containing aluminum | Decreases isoniazid (INH) absorption. |
| Carbamazepine | Increases carbamazepine effect. |
| Diazepam | Increases diazepam effect. |
| Disulfiram | Causes central-nervous-system adverse effects. |
| Folate | May decrease folate levels. |
| Laxatives | Decreases isoniazid absorption. |
| Oral contraceptives | Decreases contraceptive effectiveness. |
| Phenytoin | Decreases phenytoin effectiveness. |
| Primidone | Alters primidone metabolism. |
| Pyridoxine | Increases urinary loss of pyridoxine. Causes pyridoxine depletion. |
| Rifampin | Increases liver damage. |
| Steroids | Decreases isoniazid (INH) effect, and increases steroid effect. |
| Warfarin | Increases warfarin effect. |

### Interactions with other substances:
- Use with alcohol may produce facial flushing, difficulty breathing, fast heart rate, low blood pressure, nausea and vomiting. Life-threatening symptoms have rarely occurred.
- Use with alcohol may increase the risk of developing severe liver damage.
- Taking isoniazid (INH) with food decreases effectiveness.

*See Glossary.

# Isoproterenol

**Definition and description:** Acts as a bronchodilator* to treat asthma*, chronic bronchitis* and emphysema*.

**Other names:** Isoproterenol hydrochloride. Also see brand-name list, page 390.

 ## Dosage

### Safe dosage:
- Isoproterenol can be taken by inhalation, ingestion or injection.
- Dose is determined by person's size and route of administration.
- Usual adult dose by inhalation—2 puffs up to 5 times a day.

### Toxic dosage:
- Toxic dose is influenced by the person's condition, size and age.
- Exact toxic doses cannot be predicted.
- Deaths have occurred from excessive use by inhalation.

 ## Possible benefits

### Benefits before pregnancy:
- Relieves symptoms of asthma*, chronic bronchitis* and emphysema*.

### Benefits to mother:
- See *Benefits before pregnancy.*

### Benefits to fetus:
- Severe asthma* may have detrimental effects on the fetus. Isoproterenol relieves asthma* symptoms and improves oxygen exchange in the mother.

### Benefits during lactation:
- None reported.

 ## Possible adverse effects

### Effects before pregnancy:
- Adverse effects include nervousness, tremor, headache, increased heart rate, unusual heart rhythm, drowsiness, nausea, vomiting, sweating and muscle cramps.
- Notify your doctor of any adverse effects.
- Inhalation of isoproterenol has rarely worsened asthma* symptoms.
- Deaths have been reported from overuse of inhaled isoproterenol.

### Effects on mother:
- Pregnant women may have the same adverse effects as any other person.
- Call your doctor if you develop any new or unusual adverse effects.

### Effects on fetus:
- Hernias*, club foot* and minor malformations have been found to be more frequent after exposure to some bronchodilators. See Isoetharine, page 148.

### Effects on newborn:
- Similar medications cause low blood sugar. See Terbutaline, page 252.

### Effects during lactation:
- None reported. It is unknown if isoproterenol enters breast milk.
- Lactating women may have the same adverse effects as any other person.

 ## Additional information

- Pregnancy may affect asthma*. About 50% of pregnant asthmatic women have no change in symptoms during pregnancy, 30% improve and 20% worsen. If symptoms worsen during one pregnancy, they are more likely to worsen in other pregnancies.
- Premature delivery, low birth weight, stillbirth, newborn deaths and maternal deaths are more likely to occur in women with asthma*. Treatment of asthma* improves outcome.

# Isoproterenol, continued

 ## Recommendations for use

### Women considering pregnancy:
- Notify your doctor if you plan to become pregnant. Risks to you and your baby must be considered on an individual basis.
- Do not exceed the dose recommended by your doctor.
- Notify your doctor if symptoms worsen while using isoproterenol.
- If you have frequent asthma* attacks, it is important to work with your doctor to control your asthma* *before* pregnancy.
- Your doctor can provide the best recommendation for you. Do *not* change your medications unless your doctor tells you to do so.

### Recommendations during pregnancy:
- See your doctor regularly.
- Do not exceed the dose recommended by your doctor.
- Notify your doctor if symptoms worsen while using this medication.
- If your asthma* improves, your doctor may decrease your medication.
- If your asthma* worsens, your doctor may increase your medication.
- Do not adjust your dose without medical supervision.
- Avoid exposure to anything that worsens your asthma*.

### Recommendations during lactation:
- Your doctor can provide the best recommendation for you.
- If nursing is attempted, taking isoproterenol by inhalation produces lower levels in your blood and possibly in your breast milk.

 ## Interactions

### Interactions with medications, vitamins and minerals:

| Interacts with | Combined effect |
| --- | --- |
| Adrenergic stimulants* | Increases heart rate. |
| Beta-adrenergic blockers* | Decreases isoproterenol effectiveness. |

### Interactions with other substances:
- None reported.

*See Glossary.

153

# Isotretinoin

**Definition and description:** Acts as a retinoid to treat acne and other skin diseases. Retinoids are vitamin-A derivatives.

**Other names:** Cis-retinoic acid, Accutane®.

 ## Dosage

### Safe dosage:
• Usual adult dose—0.5 to 1mg/kg body weight/day.
• *No dose is safe during pregnancy.*

### Toxic dosage:
• Overdose has produced headache, facial flushing, vomiting, abdominal pain, dizziness and staggering.
• Serious overdose is expected to cause symptoms similar to vitamin-A toxicity. See Vitamin A, page 328.
• Contact your doctor, poison-control center or emergency room if you think you have taken an overdose of this medication.
• Changes in vision may indicate the beginning of toxicity to the cornea. Contact your doctor as soon as possible.
• Increased intercranial pressure has been reported. Symptoms include headache, vision changes, nausea and vomiting. Contact your doctor immediately.

 ## Possible benefits

### Benefits before pregnancy:
• Treats severe acne.
• Isotretinoin has been used experimentally in some severe skin diseases.

### Benefits to mother:
• *The risk of isotretinoin to the fetus outweighs any possible benefit to the mother.*
• *This medication should not be used by pregnant women.*

### Benefits to fetus:
• None reported.
• *Do not use during pregnancy.*

### Benefits during lactation:
• None reported.

 ## Possible adverse effects

### Effects before pregnancy:
• Adverse effects include dry skin, itching, bloody nose, dry mouth, cracking at the corners of the lips, eye irritation, muscle pain, joint pain, rash, temporary loss of hair, peeling of palms and soles, headache, sensitivity to sunburn, seizures, dizziness, nervousness, drowsiness, weakness, sleeplessness, tingling in extremities and depression.
• Elevation in triglyceride levels and cholesterol levels and a decrease in HDL levels occurs.
• Patients with inflammatory bowel disease* may experience worsening of symptoms.
• Notify your doctor of any adverse effects.

### Effects on mother:
• *Isotretinoin should not be used by pregnant women because of toxicity to the fetus.*

### Effects on fetus:
• *This medication produces serious malformations in exposed fetuses. Malformations include small brain and other nervous-system abnormalities, ear abnormalities, absence of the thymus, cleft lip*, cleft palate*, small eyes, serious heart abnormalities and blood-vessel abnormalities. Slow mental development is associated with small brain and other central-nervous-system abnormalities.*
• Studies indicate a malformation rate of at least 40%.

### Effects on newborn:
• *This medication should not be used by pregnant women.*

## Effects during lactation:
- It is unknown if isotretinoin is found in breast milk.
- Lactating women may have the same adverse effects as any other person.

 **Additional information**

- Risks of this medication to the fetus outweigh the benefits to the mother. This medication should *not* be used during pregnancy.
- Contraception should be continued for at least 1 month after discontinuing isotretinoin.

 **Recommendations for use**

### Women considering pregnancy:
- *Do not use this medication if you are planning to become pregnant.*
- Start using an effective form of birth control 1 month before this medication is started. Your doctor can recommend an effective method of birth control.
- Start using isotretinoin during your menstrual period, after you have a negative pregnancy test.
- Continue using an effective method of birth control for 1 month after discontinuing use of isoretinoin.

### Recommendations during pregnancy:
- *Do not use this medication during pregnancy.*
- Discontinue use *immediately* and contact your doctor if you think you might be pregnant.
- Your doctor can advise you.

### Recommendations during lactation:
- *Do not use this medication while nursing.*

 **Interactions**

### Interactions with medications, vitamins and minerals
- None reported.

### Interactions with other substances:
- None reported.

*See Glossary.

MEDICATION

# Levothyroxine

**Definition and description:** Hormone used to replace thyroid hormone in hypothyroid* persons.

**Other names:** Cytolen®, Levoid®, Noroxine®, Synthroid®.

 ## Dosage

**Safe dosage:**
- Correct dose must be established for each person.

**Toxic dosage:**
- Exact toxic dose cannot be predicted.
- Overdose produces symptoms of hyperthyroidism*, including heat intolerance, rapid heart rate, tremor*, nervousness, diarrhea, muscle cramps and sweating.

 ## Possible benefits

**Benefits before pregnancy:**
- Maintains normal thyroid condition in hypothyroid* persons.

**Benefits to mother:**
- See *Benefits before pregnancy.*

**Benefits to fetus:**
- Fetuses have been treated with amniotic or direct-intramuscular injections to prevent hypothyroidism* after use of antithyroid medications by the mother.

**Benefits during lactation:**
- None reported.

 ## Possible adverse effects

**Effects before pregnancy:**
- Adverse effects include tremor*, headache, irritability, sleeplessness, hives*, rash, chest pain, rapid heart rate, leg cramps, changes in menstrual periods, fever, heat intolerance and weight loss.
- Notify your doctor of any adverse effects.

**Effects on mother:**
- Pregnant women may have the same adverse effects as any other person, except changes in menstrual periods.
- Call your doctor if you develop any new adverse effects during pregnancy.

**Effects on fetus:**
- Adverse effects to the fetus are not expected.
- Malformations have been reported. These malformations are attributed to maternal disease, *not* to thyroid replacement medications. See *Additional information.*

**Effects on newborn:**
- None reported.

**Effects during lactation:**
- Small quantities of levothyroxine enter breast milk.
- Lactating women may have the same adverse effects as any other person.

 ## Additional information

- Infant-death and fetal-death rates are slightly higher in pregnancies of hypothyroid* women.
- Some investigators have demonstrated an increase in malformations in children of women with hypothyroidism*. Other investigators have not found increased rates of malformations. Ask your doctor to review the evidence with you.

**Recommendations for use**

## Women considering pregnancy:
- Notify your doctor if you plan to become pregnant.
- Use this medication only as directed by your doctor.
- Do not stop taking this medication unless told to do so by your doctor.

## Recommendations during pregnancy:
- See your doctor early in pregnancy.
- Continue this medication throughout your pregnancy.

## Recommendations during lactation:
- With medical supervision, nursing may be safe while using this medication.
- Your doctor or your baby's doctor can provide the best recommendation for you.

 **Interactions**

## Interactions with medications, vitamins and minerals:

| Interacts with | Combined effect |
| --- | --- |
| Cholestyramine | Decreases thyroid effect. |
| Insulin | Increases insulin requirement. |
| Oral anti-diabetic agents | Increases anti-diabetic agent requirement. |
| Phenytoin | Decreases thyroid effect. |
| Warfarin | Increases risk of bleeding. |

## Interactions with other substances:
- None reported.

*See Glossary.

Note: This page purposely left blank.

# Lindane

### Definition and description: Treats scabies*.

### Other names: Gamma benzene hexachloride, Kwell®.

 ## Dosage

### Safe dosage:
- Apply to skin and rub in well. After 8 to 12 hours, wash thoroughly.

### Toxic dosage:
- Exceeding the recommended dose or taking this medication by mouth can produce serious toxicity.

 ## Possible benefits

### Benefits before pregnancy:
- Treats scabies* infestations.

### Benefits to mother:
- See *Benefits before pregnancy*.

### Benefits to fetus:
- None reported.

### Benefits during lactation:
- None reported.

 ## Possible adverse effects

### Effects before pregnancy:
- This medication penetrates the skin. Central-nervous-system adverse effects, including convulsions, has been reported.
- Notify your doctor of any adverse effects.

### Effects on mother:
- Pregnant women may have the same adverse effects as any other person.
- Call your doctor if you develop any adverse effects.

### Effects on fetus:
- Use has been restricted because lindane is not recommended in pregnancy.
- This medication *cannot* be considered safe.

### Effects on newborn:
- Use has been restricted because lindane is not recommended in pregnancy or in children under 2.
- This medication *cannot* be considered safe.

### Effects during lactation:
- Use has been restricted because lindane is not recomended during lactation.
- This medication cannot be considered safe.

 ## Recommendations for use

### Women considering pregnancy:
- Use this medication as directed by your doctor.
- Avoid frequent use.
- Notify your doctor of any adverse effects.

### Recommendations during pregnancy:
- Do not use during pregnancy.
- Your doctor can recommend an alternative treatment.

### Recommendations during lactation:
- Do not breast-feed while using lindane.
- Your doctor can recommend an alternative treatment.
- If you use this medication, it is possible to resume breast-feeding when treatment is complete. Ask your doctor to advise you.

 ## Interactions

### Interactions with medications, vitamins and minerals:
- None reported.

### Interactions with other substances:
- None reported.

*See Glossary.

# Liothyronine

## Definition and description:
Hormone used to replace thyroid hormone in hypothyroid* persons.

**Other names:** Cytomel®.

## Dosage

### Safe dosage:
• Correct dose must be established for each person.

### Toxic dosage:
• Exact toxic dose cannot be predicted.
• Overdose produces symptoms of hyperthyroidism*, including heat intolerance, rapid heart rate, tremor*, nervousness, diarrhea, muscle cramps and sweating.

## Possible benefits

### Benefits before pregnancy:
• Maintains normal thyroid condition in hypothyroid* persons.

### Benefits to mother:
• See Benefits before pregnancy.

### Benefits to fetus:
• There are reports of using high doses of thyroid hormones to treat hypothyroidism* in the fetus. See Thyroid, page 264.

### Benefits during lactation:
• None reported.

## Possible adverse effects

### Effects before pregnancy:
• Adverse effects include tremor*, headache, irritability, sleeplessness, hives*, rash, chest pain, rapid heart rate, leg cramps, changes in menstrual periods, fever, heat intolerance and weight loss.
• Notify your doctor of any adverse effects.

### Effects on mother:
• Pregnant women may have the same adverse effects as any other person, except changes in menstrual periods.
• Call your doctor if you develop any new adverse effects during pregnancy.

### Effects on fetus:
• Adverse effects to the fetus are not expected.

### Effects on newborn:
• None reported.

### Effects during lactation:
• Very small quantities of liothyronine enter breast milk.
• Lactating women may have the same adverse effects as any other person.

## Additional information

• Infant-death and fetal-death rates are slightly higher in pregnancies of hypothyroid* women.
• Some investigators have demonstrated an increase in malformations in children of women with hypothyroidism*. Other investigators have not found increased rates of malformations. Ask your doctor to review the evidence with you.

**Recommendations for use**

### Women considering pregnancy:
- Notify your doctor if you plan to become pregnant.
- Use this medication only as directed by your doctor.
- Do not stop taking this medication unless told to do so by your doctor.

### Recommendations during pregnancy:
- See your doctor early in pregnancy.
- Continue this medication throughout your pregnancy.

### Recommendations during lactation:
- With medical supervision, nursing may be safe while using this medication.
- Your doctor or your baby's doctor can provide the best recommendation for you.

 **Interactions**

**Interactions with medications, vitamins and minerals:**

| Interacts with | Combined effect |
|---|---|
| Cholestyramine | Decreases thyroid effect. |
| Insulin | Increases insulin requirement. |
| Oral anti-diabetic agents | Increases anti-diabetic agent requirement. |
| Phenytoin | Decreases thyroid effect. |
| Warfarin | Increases risk of bleeding. |

**Interactions with other substances:**
- None reported.

*See Glossary.

MEDICATION

# Lithium

**Definition and description:** Treats and prevents manic episodes* of manic-depressive illness.

**Other names:** Cibalith®, Eskalith®, Lithane®, Lithobid®.

 **Dosage**

### Safe dosage:
- Dose is usually determined by lithium-blood levels.

### Toxic dosage:
- Serious toxicity has occurred at doses very close to a desired dose. Lithium-blood level should be monitored and doses adjusted to avoid toxicity.
- Diarrhea, drowsiness, vomiting, muscle weakness and lack of coordination may be early signs of toxicity.
- Contact your doctor, poison-control center or emergency room if you experience any symptoms of toxicity.

 **Possible benefits**

### Benefits before pregnancy:
- Treats and prevents manic episodes*.

### Benefits to mother:
- See *Benefits before pregnancy.*

### Benefits to fetus:
- None reported.

### Benefits during lactation:
- None reported.

 **Possible adverse effects**

### Effects before pregnancy:
- Adverse effects include tremor*, increased urination, increased thirst, nausea, loss of appetite, dizziness, rash, blurred vision, swelling, slurred speech, kidney damage, changes in thyroid function, itching and headache.
- Notify your doctor of any adverse effects.

### Effects on mother:
- Lithium is eliminated more rapidly during pregnancy. After pregnancy, there is an increased risk of toxicity with the dose used during pregnancy.
- Pregnant women may have the same adverse effects as any other person.
- Call your doctor if you develop any new adverse effects or if adverse effects worsen during pregnancy.

### Effects on fetus:
- Heart defects occur more frequently in infants who are exposed to lithium. One serious heart defect (Ebstein's anomaly*) occurs in 1 in 1,000 exposures. As many as 8 to 9% of exposed babies may be affected. In some cases, life expectancy is decreased by the malformation.
- Other major malformations have been reported, including brain malformations and spine malformations.
- Fetal goiter* has been reported. In some cases, Cesarean delivery is necessary due to the large size of the goiter*.

### Effects on newborn:
- Lithium toxicity occurs in newborns exposed to the medication before birth. Lithium toxicity is associated with poor muscle tone, poor sucking, abnormal heart rhythms, heart failure and breathing problems. Although deaths have been reported, symptoms of lithium toxicity usually disappear without serious permanent effects.
- Excessive urination from kidney toxicity has lasted for up to 2 months after birth.

### Effects during lactation:
- This medication enters breast milk.
- Lithium toxicity has been reported rarely.
- Nursing women may have the same adverse effects as any other person.

## Additional information

- Pregnancy may be complicated by development or recurrence of a serious mental disorder. Treatments other than medication should be tried first. If the risks of mental illness are considered serious, use of medication to treat the mother's illness is important.
- Your doctor will determine whether medication is necessary.

 ## Recommendations for use

### Women considering pregnancy:
- Notify your doctor if you plan to become pregnant. Risks to you and your baby must be considered on an individual basis.
- Follow your doctor's instructions carefully.
- If possible, your doctor may recommend discontinuing this medication.

### Recommendations during pregnancy:
- See your doctor regularly.
- Your doctor will advise you about dosage adjustment during pregnancy, labor and after delivery.
- Avoid lithium early in pregnancy, if possible.
- Your doctor can provide the best recommendation for you.
- Blood levels should be checked frequently during and after pregnancy.
- Dose may need to be changed frequently during pregnancy and for a few weeks after delivery.

### Recommendations during lactation:
- With medical supervision, nursing may be safe while using lithium.
- Your doctor or your baby's doctor can provide the best recommendation for you.

 ## Interactions

### Interactions with medications, vitamins and minerals:

| Interacts with | Combined effect |
| --- | --- |
| Carbamazepine | Increases lithium toxicity. |
| Diazepam | Decreases body temperature. |
| Diuretics | Increases lithium toxicity. |
| Haloperidol | Increases haloperidol toxicity. |
| Indomethacin | Increases indomethacin toxicity. |
| Methyldopa | Increases lithium toxicity. |
| Piroxicam | Increases lithium toxicity. |
| Phenothiazines | Alters response to either medication. |
| Phenytoin | Increases lithium toxicity. |
| Potassium iodide | Increases thyroid damage. |
| Sodium bicarbonate | Increases lithium excretion. |
| Sodium chloride | Changes in sodium intake alter lithium elimination. |
| Tetracycline | Increases lithium toxicity. |
| Theophylline | Decreases lithium effect. |

### Interactions with other substances:
- Dietary salt intake alters lithium response.

*See Glossary.

MEDICATION

# Meclizine

**Definition and description:** Antihistamine that acts as an antiemetic* to control nausea, vomiting and dizziness of motion sickness. May be effective in managing vertigo*.

**Other names:** Antivert®, Bonine®.

 ## Dosage

### Safe dosage:
- Usual adult dose—25 to 100mg/day in divided doses for vertigo*.
- Motion sickness responds to 25 to 50mg/day, given as one dose.
- This medication can be purchased without a prescription.

### Toxic dosage:
- Exact toxic dose cannot be predicted.
- Serious toxicity has occurred with antihistamine overdose. Contact your doctor, poison-control center or emergency room if you think you have taken an overdose.

 ## Possible benefits

### Benefits before pregnancy:
- Treats nausea and vomiting associated with motion sickness.
- May be beneficial in treating vertigo*.

### Benefits to mother:
- May relieve nausea and vomiting.
- Effectiveness of non-prescription antiemetics* has not been proved for nausea and vomiting in pregnancy.

### Benefits to fetus:
- None reported.

### Benefits during lactation:
- None reported.

 ## Possible adverse effects

### Effects before pregnancy:
- Adverse effects include drowsiness, dry mouth and blurred vision.

- Discontinue use if you develop any adverse effects.
- Contact your doctor if symptoms continue.

### Effects on mother:
- Pregnant women may have the same adverse effects as any other person.
- Call your doctor if you develop any adverse effects.

### Effects on fetus:
- Studies of large numbers of persons have not demonstrated an increase in malformation rates after exposure to meclizine compared to unexposed pregnancies.
- Antihistamines as a group have not been shown to increase risk of malformations compared to unexposed pregnancies.

### Effects on newborn:
- None reported.

### Effects during lactation:
- None reported in nursing infants.
- Lactating women may have the same adverse effects as any other person.

 ## Additional information

- In 1966, the FDA* required meclizine to carry warnings against use by pregnant women. The warning was based on animal studies that demonstrated increased fetal death and malformations. Since then, the warning has been removed, based on evaluation of use by pregnant women. Risk from this medication is low. See *Effects on fetus*.
- Use medication *only* if nausea and vomiting interfere with eating or daily activities, and other treatments fail. Your doctor can prescribe other treatments. He or she should determine whether medication is necessary.
- Other treatments may include eating soda crackers or dry toast and drinking hot or cold liquids as soon as you get up in the morning.

• A severe form of nausea and vomiting of pregnancy is called *hyperemesis gravidarum\**. This condition causes nutritional deficiencies, loss of electrolytes\*, weight loss and starvation. It often requires hospitalization. Treatment with antiemetics\* alone will not reverse hyperemesis gravidarum\*.

 **Recommendations for use**

### Women considering pregnancy:
• Use this medication as directed on the package.
• Use meclizine only as needed.
• Notify your doctor if you plan to become pregnant. Before pregnancy, your doctor can advise you about ways to decrease nausea and vomiting without medication.

### Recommendations during pregnancy:
• If you have severe vomiting, contact your doctor as soon as possible.
• See your doctor regularly.
• Your doctor can advise you about ways to decrease nausea and vomiting without medication.
• If other treatments fail to reduce nausea and vomiting, contact your doctor *before* using any medication.
• Use this medication only as directed by your doctor.

### Recommendations during lactation:
• Nursing is usually safe while using antihistamines.
• Your doctor or your baby's doctor can provide the best recommendation for you.

 **Interactions**

**Interactions with medications, vitamins and minerals:**

| Interacts with | Combined effect |
| --- | --- |
| Antianxiety agents | Increases drowsiness. |
| Antidepressants | Increases drowsiness. |
| Other anti-histamines | Increase drowsiness. |
| Tranquilizers | Increase drowsiness. |

**Interactions with other substances:**
• Use with alcohol increases drowsiness and slows reaction time.

\*See Glossary.

# Meclofenamate

**Definition and description:** Relieves swelling, stiffness and pain of rheumatoid arthritis* or osteoarthritis*.

**Other names:** Meclomen®.

 ## Dosage

### Safe dosage:
- Usual adult dose—200 to 400mg/day.

### Toxic dosage:
- Exact toxic dose cannot be predicted.

 ## Possible benefits

### Benefits before pregnancy:
- Relieves swelling, stiffness and joint pain of rheumatoid arthritis* or osteoarthritis*.

### Benefits to mother:
- See *Benefits before pregnancy.*

### Benefits to fetus:
- None reported.

### Benefits during lactation:
- None reported.

 ## Possible adverse effects

### Effects before pregnancy:
- Adverse effects include dizziness, headache, rash, ringing in ears, diarrhea, nausea, abdominal pain, flatulence, bruising, bleeding, swelling, fatigue, weakness, anemia*, kidney damage, liver damage and vision changes.
- Notify your doctor if you develop any adverse effects.

### Effects on mother:
- Pregnant women may have the same adverse effects as any other person.
- Call your doctor if you develop any new adverse effects or if adverse effects worsen during pregnancy.

- Anemia*, excessive bleeding during and after labor, and prolonged or delayed labor have been reported with similar medications. Experience with this medication in pregnancy is limited. See Aspirin, page 40.

### Effects on fetus:
- Serious adverse effects have been reported after exposure to similar medications. Experience with this medication in pregnancy is limited. See Aspirin, page 40, and Indomethacin, page 142.

### Effects on newborn:
- Serious adverse effects have been reported after use of similar medications. Experience with this medication in pregnancy is limited. See Aspirin, page 40, and Indomethacin, page 142.

### Effects during lactation:
- Lactating women may have the same adverse effects as any other person.
- There are no reports of use of meclofenamate during nursing.

 ## Additional information

- Use of this or similar medications may be necessary to control severe rheumatoid arthritis* or related disorders during pregnancy.

 ## Recommendations for use

### Women considering pregnancy:
- Use this medication regularly as directed by your doctor for arthritis* and related disorders.
- If you use meclofenamate regularly, notify your doctor if you plan to become pregnant. Possible risks to you and your baby must be considered on an individual basis.
- Your doctor can provide the best recommendation for you.

## Recommendations during pregnancy:
- See your doctor regularly.
- If you use meclofenamate to control rheumatoid arthritis* or related disorders, possible risks to you and your baby must be considered on an individual basis. Follow your doctor's recommendations carefully.
- Avoid use of this medication near your expected delivery date, except as directed by your doctor.
- At the time of delivery, tell your doctor you take meclofenamate.

## Recommendations during lactation:
- Safety or risk has not been established.
- Your doctor or your baby's doctor can provide the best recommendation for you.

 Interactions

### Interactions with medications, vitamins and minerals:

| Interacts with | Combined effect |
| --- | --- |
| **Warfarin** | Increases risk of bleeding. |

### Interactions with other substances:
- None reported.

*See Glossary.

MEDICATION

# Mephobarbital

**Definition and description:** Acts as an anticonvulsant to prevent epileptic seizures. Mephobarbital is converted to phenobarbital in the liver.

**Other names:** Mebaral®.

 ## Dosage

**Safe dosage:**
- Usual adult dose—400 to 600mg/day.

**Toxic dosage:**
- Exact toxic dose cannot be predicted.

 ## Possible benefits

**Benefits before pregnancy:**
- Use of medication may prevent seizures. Seizures may result in serious injury from falls and accidents. Prolonged, frequent seizures or continuous epileptic seizures may also result in brain damage or death.

**Benefits to mother:**
- See *Benefits before pregnancy.*

**Benefits to fetus:**
- Use of medication may prevent seizures in the mother. Decreased oxygen supply due to maternal seizures may cause brain damage or death.
- Injuries from the mother falling during a seizure may damage the fetus.

**Benefits during lactation:**
- None reported.

 ## Possible adverse effects

**Effects before pregnancy:**
- Adverse effects include dizziness, drowsiness, headache, staggering, vision changes, unusual eye movements, nausea, vomiting, unusual bruising, sore throat and jaundice*.
- Notify your doctor of any adverse effects.

**Effects on mother:**
- Pregnant women may have same adverse effects as any other person.
- Call your doctor if you develop any new adverse effects or if adverse effects worsen during pregnancy.

**Effects on fetus:**
- There is limited information about the effects of mephobarbital on the developing fetus. However, malformations have been reported with similar medications. See *Additional information* and Phenobarbital, page 204.

**Effects on newborn:**
- There is limited experience with mephobarbital use in pregnancy. Serious bleeding during the first day after birth has been reported with similar medications. See *Additional information* and Phenobarbital, page 204.
- Jitteriness, changes in sleep pattern and irritability during withdrawal have been reported in infants exposed to phenobarbital. See Phenobarbital, page 204.

**Effects during lactation:**
- There is limited experience with mephobarbital use during lactation. Lethargy and sedation have been reported in infants exposed to similar medications. See *Additional information* and Phenobarbital, page 204.
- Lactating women may have the same adverse effects as any other person.

 ## Additional information

- Mephobarbital is converted to phenobarbital in the liver. See Phenobarbital, page 204.
- You have a 90% chance of having a normal child if you must take medication to control epilepsy*.
- Pregnancy may increase, decrease or have no effect on the frequency and severity of seizures.
- Very severe seizures have occurred when medication is discontinued without a doctor's supervision.

- Having epilepsy and taking anticonvulsant medications increase the risk of having a miscarriage, stillbirth or child with birth defects.

 ## Recommendations for use

### Women considering pregnancy:
- Notify your doctor if you plan to become pregnant. Possible risks to you and your baby must be considered on an individual basis.
- If you have been seizure-free for many years, your doctor may recommend slowly discontinuing this medication before pregnancy.
- If you have a severe seizure disorder, it is *absolutely necessary* to continue anticonvulsant medication throughout your pregnancy.
- Your doctor can provide the best recommendation for you. Do *not* stop taking this medication unless told to do so by your doctor.

### Recommendations during pregnancy:
- See your doctor regularly.
- If seizures occur, contact your doctor immediately.
- At the time of delivery, tell your doctor you take mephobarbital.
- Take only the vitamin supplements recommended by your doctor.
- Get plenty of sleep during your pregnancy.

### Recommendations during lactation:
- With medical supervision, nursing is usually safe while using this medication.
- Notify your baby's doctor immediately if the baby is sedated or sucks poorly. It may be necessary to check the baby's blood level of phenobarbital. See *Additional information.*

 ## Interactions

**Interactions with medications, vitamins and minerals:**

| Interacts with | Combined effect |
|---|---|
| Ascorbic acid | Increases ascorbic-acid loss in urine. |
| Beta-adrenergic blockers | Decreases beta-adrenergic-blocker effect. |
| Calcium | Decreases calcium levels. |
| Carbamazepine | Alters carbamazepine effect. |
| Chloramphenicol | Alters response to both. |
| Copper | Mephobarbital may increase copper levels. |
| Cyanocobalamin | Decreases cyanocobalamine levels. |
| Folate | Increases folic-acid requirement. Excessive supplementation may increase seizures. |
| Magnesium | Decreases magnesium levels. |
| Meperidine | Increases meperidine toxicity. |
| Metronidazole | May increase metronidazole effect. |
| Monoamine oxidase (MAO) inhibitors | May increase barbiturate effect. |
| Oral contraceptives | Decreases contraceptive effect. |
| Other anticonvulsant medications | Increases likelihood of birth defects when more than one medication is needed to control seizures. |

# Mephobarbital, continued

| | |
|---|---|
| **Phenothiazines** | Decreases phenothiazine effect. |
| **Phenytoin** | Alters effect of both. |
| **Pyridoxine** | May decrease levels of mephobarbital. |
| **Quinidine** | Decreases quinidine effect. |
| **Steroids** | Decreases steroid effect. |
| **Theophylline** | Decreases theophylline effect. |
| **Tricyclic antidepressants** | Decreases antidepressant effect. |
| **Valproic acid** | Alters mephobarbital effect. |

**Interactions with other substances:**
- Maternal alcohol consumption may increase risk of malformations.
- Regular alcohol use decreases effectiveness of mephobarbital.
- Large amounts of alcohol may increase toxicity of this medication.
- Use with alcohol increases drowsiness and slows reaction time.
- Combined overdose with this medication and alcohol may cause death.

*See Glossary.

Note: This page purposely left blank.

# Metaproterenol

**Definition and description:** Acts as a bronchodilator* to treat asthma*, chronic bronchitis* and emphysema*.

**Other names:** Alupent®, Metaprel®.

 ## Dosage

### Safe dosage:
- Metaproterenol can be taken by inhalation, ingestion or injection.
- Dose is determined by person's size and route of administration.
- Usual adult dose by inhalation—2 to 3 puffs every 3 to 4 hours.
- Usual adult dose by mouth—20mg, 3 to 4 times a day.

### Toxic dosage:
- Toxic dose is influenced by the person's condition, size and age.
- Exact toxic dose cannot be predicted.
- Deaths have occurred from excessive use by inhalation.

 ## Possible benefits

### Benefits before pregnancy:
- Relieves symptoms of asthma*, chronic bronchitis* and emphysema*.

### Benefits to mother:
- See *Benefits before pregnancy.*

### Benefits to fetus:
- Severe asthma* may have detrimental effects on the fetus. Metaproterenol relieves asthma* symptoms and improves oxygen exchange in the mother.
- Metaproterenol has been investigated in treating premature labor. This use is not approved by the FDA*. Other, similar medications are preferred. See Ritodrine, page 238, and Terbutaline, page 252.

### Benefits during lactation:
- None reported.

 ## Possible adverse effects

### Effects before pregnancy:
- Adverse effects include nervousness, tremor, headache, increased heart rate, unusual heart rhythm, drowsiness, nausea, vomiting, sweating and muscle cramps.
- Notify your doctor of any adverse effects.
- Inhalation of metaproterenol has rarely worsened asthma* symptoms.
- Deaths have been reported from overuse of inhaled metaproterenol.

### Effects on mother:
- Pregnant women may have the same adverse effects as any other person.
- Call your doctor if you develop any adverse effects.

### Effects on fetus:
- Malformations have not been reported. However, experience in early pregnancy is limited. Safety or risk in early pregnancy has not been established.
- Similar medications increase heart rate and high blood sugar. See Albuterol, page 20, and Terbutaline, page 252.

### Effects on newborn:
- Similar medications have caused low blood sugar. See Terbutaline, page 252.

### Effects during lactation:
- None reported. It is unknown if metaproterenol enters breast milk.
- Lactating women may have the same adverse effects as any other person.

 ## Additional information

- Pregnancy may affect asthma*. About 50% of pregnant asthmatic women have no change in symptoms during pregnancy, 30% improve and 20% worsen. If symptoms worsen during one pregnancy, they are more likely to worsen in other pregnancies.

- Premature delivery, low birth weight, stillbirth, newborn deaths and maternal deaths are more likely to occur in women with asthma*. Treatment of asthma* improves outcome.
- Premature delivery is associated with a high infant-mortality rate. For each 2 weeks a fetus remains in the uterus between the 25th and 37th week of pregnancy, newborn mortality is cut in half.
- Premature delivery is associated with blindness, mental retardation and severe lung disease.
- Benefits to the baby from metaproterenol may outweigh the risks of using the medication.

 ## Recommendations for use

### Women considering pregnancy:

- Notify your doctor if you plan to become pregnant. Risks to you and your baby must be considered on an individual basis.
- Do not exceed the dose recommended by your doctor.
- Notify your doctor if symptoms worsen while using metaproterenol.
- If you have frequent asthma* attacks, it is important to work with your doctor to control your asthma* before pregnancy.
- Your doctor can provide the best recommendation for you. Do not change your dose unless told to do so by your doctor.

### Recommendations during pregnancy:
- See your doctor regularly.
- Do not exceed the dose recommended by your doctor.
- Notify your doctor if symptoms worsen while using this medication.
- If your asthma* improves, your doctor may decrease your medication.
- If your asthma* worsens, your doctor may increase your medication. Do not adjust your dose without medical supervision.
- Avoid exposure to anything that worsens your asthma*.

### Recommendations during lactation:
- If nursing is attempted, taking metaproterenol by inhalation produces lower levels in your blood and possibly in your breast milk.
- Your doctor or your baby's doctor can provide the best recommendation for you.

 ## Interactions

### Interactions with medications, vitamins and minerals:

| Interacts with | Combined effect |
| --- | --- |
| Adrenergic stimulants* | Increases heart rate. |
| Beta-adrenergic blockers* | Decreases metaproterenol effectiveness. |

### Interactions with other substances:
- None reported.

*See Glossary.

# Methadone

**Definition and description:** Acts as a narcotic analgesic to relieve pain. It may also be used to treat or prevent narcotic withdrawal.

**Other names:** Dolophine®.

 ## Dosage

### Safe dosage:
- Usual adult dose—2.5 to 10mg every 8 hours.
- Maintenance or treatment of narcotic withdrawal may require higher doses.

### Toxic dosage:
- Exact toxic dose cannot be predicted.
- Symptoms of overdose include slow breathing, slow heartbeat, drowsiness or loss of consciousness.
- Death occurs after severe overdose.
- Call your doctor, poison-control center or emergency room if you think you have taken an overdose.

 ## Possible benefits

### Benefits before pregnancy:
- Relieves pain.
- Prevents symptoms of narcotic withdrawal.

### Benefits to mother:
- See *Benefits before pregnancy.*

### Benefits to fetus:
- None reported.

### Benefits during lactation:
- None reported.

 ## Possible adverse effects

### Effects before pregnancy:
- Adverse effects include lightheadedness, mood change, dizziness, drowsiness, nausea, vomiting, sweating, weakness, headache, insomnia*, vision changes, disorientation, dry mouth, constipation, abdominal pain, flushing, changes in heart rate, fainting, difficulty urinating, rash, hives* and itching.
- This medication is addicting.
- Notify your doctor of any adverse effects.

### Effects on mother:
- Pregnant women may have the same adverse effects as any other person.
- Call your doctor if you develop any adverse effects.

### Effects on fetus:
- Malformations have not been reported.
- Some evidence indicates an increase in premature deliveries and stillbirths.
- There is little experience with use of methadone for pain control during pregnancy. Most experience with this medication during pregnancy is in management of addiction.
- Babies of addicted mothers are more likely to have growth retardation*.

### Effects on newborn:
- Infants of mothers addicted to narcotics are frequently addicted. Addicted infants experience withdrawal. Withdrawal symptoms include poor nursing, irritability, restlessness, continuous crying, sleeplessness, vomiting, diarrhea, nasal stuffiness, fever, tremors* and occasionally convulsions.
- Severe withdrawal symptoms are associated with higher death rates in babies of addicted mothers.
- Withdrawal symptoms in newborns are more common if maternal dose is greater than 20mg.
- Babies of mothers in methadone-maintenance programs have less evidence of distress than babies of street-medication users.
- Behavioral problems are reported in children up to 1 year of age.
- Jaundice* may be more severe in babies of methadone-addicted mothers than in heroin users.

### Effects during lactation:
- This medication is found in high concentrations in breast milk.

- Infant deaths due to methadone have been reported. High doses of methadone increase risk.
- Continued use during breast-feeding may prevent withdrawal symptoms in infants who are addicted at birth.

## Recommendations for use

### Women considering pregnancy:
- Notify your doctor if you plan to become pregnant.
- Your doctor can provide the best recommendations for you.
- Use only as directed by your doctor.
- Do not use more than the prescribed dose.

### Recommendations during pregnancy:
- See your doctor regularly.
- Avoid unnecessary use of this medication.
- Do not stop taking methadone during pregnancy without medical supervision.
- Your doctor can provide the best recommendation for you.

### Recommendations during lactation:
- With medical supervision, nursing may be safe while using this medication.
- Do not exceed dose recommended by your doctor.
- Do *not* use other narcotics or medications that can decrease breathing or cause sedation.
- Notify your doctor or your baby's doctor if the baby feeds poorly or is drowsy.
- Your doctor can provide the best recommendation for you. Follow your doctor's advice carefully.

## Interactions

### Interactions with medications, vitamins and minerals:

| Interacts with | Combined effect |
| --- | --- |
| Acetaminophen | Increases analgesic effect. |
| Antidepressants | Increases drowsiness. |
| Antihistamines | Increases drowsiness. |
| Aspirin | Increases analgesic effect. |
| Other narcotics | Increases narcotic effect. |
| Phenytoin | Decreases methadone effect. |
| Rifampin | Decreases methadone effect. |
| Tranquilizers | Increases drowsiness. |

### Interactions with other substances:
- Use with alcohol increases drowsiness and slows reaction time.

*See Glossary.

# Metoclopramide

**Definition and description:** Relieves reflux* of stomach contents into the esophagus. Treats nausea and vomiting in some persons.

**Other names:** Octamide®, Reglan®.

 ## Dosage

**Safe dosage:**
- Usual adult dose—10mg before meals and at bedtime.

**Toxic dosage:**
- Exact toxic dose cannot be predicted.
- Symptoms of overdose include drowsiness, disorientation and extrapyramidal symptoms*.
- Contact your doctor, poison-control center or emergency room if you think you may have taken an overdose.

 ## Possible benefits

**Benefits before pregnancy:**
- Treats reflux* of stomach contents into the esophagus.
- Treats nausea and vomiting associated with diabetes* and cancer therapy.

**Benefits to mother:**
- Metoclopramide has been investigated as a treatment for nausea and vomiting of pregnancy.
- This medication has been used late in pregnancy to treat heartburn caused by reflux* of stomach contents into the esophagus.

**Benefits to fetus:**
- None reported.

**Benefits during lactation:**
- None reported.

 ## Possible adverse effects

**Effects before pregnancy:**
- Adverse effects include restlessness, drowsiness, headache, sleeplessness, confusion, dizziness, absence of menstruation, abnormal milk production, changes in blood pressure, abnormal heart rhythm, nausea, diarrhea, increased urination, low blood-cell count, rash, hives*, visual changes, extrapyramidal symptoms* and tardive dyskinesia*.
- Fatal increases in body temperature have been reported.

**Effects on mother:**
- Pregnant women may have the same adverse effects as any other person.
- Call your doctor if you develop any new adverse effects or if adverse effects worsen during pregnancy.

**Effects on fetus:**
- Safety or risk has not been established. Experience with this medication in pregnancy is limited.

**Effects on newborn:**
- Methemoglobinemia* has been reported in newborns treated with this medication.

**Effects during lactation:**
- Safety or risk has not been established.
- Metoclopramide enters breast milk.
- In early lactation, it increases milk production and increases conversion from colostrum to milk.
- Lactating women may have the same adverse effects as any other person.

 ## Additional information

- Use medication *only* if nausea and vomiting interfere with eating or daily activities, and other treatments fail. Your doctor can prescribe other treatments. He or she should determine whether medication is necessary.
- Other treatments may include eating soda crackers or dry toast and drinking hot or cold liquids as soon as you get up in the morning.

- A severe form of nausea and vomiting of pregnancy is called *hyperemesis gravidarum**. This condition causes nutritional deficiencies, loss of electrolytes*, weight loss and starvation. It often requires hospitalization. Treatment with antiemetics* alone will not reverse hyperemesis gravidarum*.

 ## Recommendations for use

### Women considering pregnancy:
- Use this medication only as directed by your doctor.
- Do not exceed the dose or frequency recommended by your doctor.
- Notify your doctor if you plan to become pregnant. Before pregnancy, your doctor can advise you about ways to decrease nausea and vomiting without medication.
- If you use this medication regularly, notify your doctor if you plan to become pregnant. Possible risks to you and your baby must be considered on an individual basis.
- Your doctor can provide the best recommendation for you.

### Recommendations during pregnancy:
- If you have severe vomiting, contact your doctor as soon as possible.
- See your doctor regularly.
- Your doctor can advise you about ways to decrease nausea and vomiting without medication.
- If other treatments fail to reduce nausea and vomiting, contact your doctor *before* using any medication.
- Use this medication only as directed by your doctor.
- Do not exceed the dose recommended by your doctor. If nausea and vomiting persist, contact your doctor. Do not increase the dose without your doctor's advice.

### Recommendations during lactation:
- Your doctor or your baby's doctor can provide the best recommendation for you.

 ## Interactions

### Interactions with medications, vitamins and minerals:

| Interacts with | Combined effect |
| --- | --- |
| Antidepressants | Decreases metoclopramide effect. |
| Antihistamines | Decreases metoclopramide effect. |
| Digoxin | Decreases digoxin effect. |
| Narcotics | Increases drowsiness. |
| Sleep aids | Increases drowsiness. |
| Tranquilizers | Increases drowsiness. |

### Interactions with other substances:
- Use of alcohol increases drowsiness and slows reaction time.

*See Glossary.

# Metronidazole

**Definition and description:** Acts as an antibacterial and antiprotozoal* to treat susceptible bacterial and protozoan infections.

**Other names:** Metronidazole hydrochloride. Also see brand-name list, page 390.

 ## Dosage

**Safe dosage:**
• Dose varies with infection treated.

**Toxic dosage:**
• Exact toxic dose cannot be predicted.
• This medication is a carcinogen* in animals. Human data does not indicate an increased risk of cancer in people exposed to this medication.

 ## Possible benefits

**Benefits before pregnancy:**
• Treats susceptible infections.

**Benefits to mother:**
• Some infections may be very serious to the mother. This medication can cure susceptible infections.

**Benefits to fetus:**
• Some infections in the mother may increase risk to the fetus. This medication can cure susceptible infections.

**Benefits during lactation:**
• None reported.

 ## Possible adverse effects

**Effects before pregnancy:**
• Adverse effects include seizures, numbness, tingling in extremities, nausea, loss of appetite, vomiting, diarrhea, abdominal discomfort, metallic taste, swelling in throat, decreased blood-cell count, confusion, dizziness, rash, hives*, flushing, bladder complaints, decreased libido and increased likelihood of yeast infections in the vagina.
• Notify your doctor of any adverse effects.

**Effects on mother:**
• Pregnant women may have the same adverse effects as any other person.
• Call your doctor if you develop any adverse effects.

**Effects on fetus:**
• This medication causes cancer in mice and rats. However, after many years of use in humans, no evidence of increased risk of cancer has been found. Due to the concern metronidazole might cause cancer later in life, the manufacturer recommends avoiding this medication before the 13th week of pregnancy.
• Most evidence indicates no increased risk of malformation, miscarriage or stillbirth after exposure to metronidazole.

**Effects on newborn:**
• None reported.

**Effects during lactation:**
• This medication is found in high concentrations in breast milk.
• Diarrhea was reported in one breast-fed infant.

 ## Additional information

• Some infections may be very serious to the mother or the baby. It is important to treat these infections.
• Risks from infection or medication must be considered on an individual basis. Your doctor can advise you.

**Recommendations for use**

### Women considering pregnancy:
- Notify your doctor if you plan to become pregnant.
- Use metronidazole as directed by your doctor.
- Do not use or consume alcohol while taking this medication.

### Recommendations during pregnancy:
- Use this medication as directed by your doctor.
- Avoid unnecessary use of metronidazole.
- Risks from infection or medication must be considered on an individual basis. Your doctor can advise you.

### Recommendations during lactation:
- If possible, do not breast-feed while using this medication. Because use is short-term, interruption of breast-feeding is recommended.
- Your doctor or your baby's doctor can provide the best recommendation for you.

 **Interactions**

### Interactions with medications, vitamins and minerals:

| Interacts with | Combined effect |
| --- | --- |
| Disulfiram | Increases toxicity of both. |
| Oral contraceptives | Decreases contraceptive effect. |
| Warfarin | Increases warfarin effect. |

### Interactions with other substances:
- Use with alcohol may produce facial flushing, difficulty breathing, fast heart rate, low blood pressure, nausea and vomiting. Life-threatening symptoms have occurred rarely.

*See Glossary.

MEDICATION

# Miconazole

**Definition and description:** Acts as an antifungal to treat susceptible fungal (yeast) infections.

**Other names:** Miconazole nitrate, Monistat®, Nibustat®.

 ## Dosage

### Safe dosage:
- There are several topical preparations for use on the skin or in the vagina.
- Dose varies with preparation.
- An injectable form may be used to treat severe fungal infections.

### Toxic dosage:
- Exact toxic dose cannot be predicted.

 ## Possible benefits

### Benefits before pregnancy:
- Cures susceptible fungal (yeast) infections.

### Benefits to mother:
- Vaginal yeast infections are more common in pregnancy. These infections often cause discomfort. Miconazole cures yeast infections.

### Benefits to fetus:
- None reported.

### Benefits during lactation:
- None reported.

 ## Possible adverse effects

### Effects before pregnancy:
- Adverse effects after topical use may include itching, burning, irritation, redness, cramping and headache.
- Notify your doctor of any adverse effects.
- More serious adverse effects may be encountered after injection.

### Effects on mother:
- Pregnant women may have the same adverse effects as any other person.
- Call your doctor if you develop any adverse effects.

### Effects on fetus:
- Small amounts of this medication are absorbed from the vagina. No adverse effects to the fetus are reported after topical use.
- Much higher concentrations occur after injection. There are no reports of fetal exposure to injected miconazole.

### Effects on newborn:
- None reported.

### Effects during lactation:
- It is unknown if this medication enters breast milk after injection.
- No adverse effects have been reported with mothers using topical or vaginal preparations.
- Absorption through the skin or vagina is very low, so presence in milk is not expected.
- Lactating women may have the same adverse effects as any other person.

**Recommendations for use**

### Women considering pregnancy:
- Use this medication as directed by your doctor.
- Notify your doctor of any adverse effects.

### Recommendations during pregnancy:
- Use miconazole as directed by your doctor.
- Notify your doctor of any adverse effects.

### Recommendations during lactation:
- Nursing is usually safe while using topical or vaginal preparations.
- Your doctor or your baby's doctor can provide the best recommendation if you use the injectable form.

 **Interactions**

### Interactions with medications, vitamins and minerals:
*No interactions have been reported with topical or vaginal use.*

| Interacts with | Combined effect |
|---|---|
| **Warfarin (injectable preparation only)** | Increases warfarin effect. |

### Interactions with other substances:
- None reported.

*See Glossary.

# Mineral oil

**Definition and description:** Acts as a laxative to relieve constipation.

**Other names:** See brand-name list, page 390.

 ## Dosage

### Safe dosage:
- Usual adult dose—1 to 3 tablespoons/day.
- This medication can be purchased without a prescription.

### Toxic dosage:
- Mineral oil is well-tolerated if used for short periods in recommended doses.
- Laxative overuse can cause diarrhea, weak bones, decreased protein, liver disease, poor absorption of fats and colon problems, low blood levels of potassium, calcium and magnesium.
- Overuse of this laxative can cause poor absorption of fat-soluble vitamins.

 ## Possible benefits

### Benefits before pregnancy:
- Relieves constipation.

### Benefits to mother:
- See *Benefits before pregnancy.*

### Benefits to fetus:
- None reported.

### Benefits during lactation:
- None reported.

 ## Possible adverse effects

### Effects before pregnancy:
- Adverse effects are related to absorption of oil droplets after internal use, which may be found in many body tissues. Pneumonia* due to oil droplets can occur after use of this product.
- Liver damage has been reported when mineral oil is used in combination with docusate.

### Effects on mother:
- Pregnant women may have the same adverse effects as any other person.

### Effects on fetus:
- Decreased availability of vitamin K has been reported.

### Effects on newborn:
- Decreased levels of fat-soluble vitamins is a possibility. It has not been reported in newborns, although it is known to occur in adults. The mother is the main source of vitamin K for the fetus.
- Depletion of vitamin K could be associated with bleeding in newborns.

### Effects during lactation:
- None reported in nursing infants.
- Lactating women may have the same adverse effects as any other person.
- Possible decreased levels of fat-soluble vitamins is a concern with long-term use.

 ## Additional information

- Try non-medication therapies first. Your doctor or nurse can instruct you.
- Increasing fiber in your diet, exercise and adequate fluid intake are helpful. See Appendix 1, page 375, for fiber sources.

**Recommendations for use**

 **Interactions**

### Women considering pregnancy:
- Use as directed on the package.
- Overuse of laxatives can produce dependence on them.
- If you require a laxative for more than a few days, contact your doctor.

### Recommendations during pregnancy:
- Do *not* use mineral oil during pregnancy.
- Other laxatives are safer during pregnancy. Ask your doctor or nurse for recommendations.
- See your doctor regularly.
- Try non-medication therapies before using any laxative.

### Recommendations during lactation:
- Nursing is usually safe while using mineral oil for short periods. Prolonged use is *not* recommended.
- Contact your doctor for an alternative if you require a laxative for more than a few days.
- Your doctor can provide the best recommendation for you.

**Interactions with medications, vitamins and minerals:**

| Interacts with | Combined effect |
| --- | --- |
| **Docusate** | Increases liver damage. |
| **Fat-soluble vitamins** | Decreases absorption of fat-soluble vitamins. |
| **Oral contraceptives** | May decrease contraceptive effect. |
| **Sulfisoxazole** | May decrease sulfisoxazole absorption. |
| **Warfarin** | May increase or decrease warfarin effect. |

**Interactions with other substances:**
- None reported.

*See Glossary.

MEDICATION

# Naproxen

**Definition and description:** Relieves swelling, stiffness and pain of rheumatoid arthritis*, ankylosing spondylitis*, osteoarthritis*, bursitis*, tendonitis* and gout*. Relieves mild to moderate pain. Relieves menstrual discomfort.

**Other names:** Naproxen sodium, Anaprox®, Naprosyn®.

 ## Dosage

**Safe dosage:**
- Usual adult dose—500 to 1,250mg/day.

**Toxic dosage:**
- Exact toxic dose cannot be predicted.

 ## Possible benefits

**Benefits before pregnancy:**
- Relieves swelling, stiffness and joint pain of rheumatoid arthritis* and related disorders.
- Relieves mild to moderate pain.
- Relieves menstrual discomfort.

**Benefits to mother:**
- See *Benefits before pregnancy*, except for menstrual discomfort.

**Benefits to fetus:**
- Naproxen has been used alone or in combination with other medications to treat premature labor. This use is *experimental.* Risks and benefits should be evaluated on an individual basis. Other medications are preferred. See Ritodrine, page 238, and Terbutaline, page 252.

**Benefits during lactation:**
- None reported.

 ## Possible adverse effects

**Effects before pregnancy:**
- Adverse effects include dizziness, headache, drowsiness, depression, rash, itching, ringing in ears, nausea, heartburn*, abdominal pain, bruising, bleeding, swelling, weakness, anemia*, kidney damage and liver damage.

- Notify your doctor if you develop any adverse effects.

**Effects on mother:**
- Anemia*, excessive bleeding during and after labor, and prolonged or delayed labor have been reported with similar medications. Experience with naproxen in pregnancy is limited. See Aspirin, page 40.
- Pregnant women may have the same adverse effects as any other person.
- Notify your doctor if you develop any new adverse effects or if adverse effects worsen during pregnancy.

**Effects on fetus:**
- Serious adverse effects have been reported after exposure to similar medications. Experience with naproxen in early pregnancy is limited. See Aspirin, page 40, and Indomethacin, page 142.

**Effects on newborn:**
- Serious adverse effects have been reported after use of similar medications. See Aspirin, page 40, and Indomethacin, page 142.
- Increased respiratory distress in premature infants has been reported.
- Decreased kidney function and bleeding in the brain and other sites have been reported in newborns exposed to naproxen in management of preterm labor.
- Premature delivery, decreased blood sodium and blood sugar, swelling and fluid retention have been reported after a very large maternal overdose.

**Effects during lactation:**
- This medication is found in very low concentrations in breast milk.
- Lactating women may have the same adverse effects as any other person.

**Additional information**

- Use of naproxen or similar medication may be necessary to control severe rheumatoid arthritis* or related disorders during pregnancy.
- Premature delivery is associated with a high infant-mortality rate. For each 2 weeks a fetus remains in the uterus between the 25th and 37th week of pregnancy, newborn death rate is cut in half.
- Premature delivery is associated with blindness, mental retardation and severe lung disease.
- Benefits to the baby from medication may outweigh the risks of using medication. Your doctor will select the safest medication for you and your baby, if you need treatment for premature labor.

 **Recommendations for use**

**Women considering pregnancy:**
- Use this medication only when needed for minor pain and menstrual discomfort.
- Use this medication regularly as directed by your doctor for arthritis* and related disorders.
- If you use naproxen regularly to control arthritis* and related disorders, notify your doctor if you plan to become pregnant. Possible risks to you and your baby must be considered on an individual basis.
- Your doctor can provide the best recommendation for you.

**Recommendations during pregnancy:**
- See your doctor regularly.
- Avoid unnecessary use of this medication for mild to moderate pain in pregnancy.
- If you use naproxen to control rheumatoid arthritis* or related disorders, possible risks to you and your baby must be considered on an individual basis. Follow your doctor's recommendations carefully.

- If you require medication to treat premature labor, your doctor will choose the best medication for you and your baby. Possible risks to you and your baby must be considered on an individual basis. Follow your doctor's recommendations carefully.
- Avoid use of this medication near your expected delivery date, except as directed by your doctor.
- At the time of delivery, tell your doctor you take naproxen.

**Recommendations during lactation:**
- Nursing is usually safe while using naproxen.

 **Interactions**

**Interactions with medications, vitamins and minerals:**

| Interacts with | Combined effect |
| --- | --- |
| Beta-andrenergic blockers | Decreases betaandrenergic blockers effect. |
| Furosemide | Decreases furosemide effect. |
| Lithium | Increases lithium toxicity. |
| Methotrexate | Increases methotrexate toxicity. |
| Thiazides | Decreases thiazides effect. |
| Warfarin | May increase risk of bleeding. |

**Interactions with other substances:**
- None reported.

*See Glossary.

# Nitrofurantoin

**Definition and description:** Acts as an antibacterial to treat susceptible bacterial infections.

**Other names:** Nitrofurantoin macrocrystals. Also see brand-name list, page 390.

 ## Dosage

### Safe dosage:
- Usual adult dose—50 to 100mg every 6 hours.

### Toxic dosage:
- Exact toxic dose cannot be predicted.
- Severe damage to the nervous system has been reported in people with some kidney diseases, anemia*, electrolyte imbalance*, vitamin-B deficiency and other chronic illnesses.
- Decreased blood-cell count, nervous-system damage and allergic reactions have rarely been fatal.

 ## Possible benefits

### Benefits before pregnancy:
- Cures susceptible bacterial infections.

### Benefits to mother:
- Some bacterial infections may be very serious to the mother. This medication can cure susceptible infections.

### Benefits to fetus:
- Some bacterial infections in the mother may increase risk to the fetus. This medication can cure susceptible infections.
- Nitrofurantoin may also be used to prevent recurrence of some infections.

### Benefits during lactation:
- None reported.

 ## Possible adverse effects

### Effects before pregnancy:
- Adverse effects include loss of appetite, nausea, vomiting, diarrhea, liver damage, lung damage, shortness of breath, pain with breathing, fever, rash, hives*, itching, Stevens-Johnson syndrome*, decreased blood-cell count, headache and dizziness.
- Some persons are genetically susceptible to anemia* due to damaged red-blood cells.
- Notify your doctor of any adverse effects.

### Effects on mother:
- Pregnant women may have the same adverse effects as any other person.
- Call your doctor if you develop any adverse effects.

### Effects on fetus:
- Damage to red-blood cells could produce anemia* in fetuses who are genetically susceptible (G6PD-deficient).
- Nitrofurantoin is usually considered safe for the fetus.

### Effects on newborn:
- Anemia* from red-blood-cell damage may occur in genetically susceptible G6PD-deficient* infants after exposure before birth.

### Effects during lactation:
- This medication is found in extremely low concentrations in breast milk.
- Anemia* due to red-blood-cell damage has been reported in genetically susceptible G6PD-deficient* infants.
- Lactating women may have the same adverse effects as any other person.

 ## Additional information

- Some bacterial infections may be very serious to the mother or the baby. It is important to treat these infections.
- Risks from infection or medication must be considered on an individual basis. Your doctor can advise you.
- Blood levels of nitrofurantoin are lower in pregnant women than other women given the same dose. Your doctor will select the best dose for you.

**Recommendations for use**

## Women considering pregnancy:

• Use nitrofurantoin as directed by your doctor.

## Recommendations during pregnancy:

• Use this medication as directed by your doctor.
• Notify your doctor of any adverse effects.
• Risks from infection or medication must be considered on an individual basis. Your doctor can advise you.
• Contact your doctor if symptoms continue.

## Recommendations during lactation:

• Infants with G6PD-deficiency* could develop anemia* from red-blood-cell damage. These infants should not be exposed to nitrofurantoin in breast milk.
• Nursing is usually safe for other infants.
• Your doctor or your baby's doctor can provide the best recommendation for you.

 **Interactions**

## Interactions with medications, vitamins and minerals:

| Interacts with | Combined effect |
|---|---|
| Oral contraceptives | Decreases contraceptive effect. |
| Nalidixic acid | Decreases effectiveness of both. |
| Phenytoin | May decrease phenytoin effect. |

## Interactions with other substances:

• Taking nitrofurantoin with food delays absorption but increases amount absorbed.

*See Glossary.

MEDICATION

187

# Nortriptyline

**Definition and description:** Acts as an antidepressant to relieve symptoms of depression.

**Other names:** Pamelor®.

 ## Dosage

**Safe dosage:**
- Usual adult dose—50 to 150mg/day.

**Toxic dosage:**
- Exact toxic dose cannot be predicted.
- Overdose has produced serious, life-threatening toxicity.
- Symptoms of toxicity include confusion, hallucinations*, drowsiness, decreased or increased body temperature, muscle rigidity, dangerous heart rhythm, dilated pupils, low blood pressure and loss of consciousness.
- Contact your doctor, poison-control center or emergency room if you think you have taken an overdose.

 ## Possible benefits

**Benefits before pregnancy:**
- Controls symptoms of depression.

**Benefits to mother:**
- See *Benefits before pregnancy.*

**Benefits to fetus:**
- None reported.

**Benefits during lactation:**
- None reported.

 ## Possible adverse effects

**Effects before pregnancy:**
- Adverse effects include low blood pressure or (less often) high blood pressure, rapid heart rate, unusual heart rhythm, altered mental state, tingling, staggering, ringing in ears, seizures, dry mouth, blurred vision, constipation, difficulty urinating, rash, hives*, sensitivity to sunburn, low blood-cell count, nausea, vomiting, diarrhea, jaundice*, dizziness, headache and drowsiness.

- Notify your doctor of any new or unusual adverse effects.

**Effects on mother:**
- Pregnant women may have the same adverse effects as any other person.
- Call your doctor if you develop any new adverse effects or if adverse effects worsen during pregnancy.

**Effects on fetus:**
- Some evidence indicates no increased rate of malformations with this group of antidepressants. However, limb malformations have been reported after use by some women.
- Safety or risk has not been established in early pregnancy.
- Ask your doctor to review the evidence with you.

**Effects on newborn:**
- Use of a similar medication late in pregnancy produced withdrawal symptoms in newborns, including irritability, rapid heart rate, sweating and seizures. See Imipramine, page 140.
- Inability to urinate was reported in an infant.

**Effects during lactation:**
- This medication is found in breast milk but has not been detected in the blood of babies who nurse.
- Lactating women may have the same adverse effects as any other person.

 ## Additional information

- Pregnancy may be complicated by development or recurrence of a serious mental disorder. Treatments other than medication should be tried first. If the risks of mental illness are considered serious, use of medications to treat the mother's illness is important.
- Depression during pregnancy may threaten you or your fetus if you are suicidal, unable to eat or if you have impaired judgment.
- Your doctor will determine if medication is necessary.

## Recommendations for use

### Women considering pregnancy:
- Use nortriptyline as directed by your doctor.
- Do not exceed the dose or frequency recommended by your doctor.
- Notify your doctor if you plan to become pregnant. Possible risks to you and your baby must be considered on an individual basis.
- Your doctor can provide the best recommendation for you.

### Recommendations during pregnancy:
- See your doctor regularly.
- Use this medication as directed by your doctor.
- Do not exceed the dose recommended by your doctor.

### Recommendations during lactation:
- Your doctor or your baby's doctor can provide the best recommendation for you.

## Interactions

### Interactions with medications, vitamins and minerals:

| Interacts with | Combined effect |
| --- | --- |
| Amphetamines | Increases amphetamine toxicity. |
| Anticholinergics* | Increases toxicity of both. |
| Barbiturates | Decreases antidepressant effect. |
| Cimetidine | Increases antidepressant toxicity. |
| Clonidine | Increases blood pressure. |
| Debrisoquin | Increases blood pressure. |
| Epinephrine | Increases blood pressure. |
| Guanethidine | Increases blood pressure. |
| Methyldopa | Increases blood pressure. |
| Monoamine oxidase (MAO) inhibitors | Causes fever and seizures. |
| Phenothiazines | Increases toxicity. |
| Phenylephrine (intravenous*) | Increases blood pressure. |
| Phenytoin | Increases phenytoin toxicity. |
| Warfarin | Increases risk of bleeding. |

### Interactions with other substances:
- Use with alcohol increases drowsiness and slows reaction time.
- Smoking may decrease nortriptyline effectiveness.

*See Glossary.

MEDICATION

# Nystatin

**Definition and description:** Acts as an antifungal to treat susceptible fungal (yeast) infections.

**Other names:** Mycostatin®, Nilstat®, Nystex®, O-V Statin®.

 **Dosage**

### Safe dosage:
- There are several preparations. Dose varies with preparation.
- Nystatin may be used on the skin, in the vagina or it can be taken by mouth.

### Toxic dosage:
- Exact toxic dose cannot be predicted.

 **Possible benefits**

### Benefits before pregnancy:
- Cures susceptible fungal (yeast) infections.

### Benefits to mother:
- Vaginal yeast infections are more common in pregnancy. These infections cause discomfort. Nystatin cures yeast infections.

### Benefits to fetus:
- None reported.

### Benefits during lactation:
- None reported.

 **Possible adverse effects**

### Effects before pregnancy:
- Adverse effects include irritation at application site of topical and vaginal preparations.
- Taken by mouth, this medication may cause nausea, vomiting and diarrhea.

### Effects on mother:
- Pregnant women may have the same adverse effects as any other person.
- Call your doctor if you develop any adverse effects.

### Effects on fetus:
- No malformations have been reported after use on the skin or in the vagina.
- When used by mouth in combination with tetracycline, a possible increase in malformations was reported in one study. Malformations were found only with exposure *before* the 13th week of pregnancy. See Tetracycline, page 256.
- There is no information available regarding the use of nystatin taken orally.

### Effects on newborn:
- None reported after exposure before birth.
- Nystatin is well-tolerated when used to treat infants with thrush*.

### Effects during lactation:
- None reported.
- Absorption through the skin or vagina is very low, so presence in milk is not expected.
- Absorption when taken by mouth is low.

 **Recommendations for use**

### Women considering pregnancy:
- Use nystatin as directed by your doctor.
- Notify your doctor of any adverse effects.

### Recommendations during pregnancy:
- See *Women considering pregnancy.*

### Recommendations during lactation:
- Nursing is usually safe while using nystatin.

 **Interactions**

### Interactions with medications, vitamins and minerals:
- None reported.

### Interactions with other substances:
- None reported.

*See Glossary.

### Definition and description:
Hormonal birth-control method to prevent conception.

**Other names:** See brand-name list, page 390.

 ## Dosage

### Safe dosage:
• Take as directed on the package.

### Toxic dosage:
• Exact toxic dose cannot be predicted.
• Some women may have serious toxicity with usual doses of oral contraceptives.
• Call your doctor or emergency room if you cough up blood, have loss of vision, double vision, weakness or severe pain in an arm or leg, severe chest pains, slurred speech or tenderness in your abdomen.

 ## Possible benefits

### Benefits before pregnancy:
• Prevents pregnancy.
• Regulates unusual menstrual bleeding.
• May relieve symptoms of fibrocystic breast disease*, painful menstruation, uterine fibroids* and acne.
• Several diseases common in women of reproductive age occur less frequently in users of oral contraceptives. These include some pelvic infections, ovarian cysts*, uterine fibroids* and endometriosis*.

### Benefits to mother:
• None reported.
• Oral contraceptives should not be used during pregnancy.

### Benefits to fetus:
• None reported.
• Oral contraceptives should not be used during pregnancy.

### Benefits during lactation:
• Prevents pregnancy.

 ## Possible adverse effects

### Effects before pregnancy:
• Adverse effects include absence of menstrual periods, painful menstrual periods, abnormal spotting and bleeding, changes in breast size, increased appetite, weight gain, dark skin discoloration, swelling, dizziness, leg cramps, headache, nausea, vomiting, blood-vessel changes, depression, fatigue, acne, gallbladder disease, high blood pressure. Blood clots, stroke*, myocardial infarction* and death occur infrequently.
• Oral contraceptives decrease blood levels of pyridoxine, riboflavin, cyanocobalamin, thiamine, ascorbic acid, zinc and magnesium. However, deficiency symptoms are rare.
• Medication interactions may decrease effectiveness of oral contraceptives. See *Interactions*.
• Fertility may be delayed for a short period after discontinuing oral contraceptives.
• Notify your doctor of any adverse effects.

### Effects on mother:
• Oral contraceptives are not used during pregnancy, except in accidental exposure. Any adverse effect described above could occur while taking this medication during early pregnancy.
• Miscarriages may occur more often in women who become pregnant during the first cycles after stopping oral contraceptives.
• Blood clots in the legs or lungs occur more frequently after delivery in women who start using some oral contraceptives too quickly. Your doctor will tell you when to resume use of oral contraceptives.

### Effects on fetus:
• Most doctors and researchers believe oral contraceptives are safe. Use of oral contraceptives *before* pregnancy does *not* increase the risk of malformations.

≫→

# Oral Contraceptives, continued

- The risk from exposure to oral contraceptives *during* pregnancy is very small, if it exists at all.
- Reported malformations due to exposure during pregnancy to female sex hormones fall into two groups—genital and non-genital. Studies have shown non-genital malformations are *not* increased after exposure to oral contraceptives compared to unexposed infants.
- Genital abnormalities may be increased after exposure *during* pregnancy. Reported defects include enlargment of external female genitals to an appearance that resembles male organs. These reports have not been confirmed in large studies of oral-contraceptive users.
- Some researchers continue to express concerns that heart defects may be increased after use *during* pregnancy.
- One study found *no* association between oral-contraceptive use and stillbirth.
- One evaluation of miscarried fetuses indicates a higher incidence of fetal chromosome abnormalities in fetuses exposed to oral contraceptives early in pregnancy.

### Effects on newborn:
- None reported.

### Effects during lactation:
- Oral contraceptives may decrease breast-milk production. Protein and nitrogen content of milk is decreased.
- Decreased weight gain has been reported in nursing infants.
- Hormones in oral contraceptives are found in breast milk.
- Swelling and tenderness of breast tissue has been reported in an infant exposed to oral contraceptives in milk.
- Some oral contraceptives are less likely to produce these problems than others.
- Lactating women may have the same adverse effects as any other person.

 ## Additional information

- An estrogen hormone, diethylstilbesterol (DES), has been associated with cancer in adult women who were exposed to it before birth. These women also have more miscarriages and ectopic pregnancies. DES is *not* used in oral contraceptives.
- Some progestin hormones have been associated with spinal, heart and genital defects when used as a pregnancy test. These progestins are not used in oral contraceptives and are no longer available as pregnancy tests. Recent studies in other countries indicate no increased risk or an extremely small risk.

 ## Recommendations for use

### Women considering pregnancy:
- Use this medication as directed on the package.
- Some doctors recommend waiting for a few months after discontinuing oral contraceptives before becoming pregnant. Ask your doctor for advice.
- Read and follow the recommendations in the Patient Information that comes with your oral contraceptive.
- Many medications interact with oral contraceptives. Ask your doctor or pharmacist about drug interactions when you get a new prescription for any medication.
- Notify your doctor if you plan to become pregnant.

### Recommendations during pregnancy:
- Contact your doctor as soon as you think you may be pregnant.
- Use another method of birth control until pregnancy can be confirmed. Your doctor can recommend one. In some cases, pregnancy tests can be done immediately with results the same day.
- After delivery, ask your doctor when it is safe to resume using oral contraceptives. Some oral contraceptives should not be used in the first 2 to 4 weeks after delivery.

### Recommendations during lactation:

- Your doctor can recommend an oral contraceptive during lactation. It may not be advisable to use the same oral contraceptive you used before pregnancy.
- Notify your doctor if your baby seems unsatisfied with feedings or fails to gain weight.
- Your baby's weight gain should be checked often.
- Notify your baby's doctor if you notice swelling and tenderness of the baby's breast tissue.

 Interactions

### Interactions with medications, vitamins and minerals:

| Interacts with | Combined effect |
| --- | --- |
| Ampicillin | Decreases oral-contraceptive effect. |
| Antacids | Decreases oral-contraceptive effect. |
| Benzodiazepines | Decreases oral-contraceptive effect. |
| Carbamazepine | Decreases oral-contraceptive effect. |
| Chloral hydrate | Decreases oral-contraceptive effect. |
| Chloramphenicol | Decreases oral-contraceptive effect. |
| Chlor-diazepoxide | Increases chlordiazepoxide effect. |
| Clofibrate | Decreases oral-contraceptive effect. |
| Clomipramine | Increases depression. |
| Diazepam | Increases diazepam effect. |
| Ethosuximide | Decreases oral-contraceptive effect. |
| Insulin | Increases blood sugar. |
| Isoniazid (INH) | Decreases oral-contraceptive effect. |
| Isoproterenol | Decreases isoproterenol effect. |
| Lorazepam | Increases lorazepam effect. |
| Methyldopa | Increases fluid retention. |
| Metronidazole | Decreases oral-contraceptive effect. |
| Neomycin | Decreases oral-contraceptive effect. |
| Nitrofurantoin | Decreases oral-contraceptive effect. |
| Oral antidiabeteic agents | Increases blood sugar. |
| Oxazepam | Increases oxazepam effect. |
| Penicillin | Decreases oral-contraceptive effect. |
| Phenobarbital and other barbiturates | Decreases oral-contraceptive effect. |
| Phenothiazine | Decreases breast-milk production. |
| Phenytoin | Decreases oral-contraceptive effect. |
| Primidone | Decreases oral-contraceptive effect. |
| Rifampin | Decreases oral-contraceptive effect. |
| Sulfonamide | Decreases oral-contraceptive effect. |
| Tetracyline | Decreases oral-contraceptive effect. |

### Interactions with other substances:

- Smoking increases the risk of serious heart disease and blood-vessel disease, including stroke*, myocardial infarction* and death.

*See Glossary.

# Oxazepam

**Definition and description:** Acts as an antianxiety agent to relieve symptoms of anxiety. Also treats symptoms of acute alcohol withdrawal.

**Other names:** Serax®.

 ## Dosage

**Safe dosage:**
- Usual adult dose—30 to 120mg/day.

**Toxic dosage:**
- Exact toxic dose cannot be predicted.
- Symptoms of overdose include drowsiness, confusion and loss of consciousness.
- If you think you have taken an overdose, contact your doctor, poison-contol center or emergency room.

 ## Possible benefits

**Benefits before pregnancy:**
- Relieves anxiety.
- Relieves symptoms of alcohol withdrawal.

**Benefits to mother:**
- See *Benefits before pregnancy.*

**Benefits to fetus:**
- None reported.

**Benefits during lactation:**
- None reported.

 ## Possible adverse effects

**Effects before pregnancy:**
- Adverse effects include drowsiness, staggering, tiredness, confusion, constipation, depression, changes in vision, headache, nausea, dizziness and slurred speech.
- Anxiety has rarely worsened and hallucinations* have occurred.
- Oxazepam is addicting.
- Notify your doctor if you have any adverse effects.

**Effects on mother:**
- Pregnant women may have the same adverse effects as any other person.
- Call your doctor if you develop any adverse effects.

**Effects on fetus:**
- This medication enters fetal circulation in high concentrations.
- Similar medications are associated with malformations. See *Additional information* and Diazepam, page 94. Data with oxazepam is very limited. This data is inadequate to establish safety or risk.

**Effects on newborn:**
- Similar medications are associated with sedation and other problems in the newborn. See *Additional information* and Diazepam, page 94.

**Effects during lactation:**
- Drowsiness has been reported in nursing infants.
- Similar medications are associated with adverse effects. See *Additional information* and Diazepam, page 94.
- Lactating women may have the same adverse effects as any other person.

 ## Additional information

- Diazepam is converted to oxazepam in the liver. Both are active antianxiety agents. See Diazepam, page 94.

# Oxazepam, continued

 ## Recommendations for use

### Women considering pregnancy:
- Notify your doctor if you plan to become pregnant.
- Discontinue use of this medication, if possible. Your doctor can advise you.

### Recommendations during pregnancy:
- See your doctor regularly.
- Avoid use of this medication during early pregnancy, if possible.

### Recommendations during lactation:
- With medical supervision, nursing may be safe.
- Your doctor or your baby's doctor can provide the best recommendation for you.
- Notify the baby's doctor if the baby is drowsy.

 ## Interactions

### Interactions with medications, vitamins and minerals:

| Interacts with | Combined effect |
| --- | --- |
| Antidepressants | Increases sedation. |
| Cimetidine | Increases oxazepam effect. |
| Isoniazid (INH) | Increases oxazepam effect. |
| Lithium | Decreases body temperature. |
| Oral contraceptives | Decreases contraceptive effect. |
| Phenytoin | Increases phenytoin toxicity. |
| Valproic acid | Increases oxazepam effect. |

### Interactions with other substances:
- Use with alcohol increases drowsiness and slows reaction time.
- Food increases absorption of oxazepam.
- Smoking decreases oxazepam effectiveness.

*See Glossary.

MEDICATION

# Oxycodone

**Definition and description:** Acts as a narcotic analgesic to relieve pain. Also acts as an antitussive* to relieve cough.

**Other names:** Oxycodone hydrochloride, oxycodone terephalate.

 Dosage

### Safe dosage:
• Usual adult dose—5 to 10mg every 6 hours.

### Toxic dosage:
• Exact toxic dose cannot be predicted.
• Symptoms of overdose include slow breathing, slow heartbeat, drowsiness or loss of consciousness.
• Death occurs after severe overdose.
• Call your doctor, poison-control center or emergency room if you think you have taken an overdose.

 Possible benefits

### Benefits before pregnancy:
• Relieves moderate to moderately severe pain.
• Relieves cough.

### Benefits to mother:
• See *Benefits before pregnancy*.

### Benefits to fetus:
• None reported.

### Benefits during lactation:
• None reported.

 Possible adverse effects

### Effects before pregnancy:
• Adverse effects include depression, dizziness, drowsiness, hives*, rash, itching, flushing, blurred vision, constipation, abdominal pain, vomiting, difficulty urinating and fatigue.
• Oxycodone is addicting.
• Notify your doctor of any adverse effects.

### Effects on mother:
• Pregnant women may have the same adverse effects as any other person.
• Call your doctor if you develop any adverse effects.

### Effects on fetus:
• Similar medications have been associated with malformations. See Codeine, page 82.

### Effects on newborn:
• Withdrawal has occurred after use of similar medications. See Codeine, page 82, and Methadone, page 174.

### Effects during lactation:
• Drowsiness and poor feeding have been reported in newborns.
• Lactating women may have the same adverse effects as any other person.

**Recommendations for use**

### Women considering pregnancy:
- Notify your doctor if you plan to become pregnant.
- If you use oxycodone regularly, ask your doctor's advice about discontinuing use.
- Use only as directed by your doctor.

### Recommendations during pregnancy:
- See your doctor regularly.
- Avoid unnecessary use of this medication.
- Use only as directed by your doctor.

### Recommendations during lactation:
- Your doctor can provide the best recommendation for you.

 **Interactions**

**Interactions with medications, vitamins and minerals:**

| Interacts with | Combined effect |
| --- | --- |
| **Aspirin** | Increases analgesic effect. |
| **Acetaminophen** | Increases analgesic effect. |
| **Anti-depressants** | Increases drowsiness. |
| **Antihistamines** | Increases drowsiness. |
| **Other narcotics** | Increases narcotic effect. |
| **Tranquilizers** | Increases drowsiness. |

**Interactions with other substances:**
- Use with alcohol increases drowsiness and slows reaction time.

*See Glossary.

# Paramethadione

**Definition and description:** Acts as an anticonvulsant to prevent petit mal epileptic seizures*.

**Other names:** Paradione®.

 ## Dosage

**Safe dosage:**
- Usual adult dose—900 to 2,400mg/day.
- Your doctor can use blood levels to determine the correct dosage.
- *Not recommended for use in pregnancy.*

**Toxic dosage:**
- Exact toxic dose cannot be predicted.
- Toxic effects include kidney, liver and blood-cell damage. Call your doctor if your develop a sore throat, fever, unusual bruising or bleeding.

 ## Possible benefits

**Benefits before pregnancy:**
- Use of medication may prevent seizures. Seizures may result in serious injury from falls and accidents. However, the risk to the fetus associated with use of paramethadione outweighs the benefit.
- *This medication should be used in women of childbearing age only when other, less-toxic medications have failed. See Possible adverse effects.*

**Benefits to mother:**
- See *Benefits before pregnancy.*

**Benefits to fetus:**
- *The risk to the fetus associated with this medication outweighs the benefit. Paramethadione should be used in women of childbearing age only when other, less-toxic medications have failed.* See *Possible adverse effects.*

**Benefits during lactation:**
- None reported.

 ## Possible adverse effects

**Effects before pregnancy:**
- Adverse effects include headache, irritability, drowsiness, fatigue, insomnia*, vision changes, vomiting, nausea, loss of appetite, swollen lymph glands*, joint pain and skin rash.
- Notify your doctor of any adverse effects.

**Effects on mother:**
- Pregnant women may have the same adverse effects as any other person.
- Call your doctor if you develop any new adverse effects or if adverse effects worsen during pregnancy.

**Effects on fetus:**
- *69% of all children exposed to paramethadione were born with congenital malformations.* Malformations included abnormal ears, cleft lip*, cleft palate*, heart defects, club foot*, hand malformations, kidney abnormalities, inguinal hernias*, small brain, skin folds in the corners of the eyes, broad nasal bridge, eye abnormalities, genital abnormalities, slow mental development, and slow physical development.

**Effects on newborn:**
- None reported.

**Effects during lactation:**
- Lactating women may have the same adverse effects as any other person.

 ## Additional information

- You have a 90% chance of having a normal child if you must take medication to control epilepsy*. *However, paramethadione is much more likely to cause birth defects than other anticonvulsant medications.*
- Pregnancy may increase, decrease or have no effect on the frequency and severity of seizures.
- Very severe seizures have occurred when medication is discontinued without a doctor's supervision.

• Having epilepsy and taking anticonvulsant medications increase the risk of having a miscarriage, stillbirth or child with birth defects.

 **Recommendations for use**

### Women considering pregnancy:

• Notify your doctor if you plan to become pregnant. *This medication is not recommended for women considering pregnancy.*
• If you have a severe seizure disorder, it is *absolutely necessary* to continue an anticonvulsant medication throughout your pregnancy. If possible, your doctor will substitute another medication to control your seizures. Follow your doctor's instructions carefully.
• If you have been seizure-free for many years, your doctor may recommend slowly discontinuing this medication before pregnancy.
• Your doctor may recommend changing your medication.
• Your doctor can provide the best recommendation for you. Do not stop taking this medication unless told to do so by your doctor.

### Recommendations during pregnancy:

• See your doctor *immediately* if you suspect you are pregnant.
• Your doctor will advise you regarding use of seizure medications during pregnancy.
• Do not stop taking this medication or change your medication unless told to do so by your doctor.

### Recommendations during lactation:

• Safety or risk has not been established.

 **Interactions**

**Interactions with medications, vitamins and minerals:**

| Interacts with | Combined effect |
| --- | --- |
| **Other anticonvulsant medications** | Increases likelihood of birth defects when more than one medication is needed to control seizures. |

**Interactions with other substances:**
• None reported.

*See Glossary.

# Penicillin

**Definition and description:** Acts as an antibiotic to treat susceptible bacterial infections.

**Other names:** Penicillin G, penicillin V, benzathine penicillin G, penicillin G procaine. Also see brand-name list, page 390.

##  Dosage

### Safe dosage:
- Usual adult dose—125 to 500mg every 6 hours. Smaller or larger doses may be used for some infections.
- Larger doses given by injection may be required for serious infections.

### Toxic dosage:
- This medication is well-tolerated.
- Rare cases of seizures have occurred in kidney-failure patients receiving very high intravenous* doses.
- Life-threatening allergic reactions have occurred. Contact your doctor or emergency room immediately if you have difficulty breathing or swelling of the face, mouth or throat. Hives* sometimes precede serious reactions.
- Exact toxic dose cannot be predicted.

##  Possible benefits

### Benefits before pregnancy:
- Cures susceptible bacterial infections.

### Benefits to mother:
- Some bacterial infections may be very serious to the mother. This medication can cure susceptible infections.

### Benefits to fetus:
- Some bacterial infections in the mother may increase risk to the fetus. This medication can cure susceptible infections.

### Benefits during lactation:
- None reported.

##  Possible adverse effects

### Effects before pregnancy:
- Adverse effects include nausea, vomiting, diarrhea, rash, hives*, fever and decreased blood-cell count.
- Kidney damage and changes in reflexes occur very rarely after intravenous* use.
- Fatal allergic reactions have occurred rarely.
- Notify your doctor of any adverse effects.

### Effects on mother:
- Pregnant women may have the same adverse effects as any other person.
- Call your doctor if you develop any adverse effects.

### Effects on fetus:
- This medication is considered safe.

### Effects on newborn:
- None reported in infants exposed before birth.

### Effects during lactation:
- Penicillin is found in very low levels in breast milk.
- No adverse effects have been reported.
- Lactating women may have the same adverse effects as any other person.

##  Additional information

- Some doctors believe exposure to penicillins during breast-feeding may be associated with allergy to penicillins. There is no supporting evidence.
- Some bacterial infections may be very serious to the mother or the baby. It is important to treat these infections.
- Risks from infection or medication must be considered on an individual basis. Your doctor can advise you.
- Blood levels of penicillin are lower in pregnant women than other women given the same dose. Your doctor will select the best dose for you.

**Recommendations for use**

### Women considering pregnancy:
• Use penicillin as directed by your doctor.

### Recommendations during pregnancy:
• Use this medication as directed by your doctor.
• Notify your doctor of any adverse effects.
• Contact your doctor if symptoms continue.

### Recommendations during lactation:
• Nursing is usually safe when using penicillin.

 **Interactions**

### Interactions with medications, vitamins and minerals:

| Interacts with | Combined effect |
| --- | --- |
| Antacids | Decreases penicillin effect. |
| Chloramphenicol | Decreases penicillin effect. |
| Methotrexate | Increases methotrexate toxicity. |
| Oral contraceptives | Decreases contraceptive effect. |
| Tetracycline | Decreases penicillin effect. |

### Interactions with other substances:
• Taking penicillin with food decreases effectiveness.

*See Glossary.

# Pheniramine

**Definition and description:** Acts as an antihistamine to relieve allergy symptoms, including sneezing, runny nose, itching and tearing.

**Other names:** See brand-name list, page 390.

 ## Dosage

### Safe dosage:
- Usual adult dose—12.5 to 25mg every 4 to 6 hours.
- This medication can be purchased without a prescription. It is also found in products requiring a prescription.

### Toxic dosage:
- Exact toxic dose cannot be predicted.
- Symptoms of overdose include sedation, dry mouth, large pupils, flushing and low blood pressure.
- Serious overdose may cause convulsions and death.
- Contact your doctor, poison-control center or emergency room if you think you have taken an overdose.

 ## Possible benefits

### Benefits before pregnancy:
- Relieves allergy symptoms.

### Benefits to mother:
- See *Benefits before pregnancy.*

### Benefits to fetus:
- None reported.

### Benefits during lactation:
- None reported.

 ## Possible adverse effects

### Effects before pregnancy:
- Adverse effects include drowsiness, rash, hives*, sweating, chills, dry mouth, headache, unusual heart rhythm, low blood pressure, low blood-cell count, confusion, ringing in ears, blurred vision, nausea, vomiting and difficulty urinating.
- Notify your doctor of any adverse effects.

### Effects on mother:
- Pregnant women may have the same adverse effects as any other person.
- Call your doctor if you develop any adverse effects.

### Effects on fetus:
- Antihistamines as a group have not been shown to increase risk of malformations compared to unexposed pregnancies.
- Some evidence does not indicate an increased risk of malformations after exposure to pheniramine at any time during pregnancy. However, when use during the first 4 months of pregnancy only was studied, a possible increase in respiratory, eye or ear defects and syndromes was found.

### Effects on newborn:
- None reported.

### Effects during lactation:
- Most antihistamines enter breast milk.
- Lactating women may have the same adverse effects as any other person.

##  Additional information

- Pheniramine does not cure colds, coughs or minor allergy complaints. It provides relief for symptoms. Occasionally, when allergic reactions are very serious, using anithistamines and other medications can be life-saving.
- Viral illnesses and fever have been implicated as a cause of birth defects. This medication is often used to relieve symptoms of viral illnesses. Contact your doctor if you have a fever.
- This medication is often used in combination with other medications. Most studies did not study persons using it alone. It is difficult to determine if pheniramine caused any malformations.

##  Recommendations for use

### Women considering pregnancy:

- Notify your doctor if you plan to become pregnant.
- Use only the recommended doses of this medication.
- Use this medication only when needed.

### Recommendations during pregnancy:

- Safety or risk has not been established.
- See your doctor regularly.
- Use this medication only as directed by your doctor.
- Do not use this medication during pregnancy unless instructed by your doctor.
- Avoid unnecessary use of this medication.

### Recommendations during lactation:

- Nursing is usually safe while using antihistamines.
- Your doctor or your baby's doctor can provide the best recommendation for you.

##  Interactions

### Interactions with medications, vitamins and minerals:

| Interacts with | Combined effect |
|---|---|
| Antianxiety agents | Increases drowsiness. |
| Antidepressants | Increases drowsiness. |
| Other anti-histamines | Increases drowsiness. |
| Tranquilizers | Increases drowsiness. |

### Interactions with other substances:

- Use with alcohol increases drowsiness and slows reaction time.

*See Glossary.

MEDICATION

# Phenobarbital

**Definition and description:** Acts as an anticonvulsant to prevent epileptic seizures.

**Other names:** See brand-name list, page 390.

 **Dosage**

### Safe dosage:
• Usual adult dose—30 to 210mg/day.
• Pregnant women may require higher doses than before pregnancy. Your doctor can use blood levels to determine correct dosage.

### Toxic dosage:
• Exact toxic dose cannot be predicted.
• Call your doctor if you develop severe staggering or drowsiness.

 **Possible benefits**

### Benefits before pregnancy:
• Use of medication may prevent seizures. Seizures may result in serious injury from falls and accidents. Prolonged, frequent seizures or continuous epileptic seizures may also result in brain damage or death.

### Benefits to mother:
• Phenobarbital may be used to prevent blood reactions between mother and fetus.
• Also see *Benefits before pregnancy*.

### Benefits to fetus:
• Use of medication may prevent seizures in the mother. Decreased oxygen supply due to maternal seizures may cause brain damage or death in the fetus.
• Injuries from the mother falling during a seizure may damage the fetus.
• Phenobarbital may be used to prevent blood reactions between mother and fetus.
• Phenobarbital given to women who go into premature labor may prevent bleeding in the brain of premature infants during delivery and the first few days of life. This use is experimental.

### Benefits during lactation:
• None reported.

 **Possible adverse effects**

### Effects before pregnancy:
• Phenobarbital may cause depletion of folate and vitamin D. See Folate, page 294, and Vitamin D, page 335.
• Adverse effects include dizziness, drowsiness, headache, staggering, vision changes, unusual eye movements, nausea, vomiting, unusual bruising, sore throat and jaundice*.
• Notify your doctor of any new or unusual adverse effects.

### Effects on mother:
• Slightly lower calcium levels are found in pregnant women who use phenobarbital.
• Pregnant women may have same adverse effects as any other person.
• Call your doctor if you develop any new adverse effects or if adverse effects worsen during pregnancy.

### Effects on fetus:
• Malformations occur in 10% of children exposed to anticonvulsant medications before birth. Minor abnormalities of the hands, feet, face and head include wide nasal bridge, low-set ears, low-set forehead, malformations of eyes and ears, small or absent nails, finger-like thumbs, short fingers, skin folds in the corners of the eyes and hip dislocation*.
• Serious problems such as malformations of heart, lungs and other breathing structures, gastrointestinal defects, small brain, hernias*, oral clefts* and slow mental and physical development also occur. Deaths due to serious malformations have been reported.
• Childhood cancers have been rarely reported in children who were exposed to phenobarbital before birth. However, it is unknown whether this medication caused cancer in these children.

### Effects on newborn:

- Serious bleeding during the first day after birth can usually be prevented by specific vitamin therapy. In some cases, Cesarean delivery may be necessary to avoid trauma to the newborn.
- Newborns may be sedated for a few days after birth. Infants may develop jitteriness, changes in sleep pattern, seizures and irritability during withdrawal. In some cases, these symptoms may not be observed until a week or more after birth.

### Effects during lactation:

- Lethargy and sedation have been reported in infants.
- Lactating women may have the same adverse effects as any other person.
- Withdrawal effects occurred in one infant after nursing was abruptly discontinued. This has not been reported in infants weaned normally.

 **Additional information**

- You have a 90% chance of having a normal child if you must take medication to control epilepsy*.
- Pregnancy may increase, decrease or have no effect on the frequency and severity of seizures.
- Very severe seizures have occurred when medication is discontinued without a doctor's supervision.
- Having epilepsy and taking anticonvulsant medications increase the risk of having a miscarriage, stillbirth or child with birth defects.

 **Recommendations for use**

### Women considering pregnancy:

- Notify your doctor if you plan to become pregnant. Possible risks to you and your baby must be considered on an individual basis.

- If you have been seizure-free for many years, your doctor may recommend slowly discontinuing this medication before pregnancy.
- If you have a severe seizure disorder, it is *absolutely necessary* to continue anticonvulsant medication throughout your pregnancy.
- Your doctor can provide the best recommendation for you. Do *not* stop taking this medication unless told to do so by your doctor.

### Recommendations during pregnancy:

- See your doctor regularly.
- Blood levels should be checked frequently during pregnancy and for a few weeks after delivery to balance adverse effects and seizure control.
- Your doctor may want to adjust dose of medication frequently during and after pregnancy. It is important to follow your doctor's instructions carefully.
- Your doctor is less likely to use blood levels to monitor dose if this medication is used to treat something other than seizures.
- If seizures occur, contact your doctor immediately.
- At the time of delivery, tell your doctor you take phenobarbital.
- Take only the vitamin supplements recommended by your doctor.
- Get plenty of sleep during your pregnancy.

### Recommendations during lactation:

- With medical supervision, nursing is usually safe while using this medication.
- Notify your baby's doctor immediately if the baby is sedated or sucks poorly. It may be necessary to check the baby's blood level of phenobarbital.

# Phenobarbital, continued

 Interactions

**Interactions with medications, vitamins and minerals:**

| Interacts with | Combined effect |
| --- | --- |
| Ascorbic acid | Increases ascorbic acid loss in urine. |
| Beta-adrenergic blockers | Decreases beta-adrenergic blocker effect. |
| Calcium | Decreases blood-calcium levels. |
| Carbamazepine | Alters carbamazepine effect. |
| Chloramphenicol | Alters response to both. |
| Copper | Phenobarbital may increase copper levels. |
| Cyanocobalamin | Decreases bloodcyanocobalamine levels. |
| Doxycycline | May decrease doxycycline effect. |
| Folate | Increases requirement for folate. Excessive supplementation may increase seizures. |
| Magnesium | Decreases blood-magnesium levels. |
| Meperidine | Increases meperidine toxicity. |
| Metronidazole | May increase metronidazole effect. |
| Monoamine oxidase (MAO) inhibitors | May increase barbiturate effect. |
| Oral contraceptives | Decreases contraceptive effect. |
| Other anti-convulsant medications | Increases likelihood of birth defects when more than one medication is needed to control seizures. |
| Phenothiazines | Decreases phenothiazine effect. |
| Phenytoin | Alters effect of both. |
| Pyridoxine | May decrease levels of phenobarbital. |
| Quinidine | Decreases quinidine effect. |
| Steroids | Decreases steroid effect. |
| Theophylline | Decreases theophylline effect. |
| Tricyclic anti-depressants | Decreases anti-depressant effect. |
| Valproic acid | Alters phenobarbital effect. |
| Vitamin D | Decreases vitamin-D effect. |
| Warfarin | Increases warfarin effect. |

**Interactions with other substances:**
• Maternal alcohol consumption may increase risk of malformations.
• Regular alcohol use decreases effectiveness of this medication.
• Large amounts of alcohol may increase toxicity of this medication.
• Use of this medication with alcohol increases impairment.
• Combined overdose with this medication and alcohol may be fatal.

*See Glossary.

# Phenylephrine

**Definition and description:** Acts as a decongestant to decrease nasal secretions.

**Other names:** See brand-name list, page 390.

 Dosage

### Safe dosage:
- Usual adult dose—10mg every 4 hours by mouth.
- Nasal spray or drops can be used as directed on the package. Rebound congestion* is common.
- This medication may be purchased without a prescription.
- Phenylephrine may be used in an emergency by injection to treat very low blood pressure. It can be life-saving.

### Toxic dosage:
- Exact toxic dose cannot be determined.
- Symptoms of overdose include headache, unusual heart rhythm, slow pulse and high blood pressure.

 Possible benefits

### Benefits before pregnancy:
- Decreases nasal congestion from allergies and colds.

### Benefits to mother:
- See *Benefits before pregnancy.*

### Benefits to fetus:
- None reported.

### Benefits during lactation:
- None reported.

 Possible adverse effects

### Effects before pregnancy:
- Adverse effects include headache, slow heart rate, restlessness, unusual heart rhythm and sleeplessness.

### Effects on mother:
- Pregnant women may have the same adverse effects as any other person.
- Call your doctor if you develop any adverse effects during pregnancy.
- Severe high blood pressure has occurred when phenylephrine was used during labor with oxytocin-like medications*.

### Effects on fetus:
- Malformations have been reported after use of this medication, including club foot*, eye and ear abnormalities.

### Effects on newborn:
- None reported after exposure before birth.
- An infant treated with phenylephrine eyedrops developed poor oxygen levels and depressed heart function.

### Effects during lactation:
- Lactating women may have the same adverse effects as any other person.

 Additional information

- This medication, when used for cold or allergy symptoms, does not cure or shorten the course of an illness. It provides relief for symptoms, but otherwise it offers no benefit.
- Viral illnesses have been implicated as a cause of birth defects. It is unknown if colds or flu cause birth defects. Phenylephrine is often used to relieve symptoms of viral illnesses.
- This medication is often used in combination with other medications. Most studies did not study persons using it alone. It is difficult to determine if phenylephrine caused any malformations.

# Phenylephrine, continued

 **Recommendations for use**

### Women considering pregnancy:
- Use medication as directed on the package.
- Do not exceed the suggested dose.
- Use only when needed.
- Notify your doctor if you plan to become pregnant.

### Recommendations during pregnancy:
- Safety or risk has not been established.
- See your doctor regularly.
- Avoid unnecessary use during pregnancy. Use only if directed by your doctor.
- Avoid use of phenylephrine near the time of your delivery.

### Recommendations during lactation:
- Safety or risk has not been established.
- Your doctor or your baby's doctor can provide the best recommendation for you.

 **Interactions**

### Interactions with medications, vitamins and minerals:

| Interacts with | Combined effect |
| --- | --- |
| Antidepressants | Increases blood pressure. |
| Beta-adrenergic blockers* | Increases blood pressure, leading to death. |
| Debrisoquin | Increases blood pressure. |
| Digoxin | Causes abnormal heart rhythm. |
| Guanethidine | May increase blood pressure. Excessive reaction of the pupil to eyedrops. |
| High-blood-pressure medications | Increases blood pressure. |
| Indomethacin | Causes very high blood pressure. |
| Monoamine oxidase (MAO) inhibitor | Causes very high blood pressure and can cause death. |

### Interactions with other substances:
- None reported.

*See Glossary.

**Definition and description:** Acts as an agent mimicking the effects of certain portions of the sympathetic nervous system*. It is used to alleviate symptoms of allergic disorders or upper-respiratory infections. Phenylpropanolamine is a decongestant. It is also contained in many weight-loss products.

**Other names:** See brand-name list, page 390.

 ## Dosage

### Safe dosage:
- Phenylpropanolamine can be purchased without a prescription. It is also found in products requiring a prescription.
- No safe dose has been established during pregnancy.

### Toxic dosage:
- Any dose may have toxic effects.

 ## Possible benefits

### Benefits before pregnancy:
- Phenylpropanolamine is effective for short-term weight loss. It has not been effective in keeping weight off permanently.

### Benefits to mother:
- None reported.

### Benefits to fetus:
- None reported.

### Benefits during lactation:
- None reported.

 ## Possible adverse effects

### Effects before pregnancy:
- May cause nervousness, insomnia, increase in blood pressure, headache, dizziness, rapid and forceful heartbeats, nausea and vomiting.

### Effects on mother:
- Intracranial hemorrhage* has been associated with phenylpropanolamine use.
- Also see *Effects before pregnancy*.

### Effects on fetus:
- First-trimester use of phenylpropanolamine may increase abnormal ureter* development, eye and ear defects, extra fingers and toes, cataracts* and depression of the chest. Use any time during pregnancy was associated with hip dislocation*.
- May cause a decrease in blood flow to the placenta, decreasing oxygen supplied to the fetus. This is associated with a decreased fetal heart rate.

### Effects on newborn:
- See *Effects on fetus*.

### Effects during lactation:
- Intercranial hemorrhage in the mother has been associated with phenylpropanolamine use.
- Lactating women may have the same adverse effects as any other person.

 ## Additional information

- This medication, when used for cold or allergy symptoms, does not cure or shorten the course of an illness. It provides relief for symptoms, but otherwise it offers no benefit.

# Phenylpropanolamine, continued

 **Recommendations for use**

### Women considering pregnancy:
• Discontinue phenylpropanolamine use if you plan to become pregnant.

### Recommendations during pregnancy:
• Discontinue phenylpropanolamine use if you are pregnant.
• Inform your doctor if you took phenylpropanolamine while pregnant.

### Recommendations during lactation:
• Don't take phenylpropanolamine while you are breast-feeding. Rapid weight loss is not recommended while you breast-feed. There is a small risk of intracranial hemorrhage* in the mother.

 **Interactions**

### Interactions with medications, vitamins and minerals:

| Interacts with | Combined effect |
| --- | --- |
| Chlor- pheniramine | Two cases have been reported of infants with congenital birth defects when mothers took chlorpheniramine and phenylpro- panolamine. |

### Interactions with other substances:
• Use with caffeine increases the stimulant effect.

*See Glossary.

**Definition and description:** Acts as an anticonvulsant to prevent epileptic seizures*.

**Other names:** See brand-name list, page 390.

## Dosage

### Safe dosage:
- Usual adult dose—100 to 500mg/day.
- Pregnant women may require as much as 1,200mg/day to prevent seizures. Your doctor can use blood levels to determine correct dosage.

### Toxic dosage:
- Varies from person to person.
- Doses that may have caused adverse effects before pregnancy may not cause adverse effects during pregnancy.
- Call your doctor if you develop severe staggering or drowsiness.

## Possible benefits

### Benefits before pregnancy:
- Use of medication may prevent seizures. Seizures may result in serious injury from falls and accidents. Prolonged, frequent seizures or continuous epileptic seizures may also result in brain damage or death.

### Benefits to mother:
- See *Benefits before pregnancy.*

### Benefits to fetus:
- Use of medication may prevent seizures in the mother. Decreased oxygen supply due to maternal seizures may cause brain damage or death in the fetus.
- Injuries from the mother falling during a seizure may damage the fetus.

### Benefits during lactation:
- None reported.

## Possible adverse effects

### Effects before pregnancy:
- Phenytoin may cause depletion of folate and vitamin D. See Folate, page 294, and Vitamin D, page 335.
- Adverse effects include dizziness, drowsiness, headache, staggering, vision changes, unusual eye movements, nausea, vomiting, skin rash, unusual bruising, sore throat and jaundice*.
- Notify your doctor of any new or unusual adverse effects.

### Effects on mother:
- Slightly lower calcium levels are found in pregnant women who use phenytoin. See Calcium, page 284.
- Thyroid-hormone levels are slightly decreased in pregnant women who use this medication.
- Pregnant women may have same adverse effects as any other person.
- Call your doctor if you develop any new adverse effects or if adverse effects worsen during pregnancy.

### Effects on fetus:
- Malformations occur in 10% of children exposed to anticonvulsant medications before birth. Minor abnormalities of the hands, feet, face and head include wide nasal bridge, low-set ears, low-set forehead, malformations of eyes and ears, small or absent nails, finger-like thumbs, short fingers, skin folds in the corners of the eyes and hip dislocation*.
- Serious problems such as malformations of heart, lungs and other breathing structures, gastrointestinal defects, small brain, hernias*, oral clefts* and slow mental and physical development also occur. Deaths due to serious malformations have been reported.
- Childhood cancers have been reported rarely in children with malformations associated with phenytoin.

MEDICATION

# Phenytoin, continued

### Effects on newborn:
- Serious bleeding during the first day after birth can usually be prevented by specific vitamin therapy. In some cases, Cesarean delivery may be necessary to avoid trauma to the newborn.
- Newborns may be sedated for a few days after birth. Infants may develop jitteriness, changes in sleep pattern and irritability during withdrawal.
- Thyroid-hormone levels are slightly lower in babies exposed to phenytoin before birth.

### Effects during lactation:
- Lethargy and poor sucking have been reported in one infant.
- Lactating women may have the same adverse effects as any other person.
- Your blood levels of this medication may increase after you wean your baby.

 **Additional information**

- You have a 90% chance of having a normal child if you must take medication to control epilepsy*.
- Pregnancy may increase, decrease or have no effect on the frequency and severity of seizures.
- Very severe seizures have occurred when medication is discontinued without a doctor's supervision.
- Having epilepsy and taking anticonvulsant medications increase the risk of having a miscarriage, stillbirth or child with birth defects.

 **Recommendations for use**

### Women considering pregnancy:
- Notify your doctor if you plan to become pregnant. Possible risks to you and your baby must be considered on an individual basis.
- If you have been seizure-free for many years, your doctor may recommend slowly discontinuing this medication before pregnancy.
- If you have a severe seizure disorder, it is *absolutely necessary* to continue anticonvulsant medication throughout your pregnancy.
- Your doctor can provide the best recommendation for you. Do *not* stop taking this medication unless told to do so by your doctor.

### Recommendations during pregnancy:
- See your doctor regularly.
- Blood levels should be checked frequently during pregnancy and for a few weeks after delivery to balance adverse effects and seizure control.
- Your doctor may want to adjust dose frequently during and after pregnancy. It is important to follow your doctor's instructions carefully.
- If seizures occur, contact your doctor immediately.
- At the time of delivery, tell your doctor you take phenytoin.
- Take only the vitamin supplements recommended by your doctor.
- Get plenty of sleep during your pregnancy.

### Recommendations during lactation:
- Nursing is usually safe when using this medication.
- Notify your baby's doctor if the baby is sedated or sucks poorly.
- See your doctor regularly while you wean your baby.

Interactions

**Interactions with medications, vitamins and minerals:**

| Interacts with | Combined effect |
|---|---|
| Acetazolamide | Increases toxicity of both. |
| Antacids | Decreases phenytoin effect. |
| Antidepressants | Decreases phenytoin effect. |
| Barbiturates | Alters phenytoin effect. |
| Benzodiazepines | Alters elimination of both. |
| Carbamazepine | Alters phenytoin effect. |
| Chloramphenicol | Increases phenytoin toxicity. |
| Disulfiram | Increases phenytoin effect. |
| Calcium | Decreases blood calcium levels. |
| Copper | Phenytoin may increase blood-copper levels. |
| Cyanocobalamin | Decreases blood-cyanocobalamin levels. |
| Folate | Increases requirement for folate. Excessive supplementation may increase seizures. |
| Furosemide | Decreases furosemide effect. |
| Isoniazid (INH) | Increases phenytoin toxicity. |
| Magnesium | Decreases blood-magnesium levels. |
| Methadone | Decreases methadone effect. |
| Nitrofurantoin | Decreases phenytoin effect. |
| Oral contraceptives | Decreases effectiveness of oral contraceptives. |
| Other anti-convulsant medications | Increases likelihood of birth defects when more than one medication is needed to control seizures. |
| Para-amino salicylic acid (PAS) | May increase phenytoin toxicity. |
| Pyridoxine | May decrease blood levels of phenytoin. |
| Quinidine | Decreases quinidine effect. |
| Steroids | Decreases steroid effect. |
| Valproic acid | May decrease phenytoin effect. |
| Vitamin D | Decreases Vitamin D effect. |

**Interactions with other substances:**
- Maternal alcohol consumption may increase risk of malformations.
- Regular alcohol use decreases phenytoin effect.

*See Glossary.

# Phosphorated carbohydrate

**Definition and description:** As an antiemetic*, phosphorated carbohydrate may control nausea and vomiting. It is a combination of sugars (levolose and dextrose) and phosphoric acid. However, the FDA* does not classify this medication as proved to be effective.

**Other names:** Emetrol®.

 **Dosage**

**Safe dosage:**
* Usual adult dose—1 or 2 tablespoons, 15 minutes apart until vomiting stops. No more than 5 doses should be taken in 1 hour.
* Phosphorated carbohydrate can be purchased without a prescription.

**Toxic dosage:**
* Toxicity is related to the high sugar (levolose) content.
* Diabetics should avoid the high sugar content. If you have fructose intolerance, avoid levulose (fructose).

 **Possible benefits**

**Benefits before pregnancy:**
* May treat nausea and vomiting associated with dietary indiscretions, colds and travel discomforts.

**Benefits to mother:**
* May relieve nausea and vomiting.
* Effectiveness of non-prescription antiemetics* has not been proved for nausea and vomiting in pregnancy.

**Benefits to fetus:**
* None reported.

**Benefits during lactation:**
* None reported.

 **Possible adverse effects**

**Effects before pregnancy:**
* This product is well-tolerated. See Carbohydrates, page 372, and Phosphorus, page 310.

**Effects on mother:**
* See *Effects before pregnancy*.

**Effects on fetus:**
* None reported.

**Effects on newborn:**
* None reported.

**Effects during lactation:**
* None reported in nursing infants.
* Lactating women may have the same adverse effect as any other person.

 **Additional information**

* Use medication *only* if nausea and vomiting interfere with eating or daily activities, and other treatments fail. Your doctor can prescribe other treatments. He or she should determine whether medication is necessary.
* Other treatments may include eating soda crackers or dry toast and drinking hot or cold liquids as soon as you get up in the morning.
* A severe form of nausea and vomiting of pregnancy is called *hyperemesis gravidarum*. This condition causes nutritional deficiencies, loss of electrolytes*, weight loss and starvation. It often requires hospitalization. Treatment with antiemetics* alone will not reverse hyperemesis gravidarum*.

# Phosphorated carbohydrate, continued

 **Recommendations for use**

## Women considering pregnancy:
- Use this medication as directed on the package.
- Use phosphorated carbohydrate only as needed.
- Notify your doctor if you plan to become pregnant. Before pregnancy, your doctor can advise you about ways to decrease nausea and vomiting without medication.

## Recommendations during pregnancy:
- If you have severe vomiting, contact your doctor as soon as possible.
- See your doctor regularly.
- Your doctor can advise you about ways to decrease nausea and vomiting without medication.
- If other treatments fail to reduce nausea and vomiting, contact your doctor *before* using any medication.
- Use this medication only as directed by your doctor.
- This medication is not clearly effective.

## Recommendations during lactation:
- Your doctor or your baby's doctor can provide the best recommendation for you.

 **Interactions**

## Interactions with medications, vitamins and minerals:
- None reported.

## Interactions with other substances:
- None reported.

*See Glossary.

# Prednisone

**Definition and description:** Acts as a corticosteroid to treat asthma*, inflammatory bowel disease*, arthritis* and related disorders, severe allergic reactions and many other diseases.

**Other names:** See brand-name list, page 390.

 **Dosage**

### Safe dosage:
- Dose is determined for each person.

### Toxic dosage:
- Exact toxic dosage cannot be predicted.
- Long-term use causes osteoporosis* and decreases adrenal-gland activity.

 **Possible benefits**

### Benefits before pregnancy:
- Treats many chronic diseases, such as asthma*, inflammatory bowel disease*, arthritis* and severe allergic reactions.

### Benefits to mother:
- See *Benefits before pregnancy.*

### Benefits to fetus:
- Prednisone and similar medications have been used to increase maturity of fetal lungs when premature delivery is imminent.

### Benefits during lactation:
- None reported.

 **Possible adverse effects**

### Effects before pregnancy:
- Adverse effects include increased blood sugar, swelling, potentially dangerous decreases in adrenal activity, weight gain, discoloration of skin and cataracts*.
- Notify your doctor of any adverse effects.
- Men treated with steroids may have decreased sperm counts.

### Effects on mother:
- Pregnant women may have the same adverse effects as any other person.
- Call your doctor if you develop any new adverse effects or if adverse effects worsen during pregnancy.

### Effects on fetus:
- Several studies do not indicate an increased risk of malformations.
- One fetus developed cataracts* similar to those seen in adults receiving long-term corticosteroid treatment.
- Studies evaluating stillbirths have produced conflicting results. Some evidence indicates an increased risk of stillbirths.

### Effects on newborn:
- Immune-system suppression has been reported in one infant exposed to high doses of steroids.
- Inactivity of the adrenal gland has been reported. This is treated by administration of corticosteroids.

### Effects during lactation:
- Prednisone is found in breast milk.
- Lactating women may have the same adverse effects as any other person.

 **Recommendations for use**

### Women considering pregnancy:
- Use this medication as directed by your doctor.
- Notify your doctor if you plan to become pregnant. Risks to you and your baby must be weighed on an individual basis.
- If you have used prednisone for a long time, do *not* discontinue this medication without your doctor's advice.

### Recommendations during pregnancy:
- Contact your doctor if you think you are pregnant.
- Use this medication as directed by your doctor.
- Do not discontinue use of prednisone unless your doctor tells you to do so.

**Recommendations during lactation:**
- Nursing is usually safe while taking this medication.

 **Interactions**

**Interactions with medications, vitamins and minerals:**

| Interacts with | Combined effect |
|---|---|
| **Antacids** | May increase predni-sone absorption. |
| **Aspirin and other salicylates** | Decreases salicylate blood level. |
| **Barbiturates** | Decreases predni-sone effect, and decreases barbiturate effect. |
| **Chlorthalidone** | Increases potassium loss. |
| **Ethacrynic acid** | Increases potassium loss. |
| **Furosemide** | Increases potassium loss. |
| **Indomethacin** | Increases risk of peptic ulcer. |
| **Isoniazid (INH)** | Possibly decreases isoniazid effect. |
| **Oral antidiabetic medications** | Decreases anti-diabetic effect. |
| **Phenytoin** | Decreases phenytoin effect. |
| **Rifampin** | Decreases corti-costeroid effect. |
| **Thiazide diuretics** | Increases potassium loss. |
| **Vitamin A** | Improves wound heal-ing in steroid-treated persons. |
| **Warfarin** | Possibly decreases warfarin effect. |

**Interactions with other substances:**
- None reported.

*See Glossary.

# Primidone

**Definition and description:** Acts as an anticonvulsant to prevent epileptic seizures. Primadone is converted to phenobarbital in the liver.

**Other names:** Mysoline®, Sertan®.

 ## Dosage

### Safe dosage:
- Usual adult dose—500 to 2,000mg/day.
- Pregnant women may require higher doses than before pregnancy. Your doctor can use blood levels to determine correct dosage.

### Toxic dosage:
- Varies from person to person.

 ## Possible benefits

### Benefits before pregnancy:
- Use of medication may prevent seizures. Seizures may result in serious injury from falls and accidents. Prolonged, frequent seizures or continuous epileptic seizures may also result in brain damage or death.

### Benefits to mother:
- See *Benefits before pregnancy*.

### Benefits to fetus:
- Use of medication may prevent seizures in the mother. Decreased oxygen supply due to maternal seizures may cause brain damage or death in the fetus.
- Injuries from the mother falling during a seizure may damage the fetus.

### Benefits during lactation:
- None reported.

 ## Possible adverse effects

### Effects before pregnancy:
- Primidone may cause depletion of folate and vitamin D. See Folate, page 294, and Vitamin D, page 335.
- Adverse effects include dizziness, drowsiness, headache, staggering, vision changes, unusual eye movements, nausea, vomiting, unusual bruising, sore throat and jaundice*.
- Notify your doctor of any new or unusual adverse effects.

### Effects on mother:
- Pregnant women may have same adverse effects as any other person.
- Call your doctor if you develop any new adverse effects or if adverse effects worsen during pregnancy.

### Effects on fetus:
- Malformations occur in 10% of children exposed to anticonvulsant medications before birth. Minor abnormalities of the hands, feet, face and head include wide nasal bridge, low-set ears, low-set forehead, malformations of eyes and ears, small or absent nails, finger-like thumbs, short fingers, skin folds in the corners of the eyes and hip dislocation*.
- Serious problems such as malformations of heart, lungs, other breathing structures, gastrointestinal defects, small brain, hernias*, oral clefts* and slow mental and physical development also occur. Deaths due to serious malformations have been reported.
- Childhood cancers have been reported rarely in children who were exposed before birth.

### Effects on newborn:
- Serious bleeding during the first day after birth can usually be prevented by specific vitamin therapy. In some cases, Cesarean delivery may be necessary to avoid trauma to the newborn.
- Newborns may be sedated for a few days after birth. Infants may develop jitteriness, changes in sleep pattern and irritability during withdrawal. In some cases, symptoms may not be observed until a week or more after birth.

### Effects during lactation:
- Lethargy and sedation have been reported in infants exposed to similar medications. See *Additional information* and Phenobarbital, page 204.
- Lactating women may have the same adverse effects as any other person.

## Additional information

- Primidone is converted to phenobarbital in the liver. See Phenobarbital, page 204.
- You have a 90% chance of having a normal child if you must take medication to control epilepsy*.
- Pregnancy may increase, decrease or have no effect on the frequency and severity of seizures.
- Very severe seizures have occurred when medication is discontinued without a doctor's supervision.
- Having epilepsy and taking anticonvulsant medications increase the risk of having a miscarriage, stillbirth or child with birth defects.

## Recommendations for use

### Women considering pregnancy:

- Notify your doctor if you plan to become pregnant. Possible risks to you and your baby must be considered on an individual basis.
- Your doctor or your baby's doctor can provide the best recommendation for you.
- If you have been seizure-free for many years, your doctor may recommend slowly discontinuing this medication before pregnancy.

- If you have a severe seizure disorder, it is *absolutely necessary* to continue anticonvulsant medication throughout your pregnancy.
- Your doctor can provide the best recommendation for you. Do *not* stop taking this medication unless told to do so by your doctor.

### Recommendations during pregnancy:

- See your doctor regularly.
- Blood levels should be checked frequently during pregnancy and for a few weeks after delivery to balance adverse effects and effectiveness of medication.
- Your doctor may want to adjust dosage of medication frequently during and after pregnancy. It is important to follow your doctor's instructions carefully.
- If seizures occur, contact your doctor immediately.
- At the time of delivery, tell your doctor you take primidone.
- Take only the vitamin supplements recommended by your doctor.
- Get plenty of sleep during your pregnancy.

### Recommendations during lactation:

- With medical supervision, nursing is usually safe while using this medication.
- Notify your baby's doctor immediately if the baby is sedated or sucks poorly.
- Your doctor or your baby's doctor can provide the best recommendation for you.

# Primidone, continued

 **Interactions**

**Interactions with medications, vitamins and minerals:**

| Interacts with | Combined effect |
|---|---|
| Ascorbic acid | Increases ascorbic acid loss in urine. |
| Beta-adrenergic blockers | Decreases beta-adrenergic-blocker effect. |
| Calcium | Decreases calcium levels. |
| Carbamazepine | Alters carbamazepine effect. |
| Chloramphenicol | Alters response to both. |
| Copper | May increase blood-copper levels. |
| Cyanocobalamin | Decreases blood-cyanocobalamin levels. |
| Folate | Increases requirement for folate. Excessive supplementation may increase seizures. |
| Magnesium | Decreases blood-magnesium levels. |
| Meperidine | Increases meperidine toxicity. |
| Metronidazole | May increase metronidazole effect. |
| Monoamine oxidase (MAO) inhibitors | May increase barbiturate effect. |
| Oral contraceptives | Decreases contraceptive effect. |
| Other anti-convulsant medications | Increases likelihood of birth defects when more than one medication is needed to control seizures. |
| Phenothiazines | Decreases phenothiazine effect. |
| Phenytoin | Alters effect of both. |
| Pyridoxine | May decrease levels of primidone. |
| Quinidine | Decreases quinidine effect. |
| Steroids | Decreases steroid effect. |
| Theophylline | Decreases theophylline effect. |
| Tricyclic anti-depressants | Decreases anti-depressant effect. |
| Valproic acid | Alters phenobarbital effect. |
| Vitamin D | Decreases vitamin D effect. |
| Warfarin | Increases warfarin effect. |

**Interactions with other substances:**
- Maternal alcohol consumption may increase risk of malformations.
- Combined overdose with this medication and alcohol may be fatal.
- Regular alcohol use decreases effectiveness of this medication.
- Large amounts of alcohol may increase toxicity of this medication.
- Use of this medication with alcohol increases impairment.

*See Glossary.

**Definition and description:** Acts as a phenothiazine tranquilizer* to treat manifestations of psychiatric disorders. Also controls nausea and vomiting.

**Other names:** Compazine®.

## Dosage

### Safe dosage:
- Usual adult dose—5 to 10mg 3 or 4 times/day by mouth for nausea and vomiting.
- 25mg suppositories can be used twice daily for nausea and vomiting.

### Toxic dosage:
- Exact toxic dose cannot be predicted.
- Symptoms of overdose include agitation, restlessness, convulsions, fever, dry mouth, bowel paralysis, loss of consciousness, low blood pressure and dangerous heart rhythm.
- Extrapyramidal symptoms* occur after overdose or occasionally after usual doses.
- Contact your doctor, poison-control center or emergency room if you think you have taken an overdose.

## Possible benefits

### Benefits before pregnancy:
- Controls psychiatric disorders.
- Controls nausea and vomiting.

### Benefits to mother:
- See *Benefits before pregnancy*.

### Benefits to fetus:
- None reported.

### Benefits during lactation:
- None reported.

## Possible adverse effects

### Effects before pregnancy:
- Adverse effects include drowsiness, jaundice*, low blood-cell count, low blood pressure, unusual heart rhythm, seizures, rash, sensitivity to sunburn, dry mouth, nasal stuffiness, nausea, constipation, urinary retention, skin discoloration and eye damage. Tardive dyskinesia* occurs in some persons.
- Fatal anemia*, abnormal heart rhythm and allergic reactions have occurred.
- Abnormal milk production and absence of menstrual periods occur in some women after prolonged use. These symptoms are associated with decreased fertility.
- Notify your doctor of any new or unusual adverse effects.
- Impotence* has been reported in men.

### Effects on mother:
- Pregnant women may have the same adverse effects as any other person.
- Call your doctor if you develop any new adverse effects or if adverse effects worsen during pregnancy.

### Effects on fetus:
- Most evidence indicates that the risk of birth defects with phenothiazines is low. However, there is some controversy.
- Ask your doctor to review the data with you.

### Effects on newborn:
- Birth weight, infant mortality and intelligence at 4 years of age are *not* affected by use of phenothiazines during pregnancy.
- Adverse effects have been reported with similar medications after use throughout pregnancy. See Chlorpromazine, page 68.

### Effects during lactation:
- None reported in nursing infants.
- Lactating women may have the same adverse effects as any other person.

# Prochloperazine, continued

 **Additional information**

- Pregnancy may be complicated by development or recurrence of a serious mental disorder. Treatments other than medication should be tried first. If the risks of mental illness are considered serious, use of medication to treat the mother's illness is important.
- Your doctor will determine whether medication is necessary.
- Use medication *only* if nausea and vomiting interfere with eating or daily activities, and other treatments fail. Your doctor can prescribe other treatments. He or she should determine whether medication is necessary.
- Other treatments may include eating soda crackers or dry toast and drinking hot or cold liquids as soon as you get up in the morning.
- A severe form of nausea and vomiting of pregnancy is called *hyperemesis gravidarum**. This condition causes nutritional deficiencies, loss of electrolytes*, weight loss and starvation. It often requires hospitalization. Treatment with antiemetics* alone will not reverse hyperemesis gravidarum*.

 **Recommendations for use**

**Women considering pregnancy:**
- Use this medication only as directed by your doctor.
- Do not exceed the dose or frequency recommended by your doctor.
- If you use prochloperazine regularly, notify your doctor if you plan to become pregnant. Possible risks to you and your baby must be considered on an individual basis.
- Your doctor can provide the best recommendation for you.

**Recommendations during pregnancy:**
- If you have severe vomiting, contact your doctor as soon as possible.
- See your doctor regularly.
- Your doctor can advise you about ways to decrease nausea and vomiting without medication.
- If other treatments fail to reduce nausea and vomiting, contact your doctor *before* using any medication.
- Use this medication only as directed by your doctor.
- Do not exceed the dose recommended by your doctor. If nausea and vomiting persist, contact your doctor. Do not *increase* the dose without your doctor's consent.

**Recommendations during lactation:**
- Nursing is usually safe while using this medication.
- Your doctor or your baby's doctor can provide the best recommendation for you.

## Interactions

**Interactions with medications, vitamins and minerals:**

| Interacts with | Combined effect |
|---|---|
| **Antacids** | Decreases prochlorperazine absorption. |
| **Anti-cholinergics*** | Decreases effect on psychiatric disease. Decreases prochlorperazine absorption. Increases toxicity of both. |
| **Antidepressants** | Increases toxicity of both. Decreases effect of both. |
| **Barbiturates** | Increases prochlorperazine metabolism. |
| **Beta-adrenergic blockers** | Increases effect of both. |
| **Guanethidine** | Increases blood pressure. |
| **Insulin** | Increases blood sugar. |
| **Lithium** | Decreases prochlorperazine effect. Decreases prochlorperazine levels. |
| **Methyldopa** | Increases blood pressure. |
| **Orphenadrine** | Lowers blood-sugar levels. |
| **Phenytoin** | Alters phenytoin blood levels. |

**Interactions with other substances:**

• Use with alcohol increases drowsiness and slows reaction time.
• Smoking may increase metabolism of phenothiazine tranquilizers.

*See Glossary.

MEDICATION

# Promethazine

**Definition and description:** Acts as an antihistamine of the phenothiazine group to treat stuffy nose, allergic skin reactions and other allergic reactions. As an antiemetic*, it treats nausea and vomiting and prevents motion sickness.

**Other names:** See brand-name list, page 390.

 Dosage

**Safe dosage:**
* Usual adult dose—12.5 to 25mg every 4 to 6 hours, as needed.

**Toxic dosage:**
* Exact toxic dose cannot be predicted.
* Symptoms of overdose include agitation, restlessness, convulsions, fever, dry mouth, bowel paralysis, loss of consciousness, low blood pressure and dangerous heart rhythm.
* Extrapyramidal symptoms* occur after overdose or occasionally after usual doses.
* Contact your doctor, poison-control center or emergency room if you think you have taken an overdose.

 Possible benefits

**Benefits before pregnancy:**
* Controls symptoms of allergy.
* Controls nausea and vomiting.

**Benefits to mother:**
* Promethazine has been used to treat Rh-incompatible pregnancies*.
* See *Benefits before pregnancy.*

**Benefits to fetus:**
* Promethazine has been used to treat Rh-incompatible pregnancies*.

**Benefits during lactation:**
* None reported.

 Possible adverse effects

**Effects before pregnancy:**
* Adverse effects include drowsiness, jaundice*, low blood-cell count, changes in blood pressure, rash, sensitivity to sunburn and dry mouth. Extrapyramidal symptoms* occur in some persons.
* Fatal anemia* has occurred.
* Notify your doctor of any new or unusual adverse effects.

**Effects on mother:**
* Fast heart rate has been reported in women treated with this medication during labor.
* Pregnant women may have the same adverse effects as any other person.
* Call your doctor if you develop any new adverse effects or if adverse effects worsen during pregnancy.

**Effects on fetus:**
* Most evidence indicates the risk of birth defects with phenothiazines and antiemetics* is low. However, there is some controversy. Ask your doctor to review the data with you.

**Effects on newborn:**
* The risk to newborns is low. However, breathing problems have occasionally been reported in newborns after use of promethazine in labor. Decreased platelet activity has been reported in newborns who are exposed near the time of delivery.
* Birth weight, infant mortality and intelligence at 4 years of age are *not* affected by use of phenothiazines during pregnancy.

**Effects during lactation:**
* Lactating women may have the same adverse effects as any other person.

**Additional information**

- Use medication *only* if nausea and vomiting interfere with eating or daily activities, and other treatments fail. Your doctor can prescribe other treatments. He or she should determine whether medication is necessary.
- Other treatments may include eating soda crackers or dry toast and drinking hot or cold liquids as soon as you get up in the morning.
- A severe form of nausea and vomiting of pregnancy is called *hyperemesis gravidarum\**. This condition causes nutritional deficiencies, loss of electrolytes\*, weight loss and starvation. It often requires hospitalization. Treatment with antiemetics\* alone will not reverse hyperemesis gravidarum\*.

 **Recommendations for use**

### Women considering pregnancy:

- Use this medication only as directed by your doctor.
- Do not exceed the dose or frequency recommended by your doctor.
- Notify your doctor if you plan to become pregnant. Before pregnancy, your doctor can advise you about ways to decrease nausea and vomiting without medication.
- If you use this medication regularly, notify your doctor if you plan to become pregnant. Possible risks to you and your baby must be considered on an individual basis.
- Your doctor can provide the best recommendation for you.

### Recommendations during pregnancy:

- If you have severe vomiting, contact your doctor as soon as possible.
- See your doctor regularly.
- Your doctor can advise you about ways to decrease nausea and vomiting without medication.
- If other treatments fail to reduce nausea and vomiting, contact your doctor *before* using any medication.

- Use this medication only as directed by your doctor.
- Do not exceed the dose recommended by your doctor. If nausea and vomiting persist, contact your doctor. Do *not* increase the dose without your doctor's consent.

### Recommendations during lactation:

- Your doctor or your baby's doctor can provide the best recommendation for you.

 **Interactions**

### Interactions with medications, vitamins and minerals:

| Interacts with | Combined effect |
| --- | --- |
| Antacids | Decreases promethazine absorption. |
| Antidepressants | Increases drowsiness. |
| Beta-adrenergic blockers | Increases effect of both. |
| Guanethidine | Decreases guanethidine effect. |
| Insulin | Increases blood sugar. |
| Methyldopa | Decreases methyldopa effect. |
| Orphenadrine | Lowers blood-sugar levels. |
| Phenytoin | Alters phenytoin blood levels. |

### Interactions with other substances:

- Use with alcohol increases drowsiness and slows reaction time.

\*See Glossary.

# Propylthiouracil

**Definition and description:** Acts as an antithyroid agent to decrease thyroid function in hyperthyroid* persons.

**Other names:** Propacil®.

 ## Dosage

### Safe dosage:
- Usual adult dose—200 to 400mg/day.
- Higher doses may be used initially.

### Toxic dosage:
- Exact toxic dose cannot be predicted.

 ## Possible benefits

### Benefits before pregnancy:
- Maintains normal thyroid function.

### Benefits to mother:
- See *Benefits before pregnancy.*

### Benefits to fetus:
- None reported.

### Benefits during lactation:
- None reported.

 ## Possible adverse effects

### Effects before pregnancy:
- Adverse effects include skin rash, itching, joint pain, muscle pain, bruising and low blood-cell counts.
- Fatal anemias* have been reported.

### Effects on mother:
- Pregnant women may have the same adverse effects as any other person.
- Call your doctor if you develop any adverse effects during pregnancy.

### Effects on fetus:
- Fetal goiter* and hypothyroidism* have been reported. Careful adjustment of the mother's dose decreases risk from medication and hyperthyroidism*. See *Additional information* and Levothyroxine, page 156.
- The rate of malformations with propylthiouracil does not exceed that expected in the general population. Malformations have been reported less frequently with propylthiouracil than with other antithyroid medications.

### Effects on newborn:
- Hypothyroidism* has been reported. Hypothyroidism* usually disappears within 2 to 6 weeks. Rarely, slow mental and physical development have been reported.
- Neonatal goiter* has also occurred. Goiters* are usually small and do not interfere with breathing. However, there have been reports of very large goiters* that do interfere with breathing. One infant died.
- Careful adjustment of the mother's dose decreases risk from medication and hyperthyroidism*. See *Additional information.*
- No difference in intelligence, height or bone development was found in one study comparing children exposed to propylthiouracil before birth to unexposed brothers and sisters.

### Effects during lactation:
- Propylthiouracil is found in breast milk.
- Thyroid damage has not been reported with this medication. The infant's thyroid function should be monitored, because similar medications have caused thyroid damage.

**Additional information**

- Pregnancy does not influence severity of hyperthyroidism*.
- Most pregnant hyperthyroid women do not have complicated pregnancies. Ocassionally pre-eclampsia* or eclampsia*, miscarriage, premature labor and thyroid storm* occur in women with severe hyperthyrodism*.
- Hyperthyroidism* is associated with fetal death, prematurity and low birth weight in newborns. In these cases, control of the mother's hyperthyroidism* is important for the fetus. Treatment may be surgery or medication.

 **Recommendations for use**

### Women considering pregnancy:

- Notify your doctor if you plan to become pregnant. Risks to you and your baby must be considered on an individual basis.
- Use this medication only as directed by your doctor.
- Your doctor will balance treatment to avoid toxicity to the fetus.
- Some medications for hyperthyroidism* should not be used in pregnancy. Your doctor may want to change your medication before you become pregnant.

### Recommendations during pregnancy:

- See your doctor regularly.
- Follow your doctor's instructions carefully.
- Your doctor will adjust your dose to balance toxicity and benefit.
- Use this medication only as directed by your doctor.

### Recommendations during lactation:

- Nursing may be safe with medical supervision.
- If you breast-feed while using this medication, your doctor or your baby's doctor may want to check your baby's thyroid function periodically.
- Your doctor or your baby's doctor can provide the best recommendation for you.

 **Interactions**

### Interactions with medications, vitamins and minerals:

- None reported.

### Interactions with other substances:

- Food may change absorption of propylthiouracil.

*See Glossary.

# Pseudoephedrine

**Definition and description:** Acts as a decongestant to decrease nasal secretions.

**Other names:** See brand-name list, page 390.

 ## Dosage

**Safe dosage:**
- Usual adult dose—60mg every 6 hours, as needed.
- This medication can be purchased without a prescription.

**Toxic dosage:**
- Exact toxic dose cannot be determined.
- Symptoms of overdose include headache, unusual heart rhythm, slow pulse and increased blood pressure.

 ## Possible benefits

**Benefits before pregnancy:**
- Decreases nasal congestion from allergies and colds.

**Benefits to mother:**
- See *Benefits before pregnancy.*

**Benefits to fetus:**
- None reported.

**Benefits during lactation:**
- None reported.

 ## Possible adverse effects

**Effects before pregnancy:**
- Adverse effects include agitation, sleeplessness, dizziness, headache, nausea, vomiting, irregular heartbeat, difficulty urinating, hallucinations and seizures.
- Discontinue use, and notify your doctor if you have any adverse effects.
- Notify your doctor if symptoms persist.

**Effects on mother:**
- Pregnant women may have the same adverse effects as any other person.
- Call your doctor if you develop any adverse effects during pregnancy.

**Effects on fetus:**
- Safety of this medication has not been established in early pregnancy. However, most doctors consider it safe in later pregnancy.

**Effects on newborn:**
- None reported after exposure during pregnancy.

**Effects during lactation:**
- This medication is found in high concentrations in breast milk.
- An infant developed irritability, crying and disturbed sleep after exposure to pseudoephedrine and brompheniramine. Symptoms disappeared when nursing was discontinued.
- Lactating women may have the same adverse effects as any other person.

 ## Additional information

- This medication does not cure or shorten the course of an illness. It provides relief for symptoms, but otherwise it offers no benefit.
- Viral illnesses and fever have been implicated as a cause of birth defects. This medication is often used to relieve symptoms of viral illnesses. Contact your doctor if you have a fever.
- This medication is often used in combination with other medications. Most studies did not study persons using it alone. It is difficult to determine if pseudoephedrine caused any malformations.

**Recommendations for use**

### Women considering pregnancy:
- Use medication as directed on the package.
- Do not exceed the suggested dose.
- Use only when needed.
- Notify your doctor if you plan to become pregnant.

### Recommendations during pregnancy:
- Safety or risk has not been established in early pregnancy. Your doctor can decide when it is safe to use this medication.
- See your doctor regularly.
- Avoid unnecessary use during pregnancy. Use only if directed by your doctor.

### Recommendations during lactation:
- With medical supervision, nursing is usually safe.
- Avoid high doses or long-acting products.
- Discontinue use, and contact your baby's doctor if your baby becomes irritable or restless.
- Your doctor or your baby's doctor can provide the best recommendation for you.

 **Interactions**

### Interactions with medications, vitamins, minerals

| Interacts with | Combined effect |
|---|---|
| Ammonium chloride | May decrease pseudoephedrine effect. |
| Digoxin | Causes abnormal heart rhythm. |
| High-blood-pressure medication | Increases blood pressure. |
| Indomethacin | Causes very high blood pressure. |
| Kaolin | May decrease pseudoephedrine absorption. |
| Monoamine oxidase (MAO) inhibitor | Causes very high blood pressure, leading to death. |
| Sodium bicarbonate | May prolong pseudoephedrine effect. |

### Interactions with other substances:
- None reported.

*See Glossary.

Note: This page purposely left blank.

**Definition and description:** Used to treat lice.

**Other names:** A-200®, Rid®.

## Dosage

### Safe dosage:
- Apply to affected areas for no longer than 10 minutes, then wash with warm water and soap or shampoo. Repeat in 7 to 10 days.

### Toxic dosage:
- This medication is harmful if swallowed. Avoid contact with eyes.

## Possible benefits

### Benefits before pregnancy:
- Treats infestations of head, body and pubic lice.

### Benefits to mother:
- See *Benefits before pregnancy*.

### Benefits to fetus:
- None reported.

### Benefits during lactation:
- None reported.

## Possible adverse effects

### Effects before pregnancy:
- People allergic to ragweed may react to this medication.
- Notify your doctor of any adverse effects.

### Effects on mother:
- Pregnant women may have the same adverse effects as any other person.
- Call your doctor if you develop any adverse effects.

### Effects on fetus:
- No reports of use in pregnancy. Absorption from the skin is poor. This medication in combination with piperonyl butoxide is probably safer than other available medications for treatment of lice.

### Effects on newborn:
- None reported.

### Effects during lactation:
- It is unknown if pyrethrins enter breast milk. Because this medication is applied to the entire body, it will be on breasts and nipples. It may be wise to avoid nursing while using this medication.

## Recommendations for use

### Women considering pregnancy:
- Follow the directions on the package.
- Do not used this medication if you are allergic to ragweed.

### Recommendations during pregnancy:
- Follow the directions on the package.
- Do not used this medication if you are allergic to ragweed.
- Risks from this medication must be considered on an individual basis. Your doctor can advise you.

### Recommendations during lactation:
- Interrupt nursing while using this medication.

## Interactions

### Interactions with medications, vitamins and minerals:
- None reported.

### Interactions with other substances:
- None reported.

MEDICATION

# Pyrilamine

**Definition and description:** Acts as an antihistamine to relieve allergy symptoms, including sneezing, runny nose, itching and tearing.

**Other names:** Pyrilamine maleate, pyrilamine tannate. Also see brand-name list, page 390.

 ## Dosage

### Safe dosage:
- Usual adult dose—25 to 50mg every 6 to 8 hours, as needed for relief of symptoms.
- Smaller doses are effective in combination with other medications. Follow instructions on the package for combination products.
- This medication can be purchased without a prescription. It is also found in products requiring a prescription.

### Toxic dosage:
- Exact toxic dose cannot be predicted.
- Symptoms of overdose include sedation, dry mouth, large pupils, flushing and low blood pressure.
- Serious overdose may cause convulsions and death.
- Contact your doctor, poison-control center or emergency room if you think you have taken an overdose.

 ## Possible benefits

### Benefits before pregnancy:
- Relieves allergy symptoms.

### Benefits to mother:
- See *Benefits before pregnancy.*

### Benefits to fetus:
- None reported.

### Benefits during lactation:
- None reported.

 ## Possible adverse effects

### Effects before pregnancy:
- Adverse effects include drowsiness, rash, hives*, sweating, chills, dry mouth, headache, unusual heart rhythm, low blood pressure, low blood-cell count, confusion, ringing in ears, blurred vision, nausea, vomiting and difficulty urinating.
- Severe allergic reactions have occurred.
- Notify your doctor of any adverse effects.

### Effects on mother:
- Pregnant women may have the same adverse effects as any other person.
- Call your doctor if you develop any adverse effects.

### Effects on fetus:
- Antihistamines as a group have not been shown to increase risk of malformations compared to unexposed pregnancies.
- One study demonstrated a possible association with benign tumors* after exposure at any time during pregnancy. When exposures during the first 4 months of pregnancy only were evaluated, there was no increased risk of malformations.
- This evidence is inadequate to establish safety or risk.

### Effects on newborn:
- None reported.

### Effects during lactation:
- It is unknown if this medication is found in breast milk.
- Most antihistamines enter breast milk.
- Lactating women may have the same adverse effects as any other person.

## Additional information

- This medication does not cure colds, coughs or minor allergy complaints. It provides relief for symptoms. Occasionally, when allergic reactions are very serious, using anithistamines and other medications can be life-saving.
- Viral illnesses and fever have been implicated as a cause of birth defects. This medication is often used to relieve symptoms of viral illnesses. Contact your doctor if you have a fever.
- This medication is often used in combination with other medications. Most studies did not study persons using it alone. It is difficult to determine if pyrilamine caused any malformations.

 ## Recommendations for use

### Women considering pregnancy:
- Notify your doctor if you plan to become pregnant.
- Use only the recommended doses of this medication.
- Use this medication only when needed.

### Recommendations during pregnancy:
- Safety or risk has not been established.
- See your doctor regularly.
- Use this medication only as directed by your doctor.
- Do not use this medication during pregnancy unless instructed by your doctor.
- Avoid unnecessary use of this medication.

### Recommendations during lactation:
- Nursing while using antihistamines is usually safe.
- Your doctor or your baby's doctor can provide the best recommendation for you.

 ## Interactions

**Interactions with medications, vitamins and minerals:**

| Interacts with | Combined effect |
| --- | --- |
| Antianxiety agents | Increases drowsiness. |
| Antidepressants | Increases drowsiness. |
| Other anti-histamines | Increases drowsiness. |
| Tranquilizers | Increases drowsiness. |

**Interactions with other substances:**
- Use with alcohol increases drowsiness and slows reaction time.

*See Glossary.

# Ranitidine

**Definition and description:** Treats duodenal ulcer\*, gastric ulcer,\* reflux\* of stomach contents into the esophagus.

**Other names:** Zantac®.

 **Dosage**

**Safe dosage:**
• Usual adult dose—150mg twice/day.

**Toxic dosage:**
• Exact toxic dose cannot be predicted.

 **Possible benefits**

**Benefits before pregnancy:**
• Treats ulcer disease\*.
• Treats symptoms of reflux\*.

**Benefits to mother:**
• Ranitidine has been useful in decreasing gastric-acid secretion during labor and Cesarean delivery.
• Also see *Benefits before pregnancy*.

**Benefits to fetus:**
• None reported.

**Benefits during lactation:**
• None reported.

 **Possible adverse effects**

**Effects before pregnancy:**
• Adverse effects include dizziness, sleeplessness, confusion, agitation, depression, hallucinations\*, abnormal heart rhythms, constipation, diarrhea, nausea, vomiting, liver damage, low blood-cell count, rash and allergic reactions.

**Effects on mother:**
• Pregnant women may have the same adverse effects as any other person.

**Effects on fetus:**
• There is no experience with ranitidine in early pregnancy. Safety or risk has not been established in early pregnancy.

**Effects on newborn:**
• None reported in infants exposed during labor and Cesarean delivery.

**Effects during lactation:**
• This medication is found in very high concentrations in breast milk.
• A similar medication may decrease stomach acid and cause central-nervous-system adverse effects, such as excitation. See Cimetidine, page 72.
• Lactating women may have the same adverse effects as any other person.

**Recommendations for use**

### Women considering pregnancy:
- Safety or risk has not been established in early pregnancy.
- Use this medication as directed by your doctor.
- Notify your doctor if you plan to become pregnant. Risk to you and your baby must be considered on an individual basis.

### Recommendations during pregnancy:
- Safety or risk has not been established in early pregnancy.
- See your doctor regularly.
- Use this medication only as directed by your doctor.

### Recommendations during lactation:
- Very high levels of this medication are found in breast milk.
- Avoid nursing while using ranitidine.

 **Interactions**

### Interactions with medications, vitamins and minerals:

| Interacts with | Combined effect |
|---|---|
| **Antacids** | Decreases ranitidine effect. |
| **Theophylline** | May increase toxicity of theophylline. Risk is low. |

### Interactions with other substances:
- None reported.

See Glossary.

MEDICATION

# Rifampin

**Definition and description:** Acts as an antibiotic to treat susceptible tuberculosis* bacteria.

**Other names:** Rifadin®, Rifomycin®, Rimactane®.

 ## Dosage

**Safe dosage:**
• Usual adult dose—600mg/day.

**Toxic dosage:**
• Exact toxic dose cannot be predicted.
• Liver damage may be fatal.

 ## Possible benefits

**Benefits before pregnancy:**
• Used in combination with other medications to treat active tuberculosis*.

**Benefits to mother:**
• Some bacterial infections may be very serious to the mother. This medication can cure susceptible infections.

**Benefits to fetus:**
• Some bacterial infections in the mother may increase risk to the fetus. This medication can cure susceptible infections.

**Benefits during lactation:**
• None reported.

 ## Possible adverse effects

**Effects before pregnancy:**
• Adverse effects include heartburn*, appetite loss, nausea, vomiting, gas, cramps, diarrhea, headache, drowsiness, fatigue, dizziness, confusion, vision changes, weakness, fever, rash, hives*, itching, jaundice* kidney damage and decreased blood-cell count.
• Kidney damage is more likely if therapy is interrupted and restarted.
• May produce false-positive glucose tests.
• Notify your doctor of any adverse effects.

**Effects on mother:**
• Pregnant women may have the same adverse effects as any other person.
• Call your doctor if you develop any adverse effects.

**Effects on fetus:**
• Limited information is available regarding the use of rifampin in pregnancy. The limited evidence available does not indicate an increased risk of malformations. However, safety or risk in early pregnancy has not been established.

**Effects on newborn:**
• Serious bleeding in the newborn after birth can be prevented by specific vitamin therapy.

**Effects during lactation:**
• This medication is found in low concentrations in breast milk. No adverse effects have been reported in nursing infants.
• Lactating women may have the same adverse effects as any other person.

 ## Additional information

• Tuberculosis can be a very serious infection in mothers and newborns. It is necessary to treat pregnant women with recent positive skin tests. Your doctor will determine which medication and how many medications are needed for you.
• In some cases, it will also be necessary to treat newborns of women with tuberculosis. Your doctor or your baby's doctor can advise you.
• Some bacterial infections may be very serious to the mother or the baby. It is important to treat these infections.
• Risks from infection or medication must be considered on an individual basis. Your doctor can advise you.

**Recommendations for use**

## Women considering pregnancy:
- Notify your doctor if you plan to become pregnant. Possible risks to you and your baby must be considered on an individual basis.
- Your doctor or your baby's doctor can provide the best recommendation for you.

## Recommendations during pregnancy:
- Risks from infection or medication must be considered on an individual basis. Your doctor can advise you.
- Use this medication as directed by your doctor.
- Notify your doctor of any adverse effects.

## Recommendations during lactation:
- Your doctor can provide the best recommendation for you.

 **Interactions**

### Interactions with medications, vitamins and minerals:

| Interacts with | Combined effect |
| --- | --- |
| Aminosalicylic acid | May decrease 'rifampin absorption. |
| Corticosteroids | Decreases corticosteroid effect. |
| Diazepam | Decreases diazepam effect. |
| Disopyramide | Decreases disopyramide effect. |
| Isoniazid (INH) | Increases liver damage. |
| Metoprolol | Decreases metoprolol effect. |
| Oral contraceptives | Decreases contraceptive effect. |
| Oral antidiabetes medication | Increases blood sugar. |
| Quinidine | Decreases quinidine effect. |
| Warfarin | Decreases warfarin effect. |

### Interactions with other substances:
- None reported.

*See Glossary.

# Ritodrine

**Definition and description:** Acts as a muscle relaxant to decrease uterine activity and treat premature labor.

**Other names:** See brand-name list, page 390.

 ## Dosage

### Safe dosage:
- Dose is adjusted to person's response and tolerance.
- Therapy is started with intravenous* infusion.
- Oral therapy usually follows intravenous* therapy.

### Toxic dosage:
- Exact toxic dose cannot be predicted.
- Rarely, maternal death has been reported from fluid in the lungs.

 ## Possible benefits

### Benefits before pregnancy:
- None. Medication is used only during pregnancy

### Benefits to mother:
- Treats premature labor.

### Benefits to fetus:
- Prevents premature delivery. See *Additional information.*

### Benefits during lactation:
- None. Medication is used only during pregnancy.

 ## Possible adverse effects

### Effects before pregnancy:
- None. Medication is used only during pregnancy.

### Effects on mother:
- Adverse effects during intravenous* use include fast heart rate, blood-pressure changes, fluid in the lungs, high blood-glucose levels, tremor*, nausea, vomiting, headache, nervousness, restlessness, anxiety, chest pain, unusual heart rhythms, rash, allergic reaction with shock, constipation, diarrhea, painful or difficult breathing, sweating, chills, drowsiness and weakness. Adverse effects are more severe during intravenous* administration.
- During oral administration, adverse effects are usually limited to a slight increase in heart rate, tremor*, nausea, rash and, rarely, unusual heart rhythms.

### Effects on fetus:
- Adverse effects include fast heart rate.

### Effects on newborn:
- Newborns may have low blood sugar and decreased bowel function.
- Low blood-calcium levels and low blood pressure in newborns have been reported after use of similar medications. See Terbutaline, page 252.

### Effects during lactation:
- None reported.

**Additional information**

- *This is the only medication approved by the FDA\* for treatment of premature labor.* Other medications are effective, however. Your doctor will select the safest medication for you and your baby, if you need treatment for premature labor.
- Premature delivery is associated with a high infant-mortality rate. For each 2 weeks a fetus remains in the uterus between the 25th and 37th week of pregnancy, newborn mortality is cut in half.
- Premature delivery is associated with blindness, mental retardation and severe lung disease.
- Benefits to the baby from medication often outweigh the risks of using medication.

 **Recommendations for use**

### Women considering pregnancy:
- Ritrodine is not used before pregnancy.

### Recommendations during pregnancy:
- See your doctor regularly.
- Notify your doctor *immediately* if you think you may have begun premature labor. Premature labor should be regarded as an emergency.
- Follow your doctor's instructions carefully.

### Recommendations during lactation:
- Ritodrine is not used during lactation.

 **Interactions**

**Interactions with medications, vitamins and minerals:**

| Interacts with | Combined effect |
|---|---|
| Corticosteroids | Increases risk of fluid accumulation in lungs. |
| Magnesium sulfate | Causes low blood pressure and abnormal heart rhythms. |
| Meperidine | Causes low blood pressure and abnormal heart rhythms. |

**Interactions with other substances:**
- None reported.

\*See Glossary.

# Salsalate

**Definition and description:** Relieves swelling, stiffness and pain of rheumatoid arthritis*, osteoarthritis* and related disorders.

**Other names:** Disalcid®, Mono-Gesic®.

 ## Dosage

**Safe dosage:**
• Usual adult dose—3g/day.

**Toxic dosage:**
• Exact toxic dose cannot be predicted.

 ## Possible benefits

**Benefits before pregnancy:**
• Relieves swelling, stiffness and joint pain of rheumatoid arthritis* and related disorders.

**Benefits to mother:**
• See *Benefits before pregnancy.*

**Benefits to fetus:**
• None reported.

**Benefits during lactation:**
• None reported.

 ## Possible adverse effects

**Effects before pregnancy:**
• Adverse effects include dizziness, headache, drowsiness, confusion, ringing in ears, nausea, vomiting, heartburn*, abdominal pain.
• Notify your doctor if you develop any adverse effects.

**Effects on mother:**
• Pregnant women may have the same adverse effects as any other person.

• Call your doctor if you develop any new adverse effects or if adverse effects worsen during pregnancy.
• Anemia*, excessive bleeding during and after labor, and prolonged or delayed labor have been reported with similar medications. See Aspirin, page 40. Experience with salsalate in pregnancy is limited.

**Effects on fetus:**
• Serious adverse effects have been reported after exposure to similar medications. Experience with this medication in pregnancy is limited. See Aspirin, page 40, and Indomethacin, page 142.

**Effects on newborn:**
• Serious adverse effects have been reported after use of similar medications. Experience with this medication in pregnancy is limited. See Aspirin, page 40, and Indomethacin, page 142.

**Effects during lactation:**
• The metabolite* of this medication is found in breast milk.
• Similar medications have caused illness in infants exposed via breast milk. See Aspirin, page 40.
• Lactating women may have the same adverse effects as any other person.

 ## Additional information

• Use of salsalate or similar medications may be necessary to control severe rheumatoid arthritis* or related disorders during pregnancy.
• Salsalate is less likely to cause stomach irritation and blood loss than similar medications. See Aspirin, page 40.

**Recommendations for use**

### Women considering pregnancy:

- Use this medication regularly as directed by your doctor for arthritis* and related disorders.
- If you use salsalate regularly, notify your doctor if you plan to become pregnant. Possible risks to you and your baby must be considered on an individual basis.
- Your doctor can provide the best recommendation for you.

### Recommendations during pregnancy:

- See your doctor regularly.
- If you use salsalate to control rheumatoid arthritis* or related disorders, possible risks to you and your baby must be considered on an individual basis. Follow your doctor's recommendations carefully.
- Avoid use of salsalate near your expected delivery date, except as directed by your doctor.
- At the time of delivery, tell your doctor you take this medication.

### Recommendations during lactation:

- Safety or risk has not been established.
- Your doctor or your baby's doctor can provide the best recommendation for you.

 **Interactions**

### Interactions with other substances:

| Interacts with | Combined effect |
| --- | --- |
| Aspirin | Increases toxicity of both medications. |

### Interactions with other substances:

- None reported.

*See Glossary.

# Simethicone

**Definition and description:** Acts as a gastric defoaming agent to decrease stomach gas. This medication is often included in antacid products. Available evidence indicates it is less effective in combination with aluminum-containing antacids.

**Other names:** See brand-name list, page 390.

 ## Dosage

**Safe dosage:**
- Usual adult dose—1 or 2 tablets 4 times/day.
- Simethicone can be purchased without a prescription.

**Toxic dosage:**
- This medication is well-tolerated. Few adverse effects have been reported.

 ## Possible benefits

**Benefits before pregnancy:**
- Decreases gastrointestinal gas.

**Benefits to mother:**
- See *Benefits before pregnancy.*

**Benefits to fetus:**
- None reported.

**Benefits during lactation:**
- None reported.

 ## Possible adverse effects

**Effects before pregnancy:**
- Simethicone is well-tolerated. Few adverse effects have been reported.

**Effects on mother:**
- Pregnant women may have the same adverse effects as any other person.

**Effects on fetus:**
- None reported.

**Effects on newborn:**
- None reported.

**Effects during lactation:**
- Lactating women may have the same adverse effects as any other person.

 ## Recommendations for use

**Women considering pregnancy:**
- Follow instructions on the package.

**Recommendations during pregnancy:**
- See your doctor regularly.
- Ask your doctor or nurse for recommendations.

**Recommendations during lactation:**
- Follow instructions on the package.

 ## Interactions

**Interactions with medications, vitamins and minerals:**

| Interacts with | Combined effect |
| --- | --- |
| Warfarin | May decrease warfarin effect. |

**Interactions with other substances:**
- None reported.

**Definition and description:** Birth-control method to prevent conception by killing sperm.

**Other names:** Nonoxynol-9. Also see brand-name list, page 390.

 ## Dosage

### Safe dosage:
- May be purchased as a foam, cream, jelly, suppository, on a condom or in a sponge.
- Some commercial products are intended to be used with a diaphragm or condom. If the package specifies use with a diaphragm or condom, do not use spermicide alone.

### Toxic dosage:
- Exact toxic dose cannot be predicted.
- Do not take orally.

 ## Possible benefits

### Benefits before pregnancy:
- Prevents pregnancy.

### Benefits to mother:
- None reported.

### Benefits to fetus:
- None reported.

### Benefits during lactation:
- Prevention of pregnancy.

 ## Possible adverse effects

### Effects before pregnancy:
- Discontinue use if local irritation occurs.

### Effects on mother:
- Spermicides are not used during pregnancy except in accidental exposure.
- Local irritation can occur while using this medication during early pregnancy.

### Effects on fetus:
- Seven evaluations with obvious exposure to spermicides during pregnancy have not demonstrated any increased risk of malformations.
- An increase in miscarriages has been reported in some studies but not in others.
- One study found *no* association between spermicide use before conception and stillbirth.

### Effects on newborn:
- None reported.

### Effects during lactation:
- Spermicides are found in breast milk.

 ## Recommendations for use

### Women considering pregnancy:
- Follow instructions on package carefully.
- Incorrect use decreases effectiveness.

### Recommendations during pregnancy:
- Contact your doctor as soon as you think you may be pregnant.
- Discontinue use as soon as pregnancy is confirmed.

### Recommendations during lactation:
- Your doctor or your baby's doctor can provide the best recommendation for you.

 ## Interactions

### Interactions with medications, vitamins and minerals
- None reported.

### Interactions with other substances:
- None reported.

# Streptomycin

**Definition and description:** Acts an an antibiotic to treat susceptible bacterial infections, including tuberculosis*.

**Other names:** Trobicin®.

 ## Dosage

### Safe dosage:
- Dose varies.

### Toxic dosage:
- Toxic dose varies with the level of kidney function and person's size.
- Deafness, dizziness and loss of balance control occur with overdose.
- Doses are adjusted for each individual.

 ## Possible benefits

### Benefits before pregnancy:
- Used in combination with other medications to treat active tuberculosis*.
- May be used to treat other serious non-tuberculosis infections.

### Benefits to mother:
- Some bacterial infections may be very serious to the mother. This medication can cure susceptible infections.

### Benefits to fetus:
- Some bacterial infections in the mother may increase risk to the fetus. This medication can cure susceptible infections.

### Benefits during lactation:
- None reported.

 ## Possible adverse effects

### Effects before pregnancy:
- Adverse effects include nausea, vomiting, dizziness, unusual sensations of the face, rash, hives*, fever, deafness, severe skin reactions, decreased blood-cell counts, changes in vision, kidney damage and serious allergic reactions.

- Deafness, dizziness and loss of balance control may be permanent.
- Notify your doctor of any adverse effects.

### Effects on mother:
- Pregnant women may have the same adverse effects as any other person.
- Call your doctor if you develop any adverse effects.

### Effects on fetus:
- Deafness has occurred in some exposed infants. However, the risk of deafness is low.

### Effects on newborn:
- None reported in infants exposed before birth, except deafness.
- Ear damage, including deafness and loss of balance control, has been reported in infants and children treated with streptomycin.

### Effects during lactation:
- This medication is found in high concentrations in breast milk. Oral absorption is low, so absorption from breast milk is low.
- No adverse effects have been reported in nursing infants.
- Lactating women may have the same adverse effects as any other person.

 ## Additional information

- Some bacterial infections may be very serious to the mother or the baby. It is important to treat these infections.
- Risks from infection or medication must be considered on an individual basis. Your doctor can advise you.
- Blood levels of streptomycin are lower in pregnant women than other women given the same dose. Your doctor will select the best dose for you.

**Recommendations for use**

### Women considering pregnancy:

- Notify your doctor if you plan to become pregnant. Possible risks to you and your baby must be considered on an individual basis.
- Your doctor can provide the best recommendation for you.
- Report decreased hearing, loss of balance or dizziness to your doctor immediately.

### Recommendations during pregnancy:

- Risks from infection or medication must be considered on an individual basis. Your doctor can advise you.
- Use this medication as directed by your doctor.
- Notify your doctor of any adverse effects, especially decreased hearing, loss of balance or dizziness.
- Your doctor will monitor your dose carefully.

### Recommendations during lactation:

- Your doctor or your baby's doctor can provide the best recommendation for you.

 **Interactions**

### Interactions with medications, vitamins and minerals:

| Interacts with | Combined effect |
| --- | --- |
| **Cephalothin** | Increases kidney damage. |
| **Riboflavin** | Decreases riboflavin absorption. |
| **Warfarin** | Increases bleeding. |

### Interactions with other substances:

- None reported.

*See Glossary.

MEDICATION

# Sulfamethoxazole

**Definition and description:** Acts as an antibacterial to treat susceptible bacterial infections.

**Other names:** Gantanol®, Bactrim®, Septra®.

 **Dosage**

**Safe dosage:**
- Usual adult dose—1g every 8 hours when used alone.
- Usual adult dose—800mg every 12 hours when used in combination with trimethoprim. See *Trimethoprim*, page 272.

**Toxic dosage:**
- Exact toxic dose cannot be predicted.
- Low blood-cell count, Stevens-Johnson syndrome* and some allergic reactions have been fatal.

 **Possible benefits**

**Benefits before pregnancy:**
- Cures susceptible bacterial infections.

**Benefits to mother:**
- Some bacterial infections may be very serious to the mother. This medication can cure susceptible infections.

**Benefits to fetus:**
- Some bacterial infections in the mother may increase risk to the fetus. This medication can cure susceptible infections.

**Benefits during lactation:**
- None reported.

 **Possible adverse effects**

**Effects before pregnancy:**
- Adverse effects include decreased blood-cell count, serious allergic reactions, red eyes, rash, itching, hives*, sensitivity to sunburn, skin disease, Stevens-Johnson syndrome*, liver damage, diarrhea, nausea, vomiting, swelling in throat, kidney damage, convulsions, headache, ringing in ears,

low blood sugar, sore muscles and joints, swelling and fever.
- Notify your doctor of any adverse effects.

**Effects on mother:**
- Sulfamethoxazole interferes with folic-acid activity. See Folate, page 294.
- Pregnant women may have the same adverse effects as any other person.
- Call your doctor if you develop any adverse effects.

**Effects on fetus:**
- Most evidence does not indicate an increased risk of malformations. However, some malformations have been reported.
- One stillborn baby showed evidence of severe anemia* due to red-blood-cell damage.
- Sulfamethoxazole is often used in combination with trimethoprim. See Trimethoprim, page 272.

**Effects on newborn:**
- Anemia* from red-blood-cell damage has been reported in infants of genetically susceptible G6PD-deficient mothers*. This occurred after exposure before birth or treatment after birth with this medication.
- Jaundice* has been reported in infants exposed before birth or treated after birth with sulfamethoxazole. Premature babies are most likely to develop jaundice*.
- The risk of kernicterus* may be increased after exposure late in pregnancy or treatment after birth with this medication.

**Effects during lactation:**
- Sulfamethoxazole is found in breast milk.
- Anemia* from red-blood-cell damage is possible in genetically susceptible G6PD-deficient infants.
- There is a risk of jaundice* in the first month after birth.
- Lactating women may have the same adverse effects as any other person.

## Additional information

- Some bacterial infections may be very serious to the mother or the baby. It is important to treat these infections.
- Risks from infection or medication must be considered on an individual basis. Your doctor can advise you.
- Elimination of sulfamethoxazole is faster in pregnant women than other women given the same dose. Your doctor will select the best dose for you.

 ## Recommendations for use

### Women considering pregnancy:
- Notify your doctor if you plan to become pregnant. Possible risks to you and your baby must be considered on an individual basis.
- Use this medication as directed by your doctor.
- Notify your doctor of any adverse effects.

### Recommendations during pregnancy:
- Use this medication only as directed by your doctor. Even if your doctor prescribes this medication during pregnancy, do not use leftover pills. If symptoms recur, contact your doctor for advice.
- This medication is not recommended late in pregnancy.
- Notify your doctor of any adverse effects.
- Take the vitamin supplements recommended by your doctor.
- Contact your doctor if symptoms continue.
- Avoid unnecessary use of this medication early in pregnancy or near your delivery date.
- Your doctor can provide the best recommendation for you.

### Recommendations during lactation:
- Avoid nursing while using sulfamethoxazole if the baby is G6DP-deficient*, jaundiced*, premature or less than 1 month of age. Nursing other babies is safe with medical supervision.
- Your baby's doctor can provide the best recommendation for you.

 ## Interactions

### Interactions with medications, vitamins and minerals:

| Interacts with | Combined effect |
|---|---|
| Cyclo-phosphamide | Alters cyclo-phosphamide elimination. |
| Folate | Interferes with folic-acid activity. |
| Local anesthetics | Decreases sulfa-methoxazole effect. |
| Methotrexate | Increases methotrexate toxicity. |
| Oral contraceptives | Decreases contraceptive effect. |
| Para-aminobenzoic acid | Decreases sulfamethoxazole effect. |
| Vitamin K | May decrease vitamin-K production. |

### Interactions with other substances:
- Use of similar medications with alcohol may increase drowsiness and slow reaction time.

*See Glossary.

MEDICATION

247

# Sulfasalazine

**Definition and description:** Acts as an anti-inflammatory to treat inflammatory bowel diseases*, such as ulcerative colitis*.

**Other names:** Azulfidine®.

 ## Dosage

### Safe dosage:
- Dose is adjusted for each individual.
- Usual adult dose—2 to 4g/day.

### Toxic dosage:
- Overdose causes nausea, vomiting, stomach pain, abdominal pain, drowsiness and seizures.
- Contact your doctor, poison-control center or emergency room if you think you have take an overdose.
- Deaths have been reported from allergic reactions, decreased blood-cell count, kidney damage, liver damage, nerve damage, muscle damage, brain damage and lung damage.
- Report sore throat, fever, bruising and jaundice* to your doctor immediately.

 ## Possible benefits

### Benefits before pregnancy:
- Treats inflammatory bowel disease*.

### Benefits to mother:
- See Benefits before pregnancy.

### Benefits to fetus:
- None reported.

### Benefits during lactation:
- None reported.

 ## Possible adverse effects

### Effects before pregnancy:
- Adverse effects include loss of appetite, headache, nausea, vomiting, rash, itching, hives*, fever, anemia*, low blood-cell count, allergic reactions, liver damage, pancreas damage, kidney damage, seizures, dizziness, depression, hallucinations*, tingling in extremities and hearing loss.

- Notify your doctor of any adverse effects.
- Men *may* have decreased sperm counts and infertility.

### Effects on mother:
- Pregnant women may have the same adverse effects as any other person.
- Call your doctor if you develop any new adverse effects or if adverse effects worsen during pregnancy.

### Effects on fetus:
- This medication and its metabolite*, sulfapyridine, enter fetal circulation.
- Studies of large numbers of pregnancies have not demonstrated an increase in malformation rates after exposure to sulfasalazine.
- Isolated reports of malformations have occurred.

### Effects on newborn:
- Jaundice* has been reported in infants exposed to similar medications before birth. See Sulfamethoxazole, page 246.
- Kernicterus* occurs after exposure to similar medications before birth. See Sulfamethoxazole, page 246.

### Effects during lactation:
- This medication is found in breast milk.
- No adverse effects have been reported in nursing infants.
- Lactating women may have the same adverse effects as any other person.

 ## Additional information

- Pregnancy does not influence the likelihood of having an attack of inflammatory bowel disease*.
- Attacks during pregnancy may be more severe than attacks at other times. Attacks during pregnancy happen most often during the early months of pregnancy. Attacks also occur after delivery.

- Women with inactive inflammatory bowel disease* have the same chance of having a normal baby as the rest of the population. Women who experience an attack of inflammatory bowel disease* at the time of conception are more likely to have a miscarriage.
- The effect of infammatory bowel disease* on fertility is difficult to predict.

## Recommendations for use

### Women considering pregnancy:

- Use this medication as directed by your doctor.
- Notify your doctor if you plan to become pregnant. Risks to you and your baby must be considered on an individual basis.
- Your doctor may want to discontinue this medication before pregnancy if your disease is inactive.

### Recommendations during pregnancy:

- See your doctor regularly.
- Follow your doctor's instructions for use of this medication.
- Your doctor may want to discontinue this medication during pregnancy if your disease is inactive.
- If inflammatory bowel disease is active during pregnancy, this medication may be continued.
- Your doctor can provide the best recommendation for you.

### Recommendations during lactation:

- Nursing is usually safe while using sulfasalazine.
- Your doctor or your baby's doctor can provide the best recommendation for you.

## Interactions

### Interactions with medications, vitamins and minerals:

| Interacts with | Combined effect |
|---|---|
| Digoxin | Decreases digoxin absorption. |
| Folate | Decreases folate absorption. |
| Phenobarbital | Decreases levels of sulfasalazine. |

### Interactions with other substances:

- None reported.

*See Glossary.

# Sulindac

**Definition and description:** Relieves swelling, stiffness and pain of rheumatoid arthritis*, ankylosing spondylitis*, osteoarthritis*, bursitis*, tendonitis* and gout*. Relieves mild to moderate pain.

**Other names:** Clinoril®.

 ## Dosage

**Safe dosage:**
• Usual adult dose—300 to 400mg/day.

**Toxic dosage:**
• Exact toxic dose cannot be predicted.

 ## Possible benefits

**Benefits before pregnancy:**
• Relieves swelling, stiffness and joint pain of rheumatoid arthritis* and related disorders.
• Relieves mild to moderate pain.

**Benefits to mother:**
• See *Benefits before pregnancy.*

**Benefits to fetus:**
• None reported.

**Benefits during lactation:**
• None reported.

 ## Possible adverse effects

**Effects before pregnancy:**
• Adverse effects include dizziness, headache, depression, nervousness, seizures, rash, ringing in ears, nausea, heartburn*, abdominal pain, bruising, bleeding, swelling, anemia*, kidney damage, liver damage and vision changes.
• Notify your doctor if you develop any adverse effects.

**Effects on mother:**
• Pregnant women may have the same adverse effects as any other person.
• Call your doctor if you develop any new adverse effects or if adverse effects worsen during pregnancy.
• Anemia*, excessive bleeding during and after labor, and prolonged or delayed labor have been reported with similar medications. Experience with sulindac in pregnancy is limited. See Aspirin, page 40.

**Effects on fetus:**
• Serious adverse effects have been reported after exposure to similar medications. Experience with sulindac in pregnancy is limited. See Aspirin, page 40, and Indomethacin, page142.

**Effects on newborn:**
• Serious problems have been reported after use of similar medications. Experience with sulindac in pregnancy is limited. See Aspirin, page 40, and Indomethacin, page 142.

**Effects during lactation:**
• There are no reports of use of this medication during nursing.
• Lactating women may have the same adverse effects as any other person.

 ## Additional information

• Use of this or similar medications may be necessary to control severe rheumatoid arthritis* or related disorders during pregnancy.

## Recommendations for use

### Women considering pregnancy:
- Use this medication only when needed for mild to moderate pain.
- Use this medication regularly as directed by your doctor for arthritis* and related disorders.
- If you use sulindac regularly, notify your doctor if you plan to become pregnant. Possible risks to you and your baby must be considered on an individual basis.
- Your doctor can provide the best recommendation for you

### Recommendations during pregnancy:
- See your doctor regularly.
- Avoid unnecessary use of sulindac for mild to moderate pain in pregnancy.
- If you use this medication to control rheumatoid arthritis* or related disorders, possible risks to you and your baby must be considered on an individual basis. Follow your doctor's recommendations carefully.
- Avoid use of sulindac near your expected delivery date, except as directed by your doctor.
- At the time of delivery, tell your doctor you take sulindac.

### Recommendations during lactation:
- Safety or risk has not been established.
- Your doctor or your baby's doctor can provide the best recommendation for you.

 ## Interactions

### Interactions with medications, vitamins and minerals:

| Interacts with | Combined effect |
| --- | --- |
| **DMSO** | Decreases sulindac effectiveness, and produces tingling and numbness. |
| **Furosemide** | Decreases furosemide effectiveness. |
| **Warfarin** | Increases risk of bleeding. |

### Interactions with other substances:
- None reported.

*See Glossary.

# Terbutaline

**Definition and description:** Acts as a bronchodilator* to treat asthma*, chronic bronchitis* and emphysema*.

**Other names:** Brethaire®, Brethine®, Bricanyl®.

 **Dosage**

### Safe dosage:
- Terbutaline can be taken by inhalation, ingestion or injection.
- Dose is determined by person's size and route of administration.
- Usual adult dose by inhalation—2 puffs every 4 to 6 hours.
- Usual adult dose by mouth—2.5 to 5mg, 3 times/day.

### Toxic dosage:
- Toxic dose is influenced by person's condition, size and age.
- Exact toxic dose cannot be predicted.
- Deaths have occurred from excessive use by inhalation. See *Effects before pregnancy.*

 **Possible benefits**

### Benefits before pregnancy:
- Relieves symptoms of asthma*, chronic bronchitis* and emphysema*.

### Benefits to mother:
- See *Benefits before pregnancy.*

### Benefits to fetus:
- Severe asthma* may have detrimental effects on the fetus. Terbutaline relieves asthma* symptoms and improves oxygen exchange in the mother.
- Premature infants of mothers who take this medication may be less likely to develop lung disease associated with prematurity. See *Additional information.*
- This medication has been used to treat premature labor. This use is not approved by the FDA*.
- Initial doses for premature labor may be higher than normal doses with asthma*. Initial therapy for premature labor is usually an intravenous* infusion. Treatment with oral doses may be necessary after

contractions have been stopped.
- This medication has been used to treat abnormal fetal heart rhythm and acidosis* during labor. This use is *experimental.*

### Benefits during lactation:
- None reported.

 **Possible adverse effects**

### Effects before pregnancy:
- Adverse effects include nervousness, tremor, headache, increased heart rate, unusual heart rhythm, drowsiness, nausea, vomiting, sweating and muscle cramps.
- Inhalation of terbutaline has worsened asthma* symptoms rarely.
- Deaths have been reported from over-use of inhaled terbutaline.
- Notify your doctor of any adverse effects.

### Effects on mother:
- Adverse effects during treatment for premature labor include fast heart rate, high blood sugar, low blood potassium, low blood pressure, vomiting and fluid in the lungs. Chest pain (angina*) may occur with high doses. Low blood pressure has occurred in pregnant asthmatic women treated by injection. Decreased blood flow to the brain has been reported in some women with migraine headache* after use of this medication. See *Additional information.*
- Pregnant women may have the same adverse effects as any other person.
- Call your doctor if you develop any adverse effects.

### Effects on fetus:
- Malformations have not been reported. However, experience in early pregnancy is limited.
- During treatment of premature labor, fetal heart rate is increased.

### Effects on newborn:
- Infants exposed to high doses when the mother is treated for premature labor may have low blood sugar.

### Effects during lactation:
- None reported. It is unknown if terbutaline enters breast milk.
- Lactating women may have the same adverse effects as any other person.

 **Additional information**

- Pregnancy may affect asthma*. About 50% of pregnant asthmatic women have no change in symptoms during pregnancy, 30% improve and 20% worsen. If symptoms worsen during one pregnancy, they are more likely to worsen in other pregnancies.
- Premature delivery, low birth weight, stillbirth, newborn deaths and maternal deaths are more likely to occur in women with asthma*. Treatment of asthma* improves outcome.
- Premature delivery is associated with a high infant-mortality rate. For each 2 weeks a fetus remains in the uterus between the 25th and 37th week of pregnancy, newborn mortality is cut in half.
- Premature delivery is associated with blindness, mental retardation and severe lung disease.
- Benefits to the baby from terbutaline often outweigh the risks of using the medication.
- Terbutaline is eliminated from the body more rapidly in pregnant women than other persons. Your doctor will select the best dose for you.

 **Recommendations for use**

### Women considering pregnancy:
- Notify your doctor if you plan to become pregnant. Risks to you and your baby must be considered on an individual basis.
- Do not exceed the dose recommended by your doctor.
- Notify your doctor if symptoms worsen while using this medication.
- If you have frequent asthma* attacks, it is important to work with your doctor to control your asthma* *before* pregnancy.

- Your doctor can provide the best recommendation for you. Do *not* change your medications unless your doctor tells you to do so.

### Recommendations during pregnancy:
- See your doctor regularly.
- Do not exceed the dose recommended by your doctor.
- Notify your doctor if symptoms worsen while using this medication.
- If your asthma* improves, your doctor may decrease your medications.
- If your asthma* worsens, your doctor may increase your medications. Do not adjust your dose without medical supervision.
- Avoid exposure to anything that worsens your asthma*.
- Carefully follow your doctor's instructions for treating premature labor.

### Recommendations during lactation:
- If nursing is attempted, taking terbutaline by inhalation produces lower levels in your blood and possibly in your breast milk.
- Your doctor can provide the best recommendation for you.

 **Interactions**

### Interactions with medications, vitamins and minerals:

| Interacts with | Combined effect |
| --- | --- |
| Adrenergic stimulants* | Increases heart rate. |
| Beta-adrenergic blockers* | Decreases terbutaline effectiveness. |
| Metoprolol | Decreases terbutaline toxicity during treatment of premature labor. Decreases terbutaline effectiveness. |

### Interactions with other substances:
- None reported.

*See Glossary

# Terpin hydrate

**Definition and description:** As an expectorant, terpin hydrate may promote removal of secretions from airways. However, the FDA* does not classify this medication as effective. Increasing fluid intake to 6 to 8 glasses of water a day may be as effective.

**Other names:** See brand-name list, page 390.

## Dosage

### Safe dosage:
- Usual adult dose—200mg every 4 hours, as needed.
- This medication can be purchased without a prescription. It is also found in products requiring a prescription.

### Toxic dosage:
- Toxicity is rare when used at recommended doses.

## Possible benefits

### Benefits before pregnancy:
- May help remove secretions from the airways.

### Benefits to mother:
- See *Benefits before pregnancy.*

### Benefits to fetus:
- None reported.

### Benefits during lactation:
- None reported.

## Possible adverse effects

### Effects before pregnancy:
- Adverse effects include nausea and vomiting.

### Effects on mother:
- Pregnant women may have the same adverse effects as any other person.
- Discontinue use and call your doctor if you develop any adverse effects during pregnancy.

### Effects on fetus:
- Some malformations have been reported after use of terpin hydrate, including benign tumors*, club foot* and hernias*.
- Cough mixtures and expectorants, as separate groups, are each associated with an increased risk of eye and ear abnormalities.
- Terpin hydrate is available as an elixir, with a high alcohol content. The fetus may experience adverse effects due to alcohol. See Alcohol, page 346.

### Effects on newborn:
- Safety or risk has not been established.

### Effects during lactation:
- Lactating women may have the same adverse effects as any other person.

## Additional information

- This medication does not cure or shorten the course of an illness. It provides relief for symptoms, but otherwise it offers no benefit.
- Viral illnesses and fever have been implicated as a cause of birth defects. This medication is often used to relieve symptoms of viral illnesses. Contact your doctor if you have a fever.
- This medication is often used in combination with other medications. Most studies did not study people using it alone. It is difficult to determine if terpin hydrate caused any malformations.

**Recommendations for use**

### Women considering pregnancy:

- Use medication as directed on the package.
- Do not exceed the suggested dose.
- Use only when needed.
- Adequate fluid intake may make this medication unnecessary.
- This medication works better with adequate fluid intake.
- Notify your doctor if you plan to become pregnant.
- Drink 6 to 8 large glasses of water each day.

### Recommendations during pregnancy:

- This medication is not clearly effective, so even minimal risks outweigh benefits.
- Safety or risk has not been established.
- See your doctor regularly.
- Adequate fluid intake may make this medication unnecessary.
- Drink 6 to 8 large glasses of water each day.
- Avoid use during pregnancy. Use only if directed by your doctor.

### Recommendations during lactation:

- Safety or risk has not been established.
- Your doctor or your baby's doctor can provide the best recommendation for you.

 **Interactions**

### Interactions with medications, vitamins and minerals:

- None reported.

### Interactions with other substances:

- None reported.

*See Glossary.

# Tetracycline

**Definition and description:** Acts as an antibiotic to treat susceptible bacterial infections. It is also used to treat acne.

**Other names:** Tetracycline hydrochloride. Also see brand-name list, page 390.

 **Dosage**

### Safe dosage:
- Usual adult dose—250 to 500mg every 6 hours.
- Lower doses are occasionally used to treat acne.

### Toxic dosage:
- Exact toxic dose cannot be predicted.

 **Possible benefits**

### Benefits before pregnancy:
- Cures susceptible bacterial infections.
- Treats acne.

### Benefits to mother:
- See *Benefits before pregnancy.*

### Benefits to fetus:
- None reported.

### Benefits during lactation:
- None reported.

 **Possible adverse effects**

### Effects before pregnancy:
- Adverse effects include loss of appetite, nausea, vomiting, diarrhea, swelling in the throat, liver damage, rash, hives*, kidney damage, decreased blood-cell counts and sensitivity to sunburn.
- Serious allergic reactions have rarely occurred.
- Notify your doctor of any adverse effects.

### Effects on mother:
- Pregnant women are more likely to develop severe liver damage than other persons. Kidney damage and pancreatitis* are associated with liver toxicity. Maternal deaths have occurred. Premature delivery and stillbirths have been reported in women with severe liver damage.
- Pregnant women may have the same adverse effects as any other person.
- Call your doctor if you develop any adverse effects.

### Effects on fetus:
- Children exposed during the last half of pregnancy have later developed permanent staining of forming teeth. Abnormal development of tooth enamel has been reported.
- Hernias* and malformations of limbs and genitals have been reported rarely.

### Effects on newborn:
- Staining of developing primary and permanent teeth has been reported in children exposed in the last half of pregnancy. This effect is also noted after administration of this medication to newborns or older children up to 8 years of age.
- Bone growth is inhibited in premature infants treated with this medication.
- Bulging fontanel* has been reported in infants treated with tetracycline.

### Effects during lactation:
- This medication is found in very low levels in breast milk.
- Calcium in milk prevents absorption of tetracycline. Therefore, tooth staining is not expected from short-term use.
- No adverse effects are reported in infants exposed to this medication in breast milk.
- Lactating women may have the same adverse effects as any other person.

## Additional information

- Some bacterial infections may be very serious to the mother or the baby. It is important to treat these infections. Your doctor will select the best medication for you.
- Risks from infection or medication must be considered on an individual basis. Your doctor can advise you.

 ## Recommendations for use

### Women considering pregnancy:

- If you use tetracycline on a regular basis, ask your doctor for advice about the risks to you or your baby. Your doctor can provide the best recommendation for you.
- Discontinue use before pregnancy, if possible.
- Avoid unnecessary exposure to this medication in early pregnancy.

### Recommendations during pregnancy:

- Avoid use of tetracycline during pregnancy.
- Your doctor can provide the best recommendation for you.

### Recommendations during lactation:

- Nursing is usually safe while using this medication.
- Risk of tooth discoloration must be considered.
- Your doctor can provide the best recommendation for you.

 ## Interactions

**Interactions with medications, vitamins and minerals:**

| Interacts with | Combined effect |
| --- | --- |
| Antacids | Decreases tetracycline absorption. |
| Bismuth subsalicylate | Decreases tetracycline absorption. |
| Calcium | Decreases tetracycline absorption. |
| Diuretics | Increases kidney damage. |
| Iron | Decreases absorption of both. |
| Lithium | Increases lithium toxicity. |
| Magnesium | May decrease magnesiumabsorption |
| Oral contraceptives | Decreases contraceptive effect. |
| Penicillin | Decreases penicillin effect. |
| Riboflavin | Decreases riboflavin absorption. |
| Steroids | Increases risk of infection. |
| Zinc | Decreases tetracycline absorption. |

**Interactions with other substances:**

- Food and milk decrease tetracycline absorption.

*See Glossary.

# Theophylline

**Definition and description:** Acts as a bronchodilator* to relieve and prevent symptoms of asthma* and reversible symptoms of chronic bronchitis* and emphysema*.

**Other names:** See brand-name list, page 390.

 ## Dosage

### Safe dosage:
- Usual adult dose—400 to 1,200mg/day. Your doctor will use blood levels to determine correct dosage.
- The dose needed may be higher or lower than the range specified.

### Toxic dosage:
- Exact toxic dose cannot be predicted.
- Overdose can cause life-threatening symptoms. Toxic symptoms include nausea, vomiting, diarrhea, convulsions, fainting, fever and dehydration.
- Death may occur in severe overdose.
- Call your doctor, poison-control center or emergency room if you think you have taken an overdose.

 ## Possible benefits

### Benefits before pregnancy:
- Prevents or relieves asthma* symptoms.

### Benefits to mother:
- See *Benefits before pregnancy.*
- The incidence of pre-eclampsia* is decreased in women with asthma* who use theophylline compared to those who are left untreated.

### Benefits to fetus:
- Theophylline relieves symptoms of asthma* and improves oxygen supply to the mother and fetus.

### Benefits to newborn:
- May decrease hyaline membrane disease* in premature infants.
- Treats apnea* in newborn infants. Apnea* is a cause of infant deaths.

### Benefits during lactation:
- None reported.

 ## Possible adverse effects

### Effects before pregnancy:
- Adverse effects include nausea, vomiting, loss of appetite, dizziness, headache, nervousness, sleeplessness, agitation, fast heartbeat, flushing, unusual heart rhythm, fast breathing and rashes.
- Notify your doctor of any new or unusual adverse effects.

### Effects on mother:
- Some adverse effects are related to blood levels. Late in pregnancy, blood levels may increase in some women. Call your doctor if you develop toxic symptoms. See *Toxic dosage.*
- Pregnant women may have the same adverse effects as any other person.
- Call your doctor if you develop any new adverse effects or if adverse effects worsen during pregnancy.

### Effects on fetus:
- Available evidence does not indicate an increase in malformations.

### Effects on newborn:
- Theophylline toxicity has been reported in some infants exposed before birth. Symptoms include jitteriness, vomiting and irritability. These infants had theophylline blood levels in the therapeutic range for newborns.
- Newborns convert theophylline to caffeine in the liver. See Caffeine, page 352.
- Infants treated with this medication may develop restlessness, stomach upset and poor feeding. Serious toxicity may occur with overdose.

### Effects during lactation:
- Theophylline is found in breast milk.
- Irritability was reported in one nursing infant exposed to theophylline.
- Lactating women may have the same adverse effects as any other person.

 ## Additional information

- Pregnancy may affect asthma*. About 50% of pregnant asthmatic women have no change in symptoms during pregnancy, 30% improve and 20% worsen. If symptoms worsen during one pregnancy, they are more likely to worsen in other pregnancies.
- Premature delivery, low birth weight, stillbirth, newborn deaths and maternal deaths are more likely to occur in women with asthma*. Treatment of asthma* improves outcome.

 ## Recommendations for use

### Women considering pregnancy:
- Notify your doctor if you plan to become pregnant. Possible risks to you and your baby must be considered on an individual basis.
- Use this medication as directed by your doctor.
- If you have frequent asthma* attacks, it is important to work with your doctor to control your asthma* *before* pregnancy.
- Your doctor can provide the best recommendation for you. Do *not* change your medications unless your doctor tells you to do so.

### Recommendations during pregnancy:
- See your doctor regularly.
- Blood levels should be checked often during pregnancy and for a few weeks after delivery to balance adverse effects and effectiveness of medication.
- Your doctor may want to adjust dose of medication during and after pregnancy. Follow your doctor's instructions carefully.
- Avoid anything that worsens your asthma* symptoms.

### Recommendations during lactation:
- With close medication supervision, nursing is usually safe.
- Your baby's doctor may want to check the baby's blood level.
- Notify your baby's doctor if your baby develops irritability, sleeplessness or poor feeding.

 ## Interactions

### Interactions with medications, vitamins and minerals:

| Interacts with | Combined effect |
| --- | --- |
| Barbiturates | Decreases theophylline effect. |
| Beta-adrenergic blockers | Decreases theophylline elimination. Inhibits theophylline action. |
| Carbamazepine | Decreases theophylline effect. |
| Cimetidine | Increases theophylline toxicity. |
| Ephedrine | Increases sleeplessness and nervousness. |
| Erythromycin | Increases theophylline toxicity. |
| Lithium | Decreases lithium effect. |
| Phenytoin | Decreases theophylline effect. |
| Ranitidine | May increase theophylline toxicity. |
| Rifampin | Decreases theophylline effect. |
| Verapamil | Increases theophylline effect. |

### Interactions with other substances:
- Smoking decreases theophylline effect.
- Food alters the absorption of some long-acting theophylline products. This interaction may increase or decrease theophylline effect.

*See Glossary.

# Thioridazine

**Definition and description:** Acts as a phenothiazine tranquilizer* to treat manifestations of psychiatric disorders.

**Other names:** Thioridazine hydrochloride, Mellaril®.

 ## Dosage

### Safe dosage:
- Usual adult dose—150 to 800mg/day.

### Toxic dosage:
- Exact toxic dose cannot be predicted.
- Symptoms of overdose include agitation, restlessness, convulsions, fever, dry mouth, bowel paralysis, loss of consciousness, low blood pressure and dangerous heart rhythm.
- Extrapyramidal symptoms* occur after overdose or occasionally after usual doses.
- Contact your doctor, poison-control center or emergency room if you think you have take an overdose.

 ## Possible benefits

### Benefits before pregnancy:
- Controls psychiatric disorders.

### Benefits to mother:
- See *Benefits before pregnancy.*

### Benefits to fetus:
- None reported.

### Benefits during lactation:
- None reported.

 ## Possible adverse effects

### Effects before pregnancy:
- Adverse effects include drowsiness, jaundice*, low blood-cell count, low blood pressure, unusual heart rhythm, seizures, rash, sensitivity to sunburn, dry mouth, nasal stuffiness, nausea, constipation, urinary retention, skin discoloration and eye damage. Tardive dyskinesia* occurs in some persons.
- Fatal anemia*, heart-rhythm disturbances and allergic reactions have occurred.
- Abnormal milk production and absence of menstruation occur in some women after prolonged use. These symptoms are associated with decreased fertility.
- Notify your doctor of any new or unusual adverse effects.
- Impotence* has been reported in men.

### Effects on mother:
- Pregnant women may have the same adverse effects as any other person.
- Call your doctor if you develop any new adverse effects or if adverse effects worsen during pregnancy.

### Effects on fetus:
- No malformations were found in infants exposed to thioridazine throughout pregnancy.
- Most evidence indicates risk of birth defects is very low with phenothiazine medications. However, malformations have been found in some studies.
- Ask your doctor to review the evidence with you.

### Effects on newborn:
- An infant exposed to thioridazine and chlorpromazine developed extrapyramidal symptoms*. Symptoms included excessive crying, abnormal motion, muscle rigidity, blood-pressure changes and delayed early learning. See Chlorpromazine, page 68.
- Intelligence at 4 years of age was not shown to be affected in a group of children exposed to phenothiazines before birth.
- Phenothiazines do *not* adversely affect birth weight or infant mortality.
- Increased jaundice* was reported in premature infants after exposure before birth.

### Effects during lactation:
- This medication enters breast milk.
- Lactating women may have the same adverse effects as any other person.

##  Additional information

- Pregnancy may be complicated by development or recurrence of a serious mental disorder. Treatments other than medication should be tried first. If the risks of mental illness are considered serious, use of medications to treat the mother's illness is important.
- Your doctor will determine whether medication is necessary.

##  Recommendations for use

### Women considering pregnancy:
- Use thioridazine as directed by your doctor.
- Do not exceed the dose or frequency recommended by your doctor.
- Notify your doctor if you plan to become pregnant. Possible risks to you and your baby must be considered on an individual basis.
- Your doctor can provide the best recommendation for you.

### Recommendations during pregnancy:
- See your doctor regularly.
- Use this medication as directed by your doctor.
- Do not exceed the dose recommended by your doctor.
- Avoid use near the time of delivery, if possible.

### Recommendations during lactation:
- Nursing is usually safe while using thioridazine.
- Contact your doctor or your baby's doctor if your baby becomes drowsy or lethargic.

### Recommendations for newborn:
- If your baby develops extrapyramidal symptoms*, contact your doctor or your baby's doctor for treatment.

##  Interactions

**Interactions with medications, vitamins and minerals:**

| Interacts with | Combined effect |
| --- | --- |
| Antacids | Decreases thioridazine absorption. |
| Anticholenergics | Decreases thioridazine effect. Increases anticholinergic effect. |
| Beta-adrenergic blockers | Increases effect of both. |
| Cimetidine | May decrease thioridazine effect. |
| Guanethidine | Increases blood pressure. |
| Hydroxyzine | May decrease thioridazine effect. |
| Insulin | Increases blood sugar. |
| Lithium | Decreases thioridazine effect. Increases delirium and seizures. |
| Methyldopa | Increases blood pressure. |
| Narcotic analgesics | Increases narcotic toxicity. |
| Oral anti-diabetic agents | Decreases anti-diabetic effect. |
| Orphenadrine | Lowers blood sugar. |
| Phenobarbital | Decreases thioridazine effect. |
| Tricyclic anti-depressants | Increases toxicity of both. |

**Interactions with other substances:**
- Use with alcohol increases drowsiness and slows reaction time.
- Smoking may decrease thioridazine effectiveness.

*See Glossary.

# Thiothixine

**Definition and description:** Acts as a tranquilizer to treat manifestations of psychiatric disorders.

**Other names:** Thiothixine hydrochloride, Navane®.

 ## Dosage

**Safe dosage:**
• Usual adult dose—6 to 60mg/day.

**Toxic dosage:**
• Exact toxic dose cannot be predicted.
• Contact your doctor, poison-control center or emergency room if you think you have take an overdose.

 ## Possible benefits

**Benefits before pregnancy:**
• Controls psychiatric disorders.

**Benefits to mother:**
• See *Benefits before pregnancy.*

**Benefits to fetus:**
• None reported.

**Benefits during lactation:**
• None reported.

 ## Possible adverse effects

**Effects before pregnancy:**
• Adverse effects include drowsiness, agitation, low blood-cell count, low blood pressure, fainting, fast heart rate, seizures, rash, sensitivity to sunburn, dry mouth, nasal stuffiness, nausea, constipation, urinary retention, skin discoloration and eye damage. Tardive dyskinesia* occurs in some persons.
• Fatal anemia*, heart-rhythm disturbances and allergic reactions have occurred.

• Abnormal milk production and absence of menstruation occur in some women after prolonged use. These symptoms are associated with decreased fertility.
• Notify your doctor of any new or unusual adverse effects.
• Impotence* has been reported in men.

**Effects on mother:**
• Pregnant women may have the same adverse effects as any other person.
• Call your doctor if you develop any new adverse effects or if adverse effects worsen during pregnancy.

**Effects on fetus:**
• Safety or risk has not been established.
• Experience with this medication in early pregnancy is limited.
• This medication enters fetal circulation.

**Effects on newborn:**
• Safety or risk has not been established.
• Experience with this medication in pregnancy is limited.

**Effects during lactation:**
• The effects of this medication on nursing infants is unknown.
• Lactating women may have the same adverse effects as any other person.

 ## Additional information

• Pregnancy may be complicated by development or recurrence of a serious mental disorder. Treatments other than medication should be tried first. If the risks of mental illness are considered serious, use of medications to treat the mother's illness is important.
• Your doctor will determine whether medication is necessary.

**Recommendations for use**

### Women considering pregnancy:
- Use thiothixine as directed by your doctor.
- Do not exceed the dose or frequency recommended by your doctor.
- Notify your doctor if you plan to become pregnant. Possible risks to you and your baby must be considered on an individual basis.
- Your doctor can provide the best recommendation for you.

### Recommendations during pregnancy:
- See your doctor regularly.
- Use thiothixine as directed by your doctor.
- Do not exceed the dose recommended by your doctor.

### Recommendations during lactation:
- Your doctor can provide the best recommendation for you.

 **Interactions**

### Interactions with medications, vitamins and minerals:

| Interacts with | Combined effect |
| --- | --- |
| Guanethidine | Increases blood pressure. |

### Interactions with other substances:
- Use with alcohol increases drowsiness and slows reaction time.

*See Glossary.

MEDICATION

# Thyroid

## Definition and description:
Hormone used to replace thyroid hormone in hypothyroid* persons.

**Other names:** Dessicated thyroid. Also see brand-name list, page 390.

 ## Dosage

### Safe dosage:
- Correct dose must be established for each person.

### Toxic dosage:
- Exact toxic dose cannot be predicted.
- Overdose produces symptoms of hyperthyroidism*, including heat intolerance, rapid heart rate, tremor*, nervousness, diarrhea, muscle cramps and sweating.

 ## Possible benefits

### Benefits before pregnancy:
- Maintains normal thyroid condition in hypothyroid* persons.

### Benefits to mother:
- See *Benefits before pregnancy.*

### Benefits to fetus:
- There are reports of using very high doses of thyroid hormone to treat hypothyroidism* in the fetus.

### Benefits during lactation:
- None reported.

 ## Possible adverse effects

### Effects before pregnancy:
- Adverse effects include tremor*, headache, irritability, sleeplessness, hives*, rash, chest pain, rapid heart rate, leg cramps, changes in menstrual periods, fever, heat intolerance and weight loss.
- Notify your doctor of any adverse effects.

### Effects on mother:
- Pregnant women may have the same adverse effects as any other person.
- Call your doctor if you develop any new adverse effects during pregnancy.

### Effects on fetus:
- Adverse effects to the fetus are not expected.
- Malformations have been reported but are attributed to maternal disease, *not* to thyroid-replacement medications. See *Additional information.*

### Effects on newborn:
- None reported.

### Effects during lactation:
- Very small quantities of this medication enter breast milk.
- Lactating women may have the same adverse effects as any other person.

 ## Additional information

- Infant-death and fetal-death rates are slightly higher in pregnancies of hypothyroid* women.
- Some investigators have demonstrated an increase in malformations in children of women with hypothyroidism*. Other investigators have not found increased rates of malformations. Ask your doctor to review the evidence with you.

## Recommendations for use

### Women considering pregnancy:

- Notify your doctor if you plan to become pregnant.
- Use this medication only as directed by your doctor.
- Do not discontinue this medication unless you are instructed by your doctor.

### Recommendations during pregnancy:

- See your doctor early in pregnancy.
- Continue this medication throughout your pregnancy.

### Recommendations during lactation:

- With medical supervision, nursing may be safe while using this medication.
- Your doctor or your baby's doctor can provide the best recommendation for you.

 ## Interactions

### Interactions with medications, vitamins and minerals:

| Interacts with | Combined effect |
|---|---|
| **Cholestyramine** | Decreases thyroid effect. |
| **Insulin** | Increases insulin requirement. |
| **Oral anti-diabetic agents** | Increases anti-diabetic-agent effect. |
| **Phenytoin** | Decreases thyroid effect. |
| **Warfarin** | Increases risk of bleeding. |

### Interactions with other substances:

- None reported.

*See Glossary.

# Tolmetin

**Definition and description:** Relieves swelling, stiffness and pain of rheumatoid arthritis* or osteoarthritis*.

**Other names:** Tolectin®, Tolectin DS®.

 ## Dosage

**Safe dosage:**
- Usual adult dose—1.2 to 2g/day.

**Toxic dosage:**
- Exact toxic dose cannot be predicted.

 ## Possible benefits

**Benefits before pregnancy:**
- Relieves swelling, stiffness and joint pain of rheumatoid arthritis* or osteoarthritis*.

**Benefits to mother:**
- See *Benefits before pregnancy.*

**Benefits to fetus:**
- None reported.

**Benefits during lactation:**
- None reported.

 ## Possible adverse effects

**Effects before pregnancy:**
- Adverse effects include dizziness, headache, drowsiness, depression, nervousness, ringing in ears, diarrhea, nausea, vomiting, flatulence, heartburn*, abdominal pain, muscle cramps, bruising, bleeding, swelling, anemia*, kidney damage, liver damage and vision changes.
- Notify your doctor if you develop any adverse effects.

**Effects on mother:**
- Pregnant women may have the same adverse effects as any other person.
- Call your doctor if you develop any new adverse effects or if adverse effects worsen during pregnancy.
- Anemia*, excessive bleeding during and after labor, and prolonged or delayed labor have been reported with similar medications. Experience with this medication in pregnancy is limited. See Aspirin, page 40.

**Effects on fetus:**
- Serious adverse effects have been reported after exposure to similar medications. Experience with this medication in pregnancy is limited. See Aspirin, page 40, and Indomethacin, page 142.

**Effects on newborn:**
- Serious adverse effects have been reported after use of similar medications. See Aspirin, page 40, and Indomethacin, page 142. Experience with tolmetin in pregnancy is limited.

**Effects during lactation:**
- This medication is found in very low concentrations in breast milk.
- Lactating women may have the same adverse effects as any other person.

 ## Additional information

- Use of tolmetin or similar medications may be necessary to control severe rheumatoid arthritis* or related disorders during pregnancy.

**Recommendations for use**

### Women considering pregnancy:

- Use this medication regularly as directed by your doctor for arthritis* and related disorders.
- If you use tolmetin regularly, notify your doctor if you plan to become pregnant. Possible risks to you and your baby must be considered on an individual basis.
- Your doctor can provide the best recommendation for you.

### Recommendations during pregnancy:

- See your doctor regularly.
- If you use tolmetin to control rheumatoid arthritis* or related disorders, possible risks to you and your baby must be considered on an individual basis. Follow your doctor's recommendations carefully.
- Avoid use of tolmetin near your expected delivery date, except as directed by your doctor.
- At the time of delivery, tell your doctor you take this medication.

### Recommendations during lactation:

- Your doctor or your baby's doctor can provide the best recommendation for you.

 **Interactions**

### Interactions with medications, vitamins and minerals:

| Interacts with | Combined effect |
| --- | --- |
| **Warfarin** | Increases risk of bleeding. |

### Interactions with other substances:

- None reported.

*See Glossary.

# Trifluperazine

**Definition and description:** Acts as a phenothiazine tranquilizer* to treat manifestations of psychiatric disorders.

**Other names:** Trifluperazine hydrochloride, Temaril®.

 ## Dosage

**Safe dosage:**
- Usual adult dose—4 to 40mg/day.

**Toxic dosage:**
- Exact toxic dose cannot be predicted.
- Symptoms of overdose include dry mouth, bowel paralysis, loss of consciousness, low blood pressure and dangerous heart rhythm.
- Extrapyramidal symptoms* occur after overdose or occasionally after usual doses.
- Contact your doctor, poison-control center or emergency room if you think you have take an overdose.

 ## Possible benefits

**Benefits before pregnancy:**
- Controls psychiatric disorders.

**Benefits to mother:**
- May be used to control nausea and vomiting in pregnancy. This is not an FDA*-approved use.
- Also see *Benefits before pregnancy.*

**Benefits to fetus:**
- None reported.

**Benefits during lactation:**
- None reported.

 ## Possible adverse effects

**Effects before pregnancy:**
- Adverse effects include drowsiness, jaundice*, low blood-cell count, low blood pressure, unusual heart rhythm, seizures, rash, sensitivity to sunburn, dry mouth, nasal stuffiness, nausea, constipation, urinary retention, skin discoloration and eye damage. Tardive dyskinesia* occurs in some persons.
- Fatal anemia*, heart rhythm disturbances and allergic reactions have occurred.
- Abnormal milk production and absence of menstruation occur in some women after prolonged use. These symptoms are associated with decreased fertility.
- False-positive pregnancy tests are reported.
- Notify your doctor of any new or unusual adverse effects.
- Impotence* has been reported in men.

**Effects on mother:**
- Pregnant women may have the same adverse effects as any other person.
- Call your doctor if you develop any new adverse effects or if adverse effects worsen during pregnancy.

**Effects on fetus:**
- Most evidence indicates risk of birth defects is very low with trifluperazine.
- Most evidence indicates risk of birth defects is very low with phenothiazine medications. Only one study found an increased risk of birth defects. Malformations reported include abnormalities of the hand, fingers, feet, toes, abdominal muscles and heart.

**Effects on newborn:**
- An infant exposed to trifluperazine and chlorpromazine developed extrapyramidal symptoms*. Symptoms include excessive crying, abnormal motion, muscle rigidity, blood-pressure changes and delayed early learning. See Chlorpromazine, page 68.
- Intelligence at 4 years of age was not shown to be affected in a group of children exposed to phenothiazines before birth.
- Increased jaundice* in premature infants is reported after phenothiazine exposure.
- Phenothiazines do not adversely affect birth weight or infant mortality.

**Effects during lactation:**
- This medication enters breast milk.
- Lactating women may have the same adverse effects as any other person.

## Additional information

- Pregnancy may be complicated by development or recurrence of a serious mental disorder. Treatments other than medication should be tried first. If the risks of mental illness are considered serious, use of medications to treat the mother's illness is important.
- Your doctor will determine whether medication is necessary.
- Use medication *only* if nausea and vomiting interfere with eating or daily activities, and other treatments fail. Your doctor can prescribe other treatments. He or she should determine whether medication is necessary.
- Other treatments may include eating soda crackers or dry toast and drinking hot or cold liquids as soon as you get up in the morning.
- A severe form of nausea and vomiting of pregnancy is called *hyperemesis gravidarum**. This condition causes nutritional deficiencies, loss of electrolytes*, weight loss and starvation. It often requires hospitalization. Treatment with antiemetics* alone will not reverse hyperemesis gravidarum*.

## Recommendations for use

### Women considering pregnancy:
- Use as directed by your doctor.
- Do not exceed the dose recommended by your doctor.
- Notify your doctor if you plan to become pregnant. Possible risks to you and your baby must be considered on an individual basis.
- Your doctor can provide the best recommendation for you.

### Recommendations during pregnancy:
- See your doctor regularly.
- Use as directed by your doctor.
- Do not exceed the dose recommended by your doctor.

### Recommendations during lactation:
- Nursing is usually safe while using this medication.

- Contact your baby's doctor if your baby becomes drowsy or lethargic.

### Recommendations for newborn:
- If your baby develops extrapyramidal symptoms*, contact your baby's doctor.

## Interactions

### Interactions with medications, vitamins and minerals:

| Interacts with | Combined effect |
|---|---|
| Anticholinergic | Decreases trifluperazine effect. Increases anticholinergic effect. |
| Antacids | Decreases trifluperazine absorption. |
| Beta-adrenergic blockers | Increases effect of both. |
| Cimetidine | May decrease trifluperazine effect. |
| Guanethidine | Increases blood pressure. |
| Hydroxyzine | May decrease trifluperazine effect. |
| Insulin | Increases blood sugar. |
| Lithium | Decreases trifluperazine effect. Increases delirium and seizures. |
| Methyldopa | Increases blood pressure. |
| Narcotic analgesics | Increases narcotic toxicity. |
| Oral anti-diabetic agents | Decreases anti-diabetic effect. |
| Orphenadrine | Lowers blood sugar. |
| Phenobarbital | Decreases trifluperazine effect. |

### Interactions with other substances:
- Use with alcohol increases drowsiness and slows reaction time.
- Smoking may decrease trifluperazine effectiveness.

*See Glossary.

269

# Trimethadione

**Definition and description:** Acts as an anticonvulsant to prevent petit mal epileptic seizures*.

**Other names:** Tridione®, Troxidone®.

##  Dosage

### Safe dosage:
- Usual adult dose—900 to 2,400mg/day.
- Your doctor can use dimethadione-blood levels to determine the correct dosage.
- *Not recommended for use in pregnancy.*

### Toxic dosage:
- Exact toxic dose cannot be predicted.
- Toxic effects include kidney, liver and blood-cell damage. Call your doctor if you develop a sore throat, fever, unusual bruising or bleeding.

##  Possible benefits

### Benefits before pregnancy:
- Use of medication may prevent seizures. Seizures may result in serious injury from falls and accidents. However, the risk to the fetus associated with use of trimethadione outweighs the benefit.
- *This medication should be used in women of childbearing age only when other, less-toxic medications have failed.* See *Possible adverse effects.*

### Benefits to mother:
- See *Benefits before pregnancy.*

### Benefits to fetus:
- *The risk to the fetus associated with this medication outweighs the benefit. Trimethadione should be used in women of childbearing age only when other, less-toxic medications have failed.* See *Possible adverse effects.*

### Benefits during lactation:
- None reported.

##  Possible adverse effects

### Effects before pregnancy:
- Adverse effects include headache, irritability, drowsiness, fatigue, insomnia*, vision changes, vomiting, nausea, loss of appetite, swollen lymph glands*, joint pain and skin rash.
- Notify your doctor of any new or unusual adverse effects.

### Effects on mother:
- Pregnant women may have the same adverse effects as any other person.
- Call your doctor if you develop any new adverse effects or if adverse effects worsen during pregnancy.

### Effects on fetus:
- *69% of all children exposed to trimethadione were born with congenital malformations.* Malformations included abnormal ears, cleft lip*, or cleft palate*, heart defects, club foot*, hand malformations, kidney abnormalities, inguinal hernias*, small brain, skin folds in the corners of the eyes, broad nasal bridge, eye abnormalities, genital abnormalities, slow mental development, slow physical development and others.

### Effects on newborn:
- None reported.

### Effects during lactation:
- Lactating women may have the same adverse effects as any other person.

## Additional information

- Trimethadione is converted to dimethadione in the body.
- You have a 90% chance of having a normal child if you must take medication to control epilepsy*. *However, this medication is much more likely to cause birth defects than other anticonvulsant medications.*
- Pregnancy may increase, decrease or have no effect on the frequency and severity of seizures.
- Very severe seizures have occurred when medication is discontinued without a doctor's supervision.
- Having epilepsy and taking anticonvulsant medications increase the risk of having a miscarriage, stillbirth or child with birth defects.

 ## Recommendations for use

### Women considering pregnancy:
- Notify your doctor if you plan to become pregnant. *This medication is not recommended for women considering pregnancy.*
- If you have a severe seizure disorder, it is *absolutely necessary* to continue an anticonvulsant medication throughout your pregnancy. If possible, your doctor will substitute another medication to control your seizures. Follow your doctor's instructions carefully.
- If you have been seizure-free for many years, your doctor may recommend slowly discontinuing this medication before pregnancy.
- Your doctor may recommend changing your medication.
- Your doctor can provide the best recommendation for you. Do not stop taking this medication unless told to do so by your doctor.

### Recommendations during pregnancy:
- See your doctor immediately if you suspect you are pregnant.
- Your doctor will advise you regarding use of seizure medications during pregnancy.
- Do not stop taking this medication or change your medication unless told to do so by your doctor.

### Recommendations during lactation:
- Safety or risk has not been established.
- Your doctor or your baby's doctor can provide the best recommendation for you.

 ## Interactions

### Interactions with medications, vitamins and minerals:

| Interacts with | Combined effect |
| --- | --- |
| Folate | Decreases folic-acid levels. |
| Other anti-convulsant medications | Increases likelihood of birth defects when more than one medication is needed to control seizures. |

### Interactions with other substances:
- None reported.

*See Glossary.

# Trimethoprim

**Definition and description:** Acts as an antibacterial to treat susceptible bacterial infections.

**Other names:** Proloprim®, Trimpex®.

 ## Dosage

### Safe dosage:
- Usual adult dose—200mg/day when used alone.
- Usual adult dose—160mg every 12 hours when used in combination with sulfamethoxazole. See Sulfamethoxazole, page 246.
- Lower doses may be used for persons with some kidney diseases.

### Toxic dosage:
- Exact toxic dose cannot be predicted.

 ## Possible benefits

### Benefits before pregnancy:
- Cures susceptible bacterial infections.

### Benefits to mother:
- Some bacterial infections may be very serious to the mother. This medication can cure susceptible infections.

### Benefits to fetus:
- Some bacterial infections in the mother may increase risk to the fetus. This medication can cure susceptible infections.

### Benefits during lactation:
- None reported.

 ## Possible adverse effects

### Effects before pregnancy:
- Adverse effects include rash, itching, nausea, vomiting, swelling in the throat, decreased blood-cell count, fever, liver damage and kidney damage.
- Notify your doctor of any adverse effects.

### Effects on mother:
- Trimethoprim interferes with folic-acid activity. See Folate, page 294.
- Pregnant women may have the same adverse effects as any other person.
- Call your doctor if you develop any adverse effects.

### Effects on fetus:
- Most evidence does not indicate increased risk of malformations or other complications when trimethoprim has been used in combination with sulfamethoxazole. Sulfamethoxazole is associated with adverse effects. See Sulfamethoxazole, page 246.
- This medication interferes with folic-acid activity. See Folate, page 294.

### Effects on newborn:
- None reported in infants exposed before birth.

### Effects during lactation:
- This medication is found in low concentrations in breast milk.
- There are no reports of adverse effects in nursing infants when used alone.
- Trimethoprim is often administered in combination with sulfamethoxazole. Sulfamethoxazole is associated with adverse effects. See Sulfamethoxazole, page 246.
- Lactating women may have the same adverse effects as any other person.

 ## Additional information

- Some bacterial infections may be very serious to the mother or the baby. It is important to treat these infections.
- Risks from infection or medication must be considered on an individual basis. Your doctor can advise you.
- Elimination of this medication is faster in pregnant women than other women given the same dose. Your doctor will select the best dose for you.

## Recommendations for use

### Women considering pregnancy:
- Notify your doctor if you plan to become pregnant. Possible risks to you and your baby must be considered on an individual basis.
- Use this medication as directed by your doctor.
- Notify your doctor of any adverse effects.

### Recommendations during pregnancy:
- Use this medication as directed by your doctor.
- Notify your doctor of any adverse effects.
- Take the vitamin supplements recommended by your doctor.
- Contact your doctor if symptoms continue.

### Recommendations during lactation:
- Nursing is safe while using trimethoprim alone.
- See Sulfamethoxazole, page 246, for recommendations when trimethoprim is used in combination with sulfamethoxazole.

## Interactions

### Interactions with medications, vitamins and minerals:

| Interacts with | Combined effect |
| --- | --- |
| Folic acid | Interferes with folic-acid activity. |

### Interactions with other substances:
- None reported.

*See Glossary.

# Tripelennamine

**Definition and description:** Acts as an antihistamine to relieve allergy symptoms, including sneezing, runny nose, itching and tearing.

**Other names:** PBZ-SR®, Pyribenzamine®, Ro-Hist®.

 ## Dosage

### Safe dosage:
- Usual adult dose—25 to 50mg every 4 to 6 hours.
- This medication can be purchased without a prescription. It is also found in products requiring a prescription.

### Toxic dosage:
- Exact toxic dose cannot be predicted.
- Symptoms of overdose include sedation, dry mouth, large pupils, flushing and low blood pressure.
- Serious overdose may cause convulsions and death.
- Contact your doctor, poison-control center or emergency room if you think you have taken an overdose.

 ## Possible benefits

### Benefits before pregnancy:
- Relieves allergy symptoms.

### Benefits to mother:
- See *Benefits before pregnancy.*

### Benefits to fetus:
- None reported.

### Benefits during lactation:
- None reported.

 ## Possible adverse effects

### Effects before pregnancy:
- Adverse effects include drowsiness, rash, hives*, sweating, chills, dry mouth, headache, unusual heart rhythm, low blood pressure, low blood-cell count, confusion, ringing in ears, blurred vision, nausea, vomiting and difficulty urinating.
- Notify your doctor of any adverse effects.

### Effects on mother:
- Pregnant women may have the same adverse effects as any other person.
- Call your doctor if you develop any adverse effects.

### Effects on fetus:
- One study did not demonstrate an increased risk of malformations in some pregnancies after exposure to tripelennamine. However, this does not establish safety or risk in early pregnancy.
- Antihistamines as a group have not been shown to increase risk of malformations compared to unexposed pregnancies.

### Effects on newborn:
- Infants exposed to tripelennamine and pentazocin (Ts and Blues*) experience withdrawal after birth.
- Persistent growth retardation is reported in infants exposed to tripelennamine and pentazocin (Ts and Blues*).

### Effects during lactation:
- Most antihistamines enter breast milk.
- Lactating women may have the same adverse effects as any other person.

**Additional information**

- This medication does not cure colds, coughs or minor allergy complaints. It provides relief for symptoms. Occasionally, when allergic reactions are very serious, using anithistamines and other medications can be life-saving.
- Viral illnesses and fever have been implicated as a cause of birth defects. This medication is often used to relieve symptoms of viral illnesses. Contact your doctor if you have a fever.
- This medication is often used in combination with other medications. Most studies did not study persons using it alone. It is difficult to determine if tripelennamine caused any malformations.

 **Recommendations for use**

### Women considering pregnancy:
- Notify your doctor if you plan to become pregnant.
- Use only the recommended doses of this medication.
- Use this medication only when needed.

### Recommendations during pregnancy:
- Safety or risk has not been established.
- See your doctor regularly.
- Use this medication only as directed by your doctor.
- Do not use this medication during pregnancy unless instructed by your doctor.
- Avoid unnecessary use of this medication.

### Recommendations during lactation:
- Nursing is usually safe while using antihistamines.
- Your doctor or your baby's doctor can provide the best recommendation for you.

 **Interactions**

**Interactions with medications, vitamins and minerals:**

| Interacts with | Combined effect |
| --- | --- |
| Antianxiety agents | Increases drowsiness. |
| Antidepressants | Increases drowsiness. |
| Other anti-histamines | Increases drowsiness. |
| Tranquilizers | Increases drowsiness. |

**Interactions with other substances:**
- Use with alcohol increases drowsiness and slows reaction time.

*See Glossary.

MEDICATION

# Valproic acid

**Definition and description:**Acts as an anticonvulsant to prevent epileptic seizures.

**Other names:** Sodium valproate, Depakene®.

 ## Dosage

### Safe dosage:
• Usual adult dose—500 to 1,250mg/day.
• Your doctor can use valproate-blood levels to determine correct dosage. See *Additional information.*

### Toxic dosage:
• Exact toxic dose cannot be predicted.
• Toxic effects include liver and blood-cell damage.
• Call your doctor if you develop unusual bruising or bleeding, sore throat, fever abdominal cramps, irregular menstruation or jaundice*.

 ## Possible benefits

### Benefits before pregnancy:
• Use of medication may prevent seizures. Seizures may result in serious injury from falls and accidents. Prolonged, frequent seizures or continuous epileptic seizures may also result in brain damage or death.

### Benefits to mother:
• See *Benefits before pregnancy.*

### Benefits to fetus:
• Use of medication may prevent seizures in the mother. Decreased oxygen supply due to maternal seizures may cause brain damage or death in the fetus.
• Injuries from the mother falling during a seizure may damage the fetus.

### Benefits during lactation:
• None reported.

 ## Possible adverse effects

### Effects before pregnancy:
• Adverse effects include drowsiness, weakness, depression, lack of coordination, unsteady gait, drowsiness, headache, vision changes, nausea, vomiting and skin rash.
• Notify your doctor of any new or unusual adverse effects.

### Effects on mother:
• Pregnant women may have same adverse effects as any other person.
• Call your doctor if you develop any new adverse effects or if adverse effects worsen during pregnancy.

### Effects on fetus:
• Serious malformations of the brain and spinal cord, including meningocele*, small brain and spina bifida*, are reported more frequently in children of women who use valproic acid compared to other anticonvulsant medications. Deaths due to serious malformations have been reported.
• Malformations of the skeleton, skull and face, including cleft lip*, cleft palate*, high forehead, flat nasal bridge, small nose, widely spaced eyes, hip dislocation*, absence of ribs, absence of radius* and abnormal development of sternum* have been reported. Malformations of the digestive tract, kidneys, genital tract, liver, heart and blood vessels and hernia have also been reported.
• Fetal distress during labor may require Cesarean delivery.
• Slow mental and physical development have been reported.

### Effects on newborn:
• Liver damage has been reported in infants exposed to valproic acid in combination with other anticonvulsant medications.
• High maternal doses may be associated with poor breathing, poor muscle tone and lethargy in the newborn period. Effects of this medication may increase during the first week of life.

- Persistent growth retardation* has been reported in some children.

### Effects during lactation:

- Lactating women may have the same adverse effects as any other person.

##  Additional information

- Valproic acid is valproate in the blood.
- You have a 90% chance of having a normal child if you must take medication to control epilepsy*.
- Pregnancy may increase, decrease or have no effect on the frequency and severity of seizures.
- Very severe seizures have occurred when medication is discontinued without a doctor's supervision.
- Having epilepsy and taking anticonvulsant medications increase the risk of having a miscarriage, stillbirth or child with birth defects.

##  Recommendations for use

### Women considering pregnancy:

- Notify your doctor if you plan to become pregnant. Possible risks to you and your baby must be considered on an individual basis.
- If you have been seizure-free for many years, your doctor may recommend slowly discontinuing this medication before pregnancy.
- If you have a severe seizure disorder, it is *absolutely necessary* to continue anticonvulsant medication throughout your pregnancy.
- Your doctor may recommend changing to another anticonvulsant medication.
- Your doctor can provide the best recommendation for you. Do *not* stop taking this medication unless told to do so by your doctor.

### Recommendations during pregnancy:

- See your doctor regularly.
- Blood levels should be checked frequently during pregnancy and for a few weeks after delivery to balance adverse effects and effectiveness of medication.

- Your doctor may want to adjust dose of medication frequently during and after pregnancy. It is important to follow your doctor's instructions carefully.
- Your doctor may recommend blood screening, sonography*, amniocentesis* or other tests to diagnose spina bifida* or similar birth defects before your baby is born.
- If seizures occur, contact your doctor immediately.
- At the time of delivery, tell your doctor you take valproic acid.
- Take only the vitamin supplements recommended by your doctor.
- Get plenty of sleep during your pregnancy.

### Recommendations during lactation:

- Nursing is usually safe when using this medication.
- Notify your baby's doctor if you notice anything unusual, especially bruising, bleeding or jaundice*.

##  Interactions

### Interactions with medications, vitamins and minerals:

| Interacts with | Combined effect |
|---|---|
| Diazepam | Increases diazepam effect. |
| Other anti-convulsant medications | Increases likelihood of birth defects when more than one medication is needed to control seizures. |
| Phenobarbital | Alters phenobarbital effect. |
| Phenytoin | Alters response to both. |
| Zinc | May decrease zinc levels. |

### Interactions with other substances:

- None reported.

*See Glossary.

# Warfarin

**Definition and description:** Acts as a coumarin anticoagulant* to prevent blood clotting.

**Other names:** Antithrombin K®, Coumadin®, Marevan®, Panwarfin®.

 ## Dosage

### Safe dosage:
- Dose is adjusted for each individual.
- Blood tests are used to determine correct dose.
- *Heparin is safer during pregnancy than warfarin.* See Heparin, page 134.

### Toxic dosage:
- Exact toxic dose cannot be predicted.
- Overdose can cause serious bleeding.
- Contact your doctor, poison-control center or emergency room if you think you may have taken an overdose.

 ## Possible benefits

### Benefits before pregnancy:
- Prevents blood clotting in persons who have experienced abnormal clotting or who are at risk of developing abnormal clotting.

### Benefits to mother:
- See *Benefits before pregnancy.*

### Benefits to fetus:
- None reported.

### Benefits during lactation:
- None reported.

 ## Possible adverse effects

### Effects before pregnancy:
- Adverse effects include serious bleeding, death of skin, hair loss, hives*, rash, fever, nausea, diarrhea, abdominal pain and purple toes.

### Effects on mother:
- Pregnant women may have the same adverse effects as any other person.
- Miscarriages are more common in women who use warfarin during pregnancy.

### Effects on fetus:
- *Up to 35% of exposed infants are affected by abnormalities at birth.* A large number of fetuses die before birth. Many other abnormalities have been reported occasionally.
- Exposure early in pregnancy (before the 13th week) is associated with growth retardation, blindness and other eye defects, abnormal larynx, skeletal deformity, deafness, heart defects, facial abnormalities and death. These malformations are called *fetal warfarin syndrome*.
- At other times during pregnancy, malformations of the brain and eye, mental retardation, absence of the corpus callosum*, Dandy-Walker malformation*, spasticity*, seizures, deafness, skeletal defects, growth retardation and death can occur.

### Effects on newborn:
- Bleeding has been reported in newborns exposed to warfarin before birth.
- Stillbirth is increased after exposure to this medication.

### Effects during lactation:
- Adverse effects have not been reported in nursing infants.
- Lactating women may have the same adverse effects as any other person.

## Additional information

- 65 to 75% of exposed infants are normal at birth.
- Deep-vein thrombosis (blood clots in the legs) and pulmonary embolism (blood clots in the lung) may be fatal. Use of anticoagulants is necessary to treat these disorders. In some cases, it is necessary to continue therapy for several months. Your doctor can recommend the safest option for you.
- Artificial heart valves also require use of anticoagulants throughout pregnancy.
- *Heparin is considered safer in pregnancy than warfarin.* See Heparin, page 134. Your doctor will advise you.

 ## Recommendations for use

### Women considering pregnancy:

- Notify your doctor if you plan to become pregnant. Risks to you and your baby must be considered on an individual basis.
- Your doctor may discontinue this medication or change to a different medication.
- Your doctor can provide the best recommendation for you.
- Do not stop using warfarin without asking your doctor's advice. Seek advice *before* you become pregnant.

### Recommendations during pregnancy:

- *Contact your doctor as soon as you think you are pregnant. It is important to seek medical attention immediately.*
- Avoid this medication during pregnancy.
- Do not change your medication without medical supervision.
- Your doctor may recommend a substitute medication.
- Follow your doctor's advice.

### Recommendations during lactation:

- With careful medical supervision, nursing may be safe while using warfarin.
- Contact your doctor or your baby's doctor if you notice bruising or bleeding from the baby.

# Warfarin, continued

 **Interactions**

**Interactions with medications, vitamins and minerals:**

| Interacts with | Combined effect |
|---|---|
| Allopurinol | Increases risk of bleeding. |
| Aminosalicylic acid | Increases risk of bleeding. |
| Amiodarone | Increases risk of bleeding. |
| Aspirin | Increases risk of bleeding. |
| Chlorpropamide | Increases risk of bleeding. |
| Cimetidine | Increases risk of bleeding. |
| Clofibrate | Increases risk of bleeding. |
| Dextran | Increases risk of bleeding. |
| Diflunisal | Increases risk of bleeding. |
| Disulfiram | Increases risk of bleeding. |
| Ethacrynic acid | Increases risk of bleeding. |
| Fenoprofen | Increases risk of bleeding. |
| Ibuprofen | Increases risk of bleeding. |
| Indomethacin | Increases risk of bleeding. |
| Mefenamic acid | Increases risk of bleeding. |
| Methyldopa | Increases risk of bleeding. |
| Metronidazole | Increases risk of bleeding. |
| Monoamine oxidase (MAO) inhibitors | Increases risk of bleeding. |
| Nalidixic acid | Increases risk of bleeding. |
| Naproxen | Increases risk of bleeding. |
| Pentoxifylline | Increases risk of bleeding. |
| Phenytoin | Increases risk of bleeding. |
| Quinidine | Increases risk of bleeding. |
| Quinine | Increases risk of bleeding. |
| Sulfonamides | Increases risk of bleeding. |
| Thyroid medications | Increases risk of bleeding. |
| Tolbutamides | Increases risk of bleeding. |
| Vitamin K | Decreases effectiveness. |

**Interactions with other substances:**
• Alcohol increases risk of bleeding.

*See Glossary.

# Vitamins, Minerals & Supplements

**V**itamins and minerals are necessary for every person's good health. If you're in good health, vitamins and minerals are needed only in small amounts. They are usually found in sufficient quantities in the foods you eat.

*Vitamins* are chemical compounds necessary for normal growth, health, metabolism and physical well-being. They provide essential parts of enzymes. They also form an essential part of many hormones.

*Minerals* are required for growth, maintenance, repair and health of tissues and bones. They help regulate many body functions, including transporting oxygen to cells and providing sparks to make muscles contract.

While you're pregnant, it is essential to eat foods that provide the vitamins and minerals you need for your health and the health of your growing baby. During lactation, it is important to continue to eat foods that supply needed nutrients to you and your baby.

Be sure to check with your doctor before you take any vitamins or minerals he or she does not prescribe for you.

VITAMIN/MINERAL

# Biotin

**Definition and description:** Biotin is a sulfur-containing vitamin. It plays a role in metabolizing fats and carbohydrates and converting proteins to carbohydrates. Biotin is critically involved in maintaining normal growth, nervous tissue, skin, hair, blood cells and sex organs.

**Other names:** Vitamin H.

 ## Dosage

**Requirement:**
- The intestine manufactures part of the body's requirement for biotin.
- No specific requirement is set because of the intestine's role in manufacturing biotin.

**Safe dosage:**
- Estimated safe and adequate daily dietary intake—100 to 200mcg.

**Toxic dosage:**
- Exact toxic dose cannot be determined.

 ## Possible benefits

**Benefits before pregnancy:**
- See *Deficiency before pregnancy.*

**Benefits to mother:**
- See *Deficiency in mother.*

**Benefits to fetus:**
- See *Deficiency in fetus.*

**Benefits to newborn:**
- See *Deficiency in newborn.*

**Benefits during lactation:**
- See *Deficiency during lactation.*

 ## Possible effects of deficiency

**Deficiency before pregnancy:**
- Biotin deficiency is very rare. Deficiency symptoms include loss of appetite, nausea, vomiting, sore tongue, mental depression and a dry, scaly skin.

**Deficiency in mother:**
- See *Deficiency before pregnancy.*

**Deficiency in fetus:**
- None reported.

**Deficiency in newborn:**
- Seborrhea* in infants under 6 months old may be due to nutritional biotin deficiency. Improvement occurs with therapeutic doses given in injections.

**Deficiency during lactation:**
- None reported.

 ## Possible adverse effects

**Effects before pregnancy:**
- None reported in humans.
- Large doses of biotin can cause infertility in animals.

**Effects on mother:**
- None reported.

**Effects on fetus:**
- None reported in humans.
- Large doses of biotin increase miscarriage rates and inhibit growth of the placenta* and fetus in animals.

**Effects on newborn:**
- None reported.

**Effects during lactation:**
- None reported.

## Recommendations for use

### Women considering pregnancy:
- Eat a well-balanced diet. Good biotin sources include liver, kidney, egg yolk and vegetables.
- Supplementation is not necessary.

### Recommendations during pregnancy:
- Eat a well-balanced diet. Good biotin sources include liver, kidney, egg yolk and vegetables.
- Supplementation is not necessary.

### Recommendations during lactation:
- Eat a well-balanced diet. Good biotin sources include liver, kidney, egg yolk and vegetables.
- Supplementation is not necessary.

 ## Interactions

### Interactions with medications, vitamins and minerals:
- None reported.

### Interactions with other substances:
- Avidin, which is present in *raw* egg white, binds with biotin and makes biotin unavailable for use by the body. However, cooked eggs *are* good sources of biotin.

*See Glossary.

VITAMIN/MINERAL

# Calcium

**Definition and description:** Helps control nerves and muscles. Calcium is necessary for blood coagulation and muscle and heart function. It is also the major ingredient in bones and teeth.

**Other names:** Calcium carbonate, calcium citrate, calcium glubionate, calcium gluconate, calcium lactate. Also see brand-name list, page 390.

 ## Dosage

### Requirement:
- Non-pregnant woman—800 to 1,000mg.
- Pregnant or lactating woman—1,200mg.
- Pregnant or lactating adolescent —1,600mg.

### Safe dosage:
- Up to 1,600mg.

### Toxic dosage:
- 3 to 8g.

 ## Possible benefits

### Benefits before pregnancy:
- See *Deficiency before pregnancy.*

### Benefits to mother:
- Calcium supplementation may reduce the incidence of pre-eclampsia* and eclampsia*.
- Calcium supplementation may reduce the incidence of pregnancy-induced hypertension*.

### Benefits to fetus:
- See *Deficiency in fetus.*

### Benefits during lactation:
- See *Deficiency during lactation.*

 ## Possible effects of deficiency

### Deficiency before pregnancy:
- Inadequate calcium intake may increase the mother's risk of osteoporosis later in life.

### Deficiency in mother:
- Inadequate calcium intake may increase incidence of pre-eclampsia* and eclampsia*.
- Inadequate calcium intake may increase the incidence of pregnancy-induced hypertension*.
- Inadequate calcium intake may reduce bone density and increase the risk of osteoporosis later in life.

### Deficiency in fetus:
- Inadequate intake of calcium, protein and calories may cause decreased bone density in newborns.

### Deficiency during lactation:
- Low calcium intake doesn't affect the level of calcium in breast milk.
- Inadequate calcium intake during lactation may reduce bone density and increase the incidence of osteoporosis later in life in the mother.

## Possible adverse effects

### Effects before pregnancy:

- High calcium blood levels may occur with very large doses of calcium or if calcium is taken with large doses of vitamin D. This is associated with nausea, vomiting, high blood pressure, diarrhea, constipation, abdominal pain, dry mouth, thirst, excessive urination, muscle wasting and loss of appetite. Kidney stones and kidney damage may also occur.
- Calcium carbonate can cause constipation, diarrhea, high levels of calcium in the blood or rebound acid secretion*.
- Very high calcium intake decreases reproduction in animals.

### Effects on mother:

- High calcium blood levels may occur with very large doses of calcium or if calcium is taken with large doses of vitamin D. This is associated with nausea, vomiting, high blood pressure, diarrhea, constipation, abdominal pain, dry mouth, thirst, excessive urination, muscle wasting and loss of appetite. Kidney stones and kidney damage may also occur. See *Effects before pregnancy.*

### Effects on fetus:

- None reported in humans.
- Very high calcium intake can sharply depress growth in animals.

### Effects on newborn:

- Bowel damage is reported in newborns treated with calcium glubionate.
- Calcium gluconate is associated with slow heart rate and calcium deposits in tissues of newborns treated by injection.

### Effects during lactation:

- No specific effects reported on lactation or breast milk.
- High calcium blood levels may occur in the mother with very large doses of calcium or if calcium is taken with vitamin D. This is associated with nausea, vomiting, high blood pressure, diarrhea, constipation, abdominal pain, dry mouth, thirst, excessive urination, muscle wasting and loss of appetite. Kidney stones and kidney damage may also occur. See *Effects before pregnancy.*

 ## Additional information

- Dolomite and bone meal are *not* recommended during pregnancy and lactation. They contain toxic metals, such as aluminum, antimony, arsenic, barium, cadmium, cobalt and lead.
- Calcium citrate is one of the most absorbable forms of calcium, especially for people with reduced amounts of stomach acid.
- Calcium carbonate is the least expensive and most recommended form of calcium supplement.
- Calcium carbonate is also available in antacids.

# Calcium, continued

## Recommendations for use

**Women considering pregnancy:**
- Eat 3 servings a day of dairy products or equivalent food to equal 800 to 1,000mg of calcium or take supplements. See Appendix 1, page 375, for calcium content of food. Appendix 2, page 379, shows calcium content of selected supplements.

**Recommendations during pregnancy:**
- Eat 4 servings a day of dairy products or equivalent food to equal 1,200mg of calcium or take supplements. See Appendix 1, page 375, for calcium content of food. Appendix 2, page 379, shows calcium content of selected supplements.

**Recommendations during lactation:**
- Eat 4 servings a day of dairy products or equivalent food to equal 1,200mg of calcium or take supplements. See Appendix 1, page 375, for calcium content of food. Appendix 2, page 379, shows calcium content of selected supplements.

## Interactions

**Interactions with medications, vitamins and minerals:**

| Interacts with | Combined effect |
| --- | --- |
| Antacids containing aluminum hydroxide | Long-term use causes calcium depletion. |
| Cholestyramine | Decreases calcium absorption. |
| Corticosteroids | Decreases calcium absorption. |
| Fluoride | Decreases fluoride absorption. |
| Iron | Decreases iron absorption. |
| Lithium | Increases calcium excretion. Decreases calcium uptake by bone. |
| Manganese | Interferes with manganese absorption. |
| Oral contraceptives | May increase calcium absorption. |
| Phenobarbital | Decreases blood calcium levels. |
| Phenytoin | Decreases blood calcium levels. |
| Phosphorus | High levels may interfere with calcium absorption. Best absorption occurs when ratio is 1:1. |
| Protein, fats, magnesium | Decreases absorption and use of protein, fat and magnesium. |
| Tetracyclines | Tetracycline absorption is impaired by calcium. |
| Vitamin D | Increases calcium absorption. |
| Zinc | At low calcium levels, zinc may interfere with absorption. |

**Interactions with other substances:**
- Caffeine decreases calcium absorption. Take calcium 1/2 hour before or 1-1/2 hours after caffeine consumption.
- Certain foods, such as spinach, rhubarb, bran and whole-grain cereals, decrease calcium absorption.
- Tobacco decreases calcium absorption.
- Alcohol decreases calcium absorption.
- Meat and cola drinks contain high amounts of phosphorous and may interfere with calcium absorption.
- Meat and cola drinks contain high amounts of phosphorus and may interfere with calcium absorption.

*See Glossary.

Note: This page purposely left blank.

# Chromium

**Definition and description:** A metallic element whose role in diet is not well-defined. It may play a role in carbohydrate metabolism.

**Other names:** Chromium chloride.

 ## Dosage

**Requirement:**
- Not established.

**Safe dosage:**
- Estimated safe and adequate intake— 0.05 to 0.2mg.

**Toxic dosage:**
- Exact toxic dose cannot be determined.

 ## Possible benefits

**Benefits before pregnancy:**
- Supplementation with chromium may improve utilization of sugar and carbohydrates.

**Benefits to mother:**
- See *Benefits before pregnancy.*

**Benefits to fetus:**
- See *Deficiency in fetus.*

**Benefits to newborn:**
- See *Deficiency in newborn.*

**Benefits during lactation:**
- See *Benefits before pregnancy.*

 ## Possible effects of deficiency

**Deficiency before pregnancy:**
- Inadequate intake of chromium may cause defective response to sugar in the blood, which may lead to diabetes mellitus*.

**Deficiency in mother:**
- Deficiency may decrease utilization of sugar and carbohydrates. Mothers who develop diabetes* during pregnancy have decreased ability to metabolize sugar and carbohydrates.

**Deficiency in fetus:**
- None reported in humans.
- Deficiency of chromium can cause growth impairment in animals.

**Deficiency in newborn:**
- None reported in humans.
- Deficiency of chromium can increase death rate in young animals.

**Deficiency during lactation:**
- No specific effects reported on lactation or breast milk.

 ## Possible adverse effects

- None reported.

**Additional information**

- Chromium levels may be reduced after pregnancy and do not return to normal levels for as long as 4 years.

 **Recommendations for use**

**Women considering pregnancy:**
- Eat a varied diet and take supplements only with your doctor's supervision.

**Recommendations during pregnancy:**
- Eat a varied diet and take supplements only with your doctor's supervision.

**Recommendations during lactation:**
- Eat a varied diet and take supplements only with your doctor's supervision.

**Interactions**

**Interactions with medications, vitamins and minerals:**

| Interacts with | Combined effect |
|---|---|
| Insulin | May decrease amount of insulin needed to treat diabetes*. |

**Interactions with other substances:**
- None reported.

*See Glossary.

VITAMIN/MINERAL

# Copper

**Definition and description:** Copper is part of a number of important enzymes. One enzyme, superoxide dismutase, is a detoxifying agent. Another enzyme assists in making hemoglobin. Copper aids in promoting connective-tissue formation. It is also involved in energy production.

**Other names:** Copper sulfate.

 ## Dosage

**Requirement:**
• No RDA established.

**Safe dosage:**
• Estimated safe and adequate intake— 2 to 3mg.

**Toxic dosage:**
• 15mg causes symptoms of toxicity.
• Exact toxic dose cannot be predicted.

 ## Possible benefits

**Benefits before pregnancy:**
• See *Deficiency before pregnancy.*

**Benefits to mother:**
• See *Deficiency in mother.*

**Benefits to fetus:**
• See *Deficiency in fetus.*

**Benefits to newborn:**
• See *Deficiency in newborn.*

**Benefits during lactation:**
• See *Deficiency during lactation.*

 ## Possible effects of deficiency

**Deficiency before pregnancy:**
• Severe copper deficiency is very rare. When it occurs, it can lead to infertility. Copper supplementation prevents this.

**Deficiency in mother:**
• None reported.

**Deficiency in fetus:**
• None reported.

**Deficiency in newborn:**
• Premature babies fed low-copper diets are at high risk of developing copper deficiency. Copper deficiency is associated with edema* and anemia*.

**Deficiency during lactation:**
• No specific effects reported on lactation or breast milk.

 ## Possible adverse effects

**Effects before pregnancy:**
• Excessive doses produce nausea, vomiting, diarrhea, abdominal cramps, destruction of blood cells, liver damage, kidney damage, gastric and intestinal ulceration, coma* and uremia*.

**Effects on mother:**
• See *Effects before pregnancy.*

**Effects on fetus:**
• None reported.

**Effects on newborn:**
• None reported.

**Effects during lactation:**
• No specific effects reported on lactation or breast milk.
• See *Effects before pregnancy.*

 ## Additional information

• Avoid acidic foods or drinks that have had prolonged contact with copper bowls or containers. Excessive amounts of copper can be absorbed into your food or beverage, causing adverse effects. See information above.

## Recommendations for use

### Women considering pregnancy:
- Eat a balanced diet containing shellfish, organ meats, nuts, legumes and dried fruits.
- No need for supplementation in most diets.
- *Absolutely do not supplement if you have Wilson's Disease\*.*

### Recommendations during pregnancy:
- Eat a balanced diet containing shellfish, organ meats, nuts, legumes and dried fruits.
- No need for supplementation in most diets.
- *Absolutely do not supplement if you have Wilson's Disease\*.*

### Recommendations during lactation:
- Eat a balanced diet containing shellfish, organ meats, nuts, legumes and dried fruits.
- No need for supplementation in most diets.
- *Absolutely do not supplement if you have Wilson's Disease\*.*

 ## Interactions

**Interactions with medications, vitamins and minerals:**

| Interacts with | Combined effect |
| --- | --- |
| Cadmium | Can interfere with copper absorption and use. |
| Molybdenum | Excess molybdenum causes urinary loss of copper. |
| Oral contraceptives | Increases blood-copper levels. |
| Phenobarbital | May increase blood-copper levels. |
| Phenytoin | May increase blood-copper levels. |
| Vitamin C | High intake interferes with copper absorption. |
| Zinc | High intake interferes with copper absorption. |

**Interactions with other substances:**
- Fiber in cereal and vegetables can interfere with copper absorption and use.

*See Glossary.

# Fluoride

**Definition and description:** Mineral necessary for development of healthy bones and teeth. It is considered an essential element for growth. Fluoride is incorporated into the crystalline structure of fetal tooth enamel before the teeth emerge from the gums.

**Other names:** Sodium fluoride and acidulated phosphate fluoride for oral intake. Sodium monofluorophosphate and stannous fluoride for oral gels, toothpastes and rinsing solutions only.

 ## Dosage

### Requirement:
• No RDA has been established.

### Safe dosage:
• Estimated safe and adequate intake—1.5 to 4mg/day.

### Toxic dosage:
• 2mg/liter of drinking water can produce mild fluorosis*.
• 2.5mg/liter or 20mg/day may produce moderate to severe fluorosis*.
• 2.5 to 10 parts/million fluoride in water produces various levels of fluorosis*.
• Your water company can provide information on the fluoride content of water in your area.

 ## Possible benefits

### Benefits before pregnancy:
• Oral rinses or gels may be beneficial in reducing tooth decay.

### Benefits to mother:
• See *Benefits before pregnancy.*

### Benefits to fetus:
• See *Deficiency in fetus.*

### Benefits to newborn:
• See *Deficiency in newborn.*

### Benefits during lactation:
• An increase in dietary fluoride can increase breast-milk-fluoride levels.
• Increasing fluoride intake in the mother is not an effective way of assuring adequate fluoride for infant.

 ## Possible effects of deficiency

### Deficiency before pregnancy:
• None reported.

### Deficiency in mother:
• None reported.

### Deficiency in fetus:
• Inadequate fluoride intake may cause defective tooth formation. Children may have stronger teeth if the mother takes prenatal fluoride supplements. Effective amount depends on the fluoride content of your local water supply.

### Deficiency in newborn:
• Inadequate fluoride intake may cause defective tooth formation. Fluoride supplementation may benefit tooth formation.

### Deficiency during lactation:
• None reported.

 ## Possible adverse effects

### Effects before pregnancy:
• Possible joint pain at levels above 20mg/day.

### Effects on mother:
• See *Effects before pregnancy.*

### Effects on fetus:
• Fluorosis* has occurred in infants whose mothers took supplements containing greater than 4mg of fluoride. Fluorosis* has also occurred in infants whose mothers lived in areas that had large amounts of fluoride in the water.

### Effects on newborn:
• None reported.

### Effects during lactation:
• No specific effects reported on lactation or breast milk.
• Possible joint pain in the mother at levels above 20mg/day.

**Additional information**

• 1 part/million of fluoride provides 1mg fluoride/liter (approximately 1 quart).

 **Recommendations for use**

**Women considering pregnancy:**
• Drink fluoridated water.

**Recommendations during pregnancy:**
• Drink fluoridated water. Your doctor will recommend appropriate fluoride supplementation for your area.
• Consider taking prenatal vitamin with 1mg fluoride in areas with moderate fluoride content in water. Check first with your doctor.
• Consider taking prenatal vitamins with 2mg fluoride in areas with low fluoride content in water. Check first with your doctor.

**Recommendations during lactation:**
• Your baby's doctor will recommend appropriate fluoride supplementation for your area.

 **Interactions**

**Interactions with medications, vitamins and minerals:**

| Interacts with | Combined effect |
| --- | --- |
| Antacids containing aluminum | Decreases fluoride absorption. |
| Calcium | Decreases fluoride absorption. |
| Magnesium | Decreases fluoride absorption. |
| Phosphates | Decreases fluoride absorption. |

**Interactions with other substances:**
• None reported.

*See Glossary.

VITAMIN/MINERAL

# Folate

**Definition and description:** Group of compounds that function as a coenzyme for five different enzyme systems. Folate is essential for making nucleic acids for RNA and DNA, the building blocks of cells. It is also involved in the metabolism of amino acids. Pregnancy is a time of rapid cell growth and multiplication; the need for folate increases dramatically.

**Other names:** Vitamin B-9, folic acid, folacin, pteroylglutamic acid (PGA).

 ## Dosage

**Requirement:**
- Non-pregnant woman—400mcg.
- Pregnant woman—800mcg.
- Lactating woman—500mcg.

**Safe dosage:**
- 1mg or less. May cover underlying $B_{12}$ deficiency at levels higher than 1mg.

**Toxic dosage:**
- 15mg.

 ## Possible benefits

**Benefits before pregnancy:**
- See *Deficiency before pregnancy.*

**Benefits to mother:**
- See *Deficiency in mother.*

**Benefits to fetus:**
- Neural-tube defects* may be prevented if the mother is supplemented with folate. Prevention is greatest when folate supplementation is started before conception.

**Benefits to newborn:**
- See *Deficiency in newborn.*

**Benefits during lactation:**
- See *Deficiency during lactation.*

 ## Possible effects of deficiency

**Deficiency before pregnancy:**
- A deficiency can cause sterility in men and women.
- Inadequate folate intake causes megaloblastic anemia*. Problems associated with megaloblastic anemia* include lip infections, ulcers in the mouth and vagina, weakness, shortness of breath, headaches, faintness, malabsorption and fatty stools. Folate supplementation prevents megaloblastic anemia*.
- Neural-tube defects* may be prevented if the mother is supplemented with folate. Prevention is greatest when folate supplementation is started before conception.

**Deficiency in mother:**
- See *Deficiency before pregnancy.*

**Deficiency in fetus:**
- Drugs that interfere with folate metabolism may increase miscarriage rate. These include aminopterin, chlorambucil and methotrexate.
- Infants born to mothers who have epilepsy* and take medication for seizures, especially phenytoin and phenobarbital combinations, may benefit from folate supplementation.
- Folate supplementation has been found to reduce miscarriage and fetal malformations in women with low blood-folate levels.
- Folate deficiency may increase miscarriages, pre-eclampsia*, abruptio placenta*, fetal malformations and abnormal infant development.

**Deficiency in newborn:**
- Folate supplementation of the mother has been found to be beneficial in preventing some complications in newborns.
- Infants born to mothers with folate deficiency that has progressed to megaloblastic anemia* may have delayed physical and intellectual development.

## Deficiency during lactation:

- Low folate intake in the mother may decrease breast-milk folate enough to cause folate deficiency and megaloblastic anemia* in the infant.
- Dietary supplements for mother increase folate content of breast milk and prevent folate deficiency.

 **Possible adverse effects**

### Effects before pregnancy:

- Folate is relatively non-toxic.
- Doses above 1mg may hide $B_{12}$ deficiency. Hidden $B_{12}$ deficiency can result in permanent nervous-system damage.

### Effects on mother:

- See *Effects before pregnancy.*

### Effects on fetus:

- None reported.

### Effects on newborn:

- None reported.

### Effects during lactation:

- See *Effects before pregnancy.*

 **Additional information**

- Folate deficiency increases when the third trimester of pregnancy occurs in winter months because the quantity of fruits and vegetables is more limited.
- Folate monitoring is suggested in women with high blood concentrations of phenytoin or phenobarbital because of the risk of megaloblastic anemia*.
- Before prenatal vitamins with folate were prescribed, the incidence of megaloblastic anemia* was 25%. Statistics suggest this rate has declined.
- Folate deficiency is one of the most common vitamin deficiencies in the world.

 **Recommendations for use**

### Women considering pregnancy:

- Eat a well-balanced diet. See Appendix 1, page 375, for a list of foods that contain high amounts of folate.
- If you have a history of babies born with neural-tube defects*, consult your doctor about preconception supplementation.
- Consult your doctor about a preconception supplement if you take seizure medications.

### Recommendations during pregnancy:

- Eat a well-balanced diet. See Appendix 1, page 375, for a list of foods that contain high amounts of folate.
- Supplement your diet with a prenatal vitamin containing 800 to 1,000mcg (1mg) of folate. Check first with your doctor.
- If you take anticonvulsant medications, your doctor may monitor blood-folate levels while you are pregnant.

### Recommendations during lactation:

- Eat a well-balanced diet. See Appendix 1, page 375, for a list of foods that contain high amounts of folate.
- Consult your doctor about continuing to supplement with a prenatal vitamin while you breast-feed.
- If you take anticonvulsant medications, consult your doctor about monitoring blood-folate levels during lactation.

# Folate, continued

 **Interactions**

**Interactions with medications, vitamins and minerals:**

| Interacts with | Combined effect |
|---|---|
| **Adrenal corti-costeroids** | Increases need for folate. |
| **Aminopterin** | Interferes with folate metabolism. May increase miscarriage rate. |
| **Barbiturates** | Increases need for folate. |
| **Chlorambucil** | Interferes with folate metabolism. May increase miscarriage rate. |
| **Isoniazid (INH)** | May decrease blood-folate levels. |
| **Methotrexate** | Decreases folate absorption. Interferes with folate metabolism. May increase miscarriage rate. |
| **Nitrofurantoin** | Decreases blood-folate levels. Can cause megaloblastic anemia*. |
| **Oral contraceptives** | Decreases blood-folate levels. May rarely cause megaloblastic anemia*. |
| **Phenytoin** | Decreases blood-folate levels. Can cause megaloblastic anemia*. Folate interferes with effectiveness of anticonvulsants. |
| **Riboflavin** | Decreases riboflavin blood levels in mother and fetus. |
| **Salicylates** | Decreases blood-folate levels in people with rheumatoid arthritis*. |
| **Salicylazo-sulfapyridine** | Decreases blood-folate levels. Decreases absorption of folate. Interferes with utilization of folate. May cause megaloblastic anemia*. |
| **Sulfonamides** | Decreases blood-folate levels. Decreases folate absorption. Interferes with utilization of folate. May cause megaloblastic anemia*. |
| **Trimethadione** | Decreases blood-folate levels. Has caused malformations in infants of mothers who did not receive folate supplementation during pregnancy. |
| **Trimethoprim** | May decrease folate absorption. Decreases blood-folate levels. May cause megaloblastic anemia*. |
| **Zinc** | High folate levels interfere with zinc absorption. Folate deficiency increases blood-zinc levels. |

**Interactions with other substances:**
• Alcohol decreases folate absorption.

*See Glossary.

**Definition and description:** An important component of thyroid hormones, which play an important role in metabolism.

**Other names:** Iodized salt.

## Dosage

### Requirement:
- Non-pregnant woman—0.150mg.
- Pregnant woman—0.175mg.
- Lactating woman—0.200mg.

### Safe dosage:
- Up to 0.300mg for short periods of time.

### Toxic dosage:
- 2mg.

## Possible benefits

### Benefits before pregnancy:
- See *Deficiency before pregnancy.*

### Benefits to mother:
- See *Deficiency in mother.*

### Benefits to fetus:
- See *Deficiency in fetus.*

### Benefits to newborn:
- See *Deficiency in newborn.*

### Benefits during lactation:
- See *Deficiency during lactation.*

## Possible effects of deficiency

### Deficiency before pregnancy:
- Inadequate intake of iodine leads to thyroid enlargement or goiter* and possibly hypothyroidism*.

### Deficiency in mother:
- See *Deficiency before pregnancy.*

### Deficiency in fetus:
- Inadequate intake of iodine may cause thyroid enlargement or goiter*.

### Deficiency in newborn:
- Severe iodine deficiency in mother can cause death in newborn.

### Deficiency during lactation:
- Dietary iodine can increase or decrease breast-milk-iodine levels.
- Inadequate intake of iodine may cause thyroid enlargement or goiter* in the infant.

## Possible adverse effects

### Effects before pregnancy:
- Iodine at high doses may cause thyrotoxicosis*, which is a cause of infertility.

### Effects on mother:
- Iodine at high doses may cause thyrotoxicosis*.

### Effects on fetus:
- Overconsumption of iodine by mother during pregnancy may cause thyroid enlargement, hypothyroidism*, dwarfism* or mental deficiency.

### Effects on newborn:
- See *Effects on fetus.*

### Effects during lactation:
- Overconsumption of iodine while nursing may cause skin rash and change the normal thyroid function of the infant.

## Additional information

- Iodine is often found in over-the-counter cough and cold preparations. Read all labels carefully.

**Recommendations for use**

### Women considering pregnancy:

- Eat a diet adequate in iodine. Include seafood and iodized salt. This is especially important if you live in a non-coastal region.
- No need for additional supplementation.
- Take supplements only under your doctor's supervision.

### Recommendations during pregnancy:

- Eat a diet adequate in iodine. Include seafood and iodized salt. This is especially important if you live in a non-coastal region.
- No need for additional supplementation.
- Take supplements only under your doctor's supervision.
- Avoid over-the-counter medications containing iodine and topic preparations, such as povidone-iodine.

### Recommendations during lactation:

- Eat a diet adequate in iodine. Include seafood and iodized salt. This is especially important if you live in a non-coastal region.
- No need for additional supplementation.
- Take supplements only under your doctor's supervision.
- If you are breast-feeding, do not ingest radioactive iodine.
- Avoid over-the-counter medications containing iodine and topic preparations, such as povidone-iodine.

 **Interactions**

### Interactions with medications, vitamins and minerals:

| Interacts with | Combined effect |
|---|---|
| Lithium | Increases thyroid toxicity. |

### Interactions with other substances:

- None reported.

*See Glossary.

**Definition and description:** Very important trace element in the body that is present in all cells. Plays a key role in metabolism and transportation of oxygen to the body. Need for iron is greatly increased in pregnancy because of increased production of blood cells for baby and mother.

**Other names:** Ferrous sulfate (most concentrated), ferrous gluconate, ferrous fumerate, polysaccharide-iron complex. Also see brand-name list, page 390.

 ## Dosage

### Requirement:
- Non-pregnant or breast-feeding woman—18mg.
- Pregnant woman—30 to 60mg. Supplementation is recommended.

### Safe dosage:
- Up to 190mg/day for short-term treatment of anemia*.

### Toxic dosage:
- Overdose can be fatal.
- Prolonged doses of 100mg may cause adverse symptoms.

 ## Possible benefits

### Benefits before pregnancy:
- See *Deficiency before pregnancy.*

### Benefits to mother:
- See *Deficiency in mother.*

### Benefits to fetus:
- See *Deficiency in fetus.*

### Benefits to newborn:
- See *Deficiency in newborn.*

### Benefits during lactation:
- See *Deficiency during lactation.*

 ## Possible effects of deficiency

### Deficiency before pregnancy:
- Inadequate iron intake causes iron-deficiency anemia*. Symptoms of iron-deficiency anemia* may include coldness in the hands or feet, craving for non-foods (dirt, clay, ice, starch), irritability, fatigue and shortness of breath.
- Iron depletion may decrease tolerance to cold.
- Most women's dietary intake of iron is 50% or less of the RDA.

### Deficiency in mother:
- See *Deficiency before pregnancy.*
- Inadequate iron intake decreases the number of red blood cells and iron stores in mother. This increases lethargy and tiredness and decreases ability to tolerate physical activity, labor and delivery. Iron supplementation can prevent this from occurring.

### Deficiency in fetus:
- If mother has severe anemia*, the fetus will have decreased iron stores.
- Increased incidence of premature birth has been reported with maternal iron deficiency.

### Deficiency in newborn:
- If mother has severe anemia*, the baby will have decreased iron stores. Premature infants have been born with decreased iron stores. Supplementation starting at birth prevents iron-deficiency anemia*.

### Deficiency during lactation:
- Inadequate iron intake during pregnancy increases the incidence of iron-deficiency anemia*.
- Supplementation helps replace iron lost or decreased during pregnancy.
- Supplemental iron does not change the quantity of iron in breast milk unless the mother is severely anemic.

**Possible adverse effects**

**Effects before pregnancy:**
- Adverse effects are dose-related. Nausea, gastrointestinal distress, constipation and diarrhea may increase as dose is increased.
- Long-term, excessive iron intake is associated with abdominal or joint pain, bronze-colored skin, fatigue, weight loss, excessive thirst and excessive urination.
- Overdose can be fatal.

**Effects on mother:**
- May contribute to nausea, stomach distress, constipation or diarrhea.
- See *Effects before pregnancy*.

**Effects on fetus:**
- None reported.

**Effects on newborn:**
- None reported.

**Effects during lactation:**
- No specific effects reported on lactation or breast milk.
- See *Effects before pregnancy*.

 **Additional information**

- Iron toxicity is the most common medication poisoning in young children. Prenatal vitamins are especially dangerous because of the high levels of iron they contain. Keep prenatal vitamins and iron supplements out of reach of children.
- All doses are listed as elemental (pure) iron. Ferrous sulfate (the most common form) is 19% elemental iron; 325mg of ferrous sulfate contains 62.5mg of elemental iron.

 **Recommendations for use**

**Women considering pregnancy:**
- Eat a diet with 18mg of iron/day, or supplement with a multivitamin/mineral supplement that contains at least 18mg of iron. Ask your doctor for recommendations. See dietary iron list, Appendix 1, page 375.

**Recommendations during pregnancy:**
- Supplement diet with prenatal vitamin containing 30 to 60mg of iron, especially in the last half of pregnancy. Your doctor will recommend additional iron if it is indicated.
- If iron supplementation is associated with gastrointestinal distress, take more tablets containing smaller amounts of iron.
- Take iron tablets with meals and orange juice to increase absorption.
- If nausea and vomiting in early pregnancy are severe, iron supplementation may be delayed until second trimester.
- Consult your doctor if you are unable to tolerate supplements.
- Cook foods in cast-iron cookware to increase iron content.

**Recommendations during lactation:**
- Supplement diet with multivitamin/mineral supplement with 30 to 60mg of iron for first 2 to 3 months of lactation.
- Premature infants need additional iron supplementation. See your baby's doctor.

**Interactions**

**Interactions with medications, vitamins and minerals:**

| Interacts with | Combined effect |
| --- | --- |
| **Antacids** | Decreases iron absorption. |
| **Aspirin** | High doses of aspirin may increase iron needs. |
| **Cholestyramine** | Decreases iron absorption. |
| **Magnesium** | Interferes with iron absorption at levels above 100mg. |
| **Neomycin** | Decreases iron absorption. |
| **Riboflavin** | High levels of iron decrease riboflavin levels in the mother and fetus. |
| **Tetracycline** | Decreases iron absorption. Iron supplements decrease tetracycline absorption. |
| **Vitamin C** | Increases iron absorption. |
| **Zinc** | 50+mg/day of iron decreases zinc absorption. Zinc may decrease iron absorption. |

**Interactions with other substances:**
- Fiber interferes with iron absorption.
- Orange juice increases iron absorption.
- Alcohol greatly increases iron absorption.
- Dairy products interfere with iron absorption.

*See Glossary.

# Magnesium

**Definition and description:** Major body mineral that is part of every cell. Involved in transmitting nerve impulses. It is also a component of many enzyme* systems.

**Other names:** Magnesium gluconate, magnesium amino acid chelate, dolomite (bone mineral). Magnesium carbonate, magnesium hydroxide, magnesium oxide, magnesium trisilicate (antacids). Magnesium citrate, magnesium sulfate (laxatives).

 **Dosage**

**Requirement:**
- Non-pregnant woman—300mg.
- Pregnant or lactating woman—450mg.

**Safe dosage:**
- Up to 1.7g.

**Toxic dosage:**
- 1.7g.
- 600mg, if kidneys do not function properly.

 **Possible benefits**

**Benefits before pregnancy:**
- Heart disease and osteoporosis* may be less common with higher magnesium intake.

**Benefits to mother:**
- See *Benefits before pregnancy.*
- Large doses of magnesium sulfate are given intramuscularly and intravascularly to treat pre-eclampsia*.

**Benefits to fetus:**
- Recently magnesium has been found to be as effective as ritodrine for treating premature labor.

**Benefits to newborn:**
- See *Benefits to fetus.*

**Benefits during lactation:**
- See *Benefits before pregnancy.*

 **Possible effects of deficiency**

**Deficiency before pregnancy:**
- Magnesium deficiency is usually seen only in disease states. Symptoms include tremor, convulsions and sometimes behavioral changes.

**Deficiency in mother:**
- See *Deficiency before pregnancy.*

**Deficiency in fetus:**
- Magnesium deficiency can cause fetal defects including skeletal deformities, cleft lip*, heart and lung abnormalities, hydrocephalus* and urogenital abnormalities.

**Deficiency in newborn;**
- See *Deficiency in fetus.*

**Deficiency during lactation:**
- Magnesium level in diet does not affect magnesium level in breast milk.
- Magnesium in antacids may increase magnesium level in breast milk.
- See *Deficiency befrore pregnancy.*

 **Possible adverse effects**

**Effects before pregnancy:**
- No adverse effects reported from magnesium supplementation.
- Magnesium contained in antacids may cause adverse effects including low blood pressure, lethargy, unsteadiness, changes in mental status, nausea, vomiting, flushing of the skin, urinary retention, heart attack and loss of consciousness.
- See Appendix 2, page 379, for magnesium content of antacids.

**Effects on mother:**
- See *Effects before pregnancy.*

**Effects on fetus:**
- Large doses of magnesium sulfate given intramuscularly or intravascularly to women with decreased kidney function may cause slowed heart rate and neonatal depression*. Calcium may be administered to reverse these effects.

- Large doses of magnesium may cause kidney damage in the fetus.

### Effects on newborn:
- None reported.

### Effects during lactation:
- No specific effects reported on lactation or breast milk.
- See *Effects before pregnancy.*

## Additional information

- Dolomite is not recommended during pregnancy or lactation. It contains toxic metals such as aluminum, antimony, arsenic, barium, cadmium, cobalt and lead.
- Magnesium is also available in antacids and laxatives.

## Recommendations for use

### Women considering pregnancy:
- Eat a well-balanced diet rich in whole grains, nuts and beans. See Appendix 1, page 375, for food sources of magnesium.
- Supplementation is unnecessary.

### Recommendations during pregnancy:
- Eat a well-balanced diet rich in whole grains, nuts and beans. See Appendix 1, page 375, for food sources of magnesium.
- Supplementation is unnecessary.
- Avoid large doses of magnesium-containing antacids. See Appendix 2, page 379, for magnesium content of various antacids.

### Recommendations during lactation:
- Eat a well-balanced diet rich in whole grains, nuts and beans. See Appendix 1, page 375, for food sources of magnesium.
- Supplementation is unnecessary.

## Interactions

**Interactions with medications, vitamins and minerals:**

| Interacts with | Combined effect |
| --- | --- |
| Fluoride | Magnesium decreases fluoride absorption. |
| Iron | Magnesium levels above 100mg in supplements decrease iron absorption. |
| Phenobarbital | Decreases blood magnesium levels. |
| Phenytoin | Decreases blood magnesium levels. |
| Phosphorus | May increase effects of magnesium deficiency. |
| Tetracycline | May decrease magnesium absorption. |
| Vitamin D | May increase magnesium absorption. |

**Interactions with other substances:**
- Fiber in bread and cereals may delay and decrease magnesium absorption.
- Excessive alcohol intake increases amount of magnesium lost in urine. It may also increase intestinal loss from vomiting and diarrhea.

*See Glossary.

VITAMIN/MINERAL

# Manganese

**Definition and description:** Acts as an essential part of several enzyme systems involved in protein and calorie metabolism. Aids normal growth and development.

**Other names:** Manganese chloride, manganese sulfate.

 ## Dosage

**Requirement:**
- Not established.

**Safe dosage:**
- Estimated safe and adequate intake—2.5 to 5mg/day.

**Toxic dosage:**
- Toxicity has been observed mainly with high concentrations of manganese dust in the air. Only one report is known of an excessive oral intake; dose was unknown.

 ## Possible benefits

- None reported.

 ## Possible effects of deficiency

- None reported.

 ## Possible adverse effects

**Effects before pregnancy:**
- Toxicity is known only in workers exposed to high concentrations of manganese dust in the air. Toxicity has not been observed as a consequence of dietary intake.
- Inhaled toxic doses produce adverse effects on the central nervous system.

**Effects on mother:**
- See *Effects before pregnancy.*

**Effects on fetus:**
- None reported.

**Effects on newborn:**
- None reported.

**Effects during lactation:**
- See *Effects before pregnancy.*

 ## Recommendations for use

**Women considering pregnancy:**
- Eat a well-balanced diet rich in nuts and cereal grains.
- Supplements are not recommended.

**Recommendations during pregnancy:**
- Eat a well-balanced diet rich in nuts and cereal grains.
- Supplements are not recommended.

**Recommendations during lactation:**
- Eat a well-balanced diet rich in nuts and cereal grains.
- Supplements are not recommended.

 ## Interactions

**Interactions with medications, vitamins and minerals:**

| Interacts with | Combined effect |
| --- | --- |
| Calcium (over 1g) | Decreases manganese absorption. |
| Iron | May decrease iron absorption. |
| Magnesium | May decrease manganese absorption. |
| Phosphate | May decrease manganese absorption. |

**Interactions with other substances:**
- Iron-deficiency anemia* increases intestinal absorption of manganese.

*See Glossary.

**Definition and description:** Essential for function of important enzymes involved in metabolism. Promotes normal growth and development. Promotes normal cell function.

**Other names:** None.

 ## Dosage

### Requirement:
• Not established.

### Safe dosage:
• Estimated safe and adequate intake—0.1 to 0.5mg/day.

### Toxic dosage:
• 10 to 15mg/day.

 ## Possible benefits

• None reported.

 ## Possible effects of deficiency

• None reported.

 ## Possible adverse effects

### Effects before pregnancy:
• Excess intake may cause gout*.

### Effects on mother:
• See *Effects before pregnancy.*

### Effects on fetus:
• None reported.

### Effects on newborn:
• None reported.

### Effects during lactation:
• See *Effects before pregnancy.*

 ## Recommendations for use

### Women considering pregnancy:
• Eat a balanced diet containing meat, grains and legumes.
• Supplements are not recommended.

### Recommendations during pregnancy:
• Eat a balanced diet containing meat, grains and legumes.
• Supplements are not recommended.

### Recommendations during lactation:
• Eat a balanced diet containing meat, grains and legumes.
• Supplements are not recommended.

 ## Interactions

### Interactions with medications, vitamins and minerals:

| Interacts with | Combined effect |
| --- | --- |
| Copper | Excess molybdenum causes urinary loss of copper. |

### Interactions with other substances:
• None reported.

*See Glossary.

# Niacin

**Definition and description:** Functions in the body as two very important coenzymes, nicotinamide adenine dinucleotide and nicotinamide adenine dinucleotide phosphate. Participates in many functions including carbohydrate, fat and protein metabolism. It is essential for growth and aids in the synthesis of hormones. Tryptophan is converted to niacin in the body.

**Other names:** Vitamin B-3, niacin is a generic term referring to nicotinic acid, niacinamide and nicotinamide.

 ## Dosage

**Requirement:**
- Non-pregnant woman (15 to 22 years) —14mg.
- Non-pregnant woman (23 to 50+years) —13mg.
- Pregnant woman—15 to 16mg.
- Lactating woman—18 to 19mg.

**Safe dosage:**
- Up to 300mg.

**Toxic dosage:**
- Niacinamide is relatively non-toxic. It may cause flushing in doses of 1g.
- Nicotinic acid may cause adverse effects above 300mg.

 ## Possible benefits

**Benefits before pregnancy:**
- High doses of niacin (nicotinic acid) are effective in reducing blood cholesterol.

**Benefits to mother:**
- See *Benefits before pregnancy.*

**Benefits to fetus:**
- None reported.

**Benefits to newborn:**
- None reported.

**Benefits during lactation:**
- See *Benefits before pregnancy.*

 ## Possible effects of deficiency

**Deficiency before pregnancy:**
- In communities where maize or sorghum make up major portions of the diet, pellagra*, a niacin-deficiency disease, may occur.
- Symptoms of deficiency are weakness, loss of appetite, indigestion, skin changes, diarrhea and dementia*

**Deficiency in mother:**
- See *Deficiency before pregnancy.*

**Deficiency in fetus:**
- None reported.

**Deficiency in newborn:**
- None reported.

**Deficiency during lactation:**
- Mother's niacin intake affects niacin levels in breast milk.
- See *Deficiency before pregnancy.*

 ## Possible adverse effects

**Effects before pregnancy:**
- Excessive doses of nicotinic acid may cause skin flushing, increased blood flow in the hands and forearms, itching, skin discoloration, chronic nausea, diarrhea, vomiting, change in liver function, high blood-glucose levels and increased blood-uric-acid levels. Liver damage may also occur.

**Effects on mother:**
- See *Effects before pregnancy.*

**Effects on fetus:**
- None reported.

**Effects on newborn:**
- None reported in humans.
- Rats developed fatty livers and a growth decrease on very high doses of niacin.

**Effects during lactation:**
- None reported.

## Additional information

- Tryptophan, an amino acid, is converted to niacin. If tryptophan or protein intake is low, niacin requirement increases.

 ## Recommendations for use

### Women considering pregnancy:
- Eat a well-balanced diet containing fortified cereals, veal, tuna, chicken, turkey, salmon, cheese, peanuts and beef.
- Additional supplementation is unnecessary.

### Recommendations during pregnancy:
- Eat a well-balanced diet containing fortified cereals, veal, tuna, chicken, turkey, salmon, cheese, peanuts and beef.
- Additional supplementation is unnecessary.

### Recommendations during lactation:
- Eat a well-balanced diet containing fortified cereals, veal, tuna, chicken, turkey, salmon, cheese, peanuts and beef.
- Additional supplementation is unnecessary.

 ## Interactions

### Interactions with medications, vitamins and minerals:

| Interacts with | Combined effect |
| --- | --- |
| Isoniazide (INH) | May increase need for niacin. |
| Oral contraceptives | May increase need for niacin. |
| Pyridoxine | High doses of niacin interfere with pyridoxine metabolism and increase pyridoxine requirement. Pyridoxine deficiency may increase niacin requirement. |
| Tryptophan | Tryptophan deficiency increases niacin requirement. |

### Interactions with other substances:
- Niacin interferes with testing for sugar with Benedict's reagent.

*See Glossary.

# Pantothenic acid

**Definition and description:** Part of coenzyme A, which is involved in the release of energy from carbohydrates and fats. Helps manufacture hormones and other vital compounds.

**Other names:** Vitamin B5.

 ## Dosage

### Requirement:
• Not established.

### Safe dosage:
• Estimated safe and adequate intake—4 to 7mg.
• Level may be higher during pregnancy and lactation.

### Toxic dosage:
• Relatively non-toxic.
• Diarrhea reported at 7g.

 ## Possible benefits

### Benefits before pregnancy:
• See *Deficiency before pregnancy.*

### Benefits to mother:
• See *Deficiency before pregnancy.*

### Benefits to fetus:
• None reported.

### Benefits to newborn:
• None reported.

### Benefits during lactation:
• See *Deficiency during lactation.*

 ## Possible effects of deficiency

### Deficiency before pregnancy:
• Dietary deficiencies in humans are unlikely. In malnutrition, however, multiple deficiencies usually exist, and pantothenic acid may be deficient.

### Deficiency in mother:
• See *Deficiency before pregnancy.*

### Deficiency in fetus:
• None reported.

### Deficiency in newborn:
• None reported.

### Deficiency during lactation:
• Pantothenic-acid content of breast milk varies proportionately with pantothenic-acid content of the diet.

 ## Possible adverse effects

### Effects before pregnancy:
• Studies indicate pantothenic acid is relatively non-toxic. High doses may result in occasional diarrhea and water retention.

### Effects on mother:
• See *Effects before pregnancy.*

### Effects on fetus:
• None reported.

### Effects on newborn:
• None reported.

### Effects during lactation:
• None reported.

# Pantothenic acid, <sub>continued</sub>

 **Recommendations for use**

### Women considering pregnancy:

- Eat a well-balanced diet. Pantothenic acid is widely distributed in foods, especially whole-grain cereals, eggs, wheat bran and legumes, and in lesser amounts in milk, vegetables and fruits.
- Additional supplementation is unnecessary.

### Recommendations during pregnancy:

- Eat a well-balanced diet. Pantothenic acid is widely distributed in foods, especially whole-grain cereals, eggs, wheat bran and legumes, and in lesser amounts in milk, vegetables and fruits.
- Additional supplementation is unnecessary.

### Recommendations during lactation:

- Eat a well-balanced diet. Pantothenic acid is widely distributed in foods, especially whole-grain cereals, eggs, wheat bran and legumes, and in lesser amounts in milk, vegetables and fruits.
- Additional supplementation is unnecessary.

 **Interactions**

### Interactions with medications, vitamins and minerals:

- None reported.

### Interactions with other substances:

- None reported.

*See Glossary.

# Phosphorus

**Definition and description:** Essential mineral for healthy bones, normal muscle contraction and function of B vitamins. It is an important component inside cells.

**Other names:** Sodium phosphate, calcium phosphate, yellow or white phosphorus (in prepared forms).

##  Dosage

**Requirement:**
- Non-pregnant woman—800mg.
- Pregnant or lactating woman—1,200mg.
- Pregnant or lactating adolescent—1,600mg.

**Safe dosage:**
- Safe dose is only exceeded when phosphorus intake greatly exceeds calcium intake.
- Calcium-to-phosphorus intake ratio should be 1:1.

**Toxic dosage:**
- Toxic only in yellow-prepared form.

##  Possible benefits

**Benefits before pregnancy:**
- See *Deficiency before pregnancy.*

**Benefits to mother:**
- None reported.

**Benefits to fetus:**
- None reported.

**Benefits to newborn:**
- None reported.

**Benefits during lactation:**
- None reported.

##  Possible effects of deficiency

**Deficiency before pregnancy:**
- Dietary intake is almost always adequate or excessive.
- Phosphorus deficiency can occur with excessive intake of antacids. Symptoms of deficiency include weakness, loss of appetite, lethargy and pain in bones.

**Deficiency in mother:**
- See *Deficiencies before pregnancy.*

**Deficiency in fetus:**
- None reported.

**Deficiency in newborn:**
- None reported.

**Deficiency during lactation:**
- None reported.

##  Possible adverse effects

**Effects before pregnancy:**
- At high ratios of phosphorus to calcium (2.5:1), interference with calcium and magnesium levels in bones may occur.

**Effects on mother:**
- See *Effects before pregnancy.*

**Effects on fetus:**
- None reported.

**Effects on newborn:**
- None reported.

**Effects during lactation:**
- No specific effects reported on lactation or breast milk.
- See *Effects before pregnancy.*

## Recommendations for use

### Women considering pregnancy:
- Eat a well-balanced diet.
- Avoid excessive intake of cola drinks.
- Supplementation is unnecessary.

### Recommendations during pregnancy:
- Eat a well-balanced diet.
- Avoid excessive intake of cola drinks.
- Supplementation is unnecessary.

### Recommendations during lactation:
- Eat a well-balanced diet.
- Avoid excessive intake of cola drinks.
- Supplementation is unnecessary.

 ## Interactions

### Interactions with medications, vitamins and minerals:

| Interacts with | Combined effect |
| --- | --- |
| **Antacids containing aluminum** | Decreases phosphorus absorption. |
| **Antacids containing magnesium** | Decreases phosphorus absorption. |
| **Calcium** | May increase amount of calcium lost in urine. |
| **Magnesium** | Increases effects of magnesium deficiency. |
| **Manganese** | Phosphorus may decrease manganese absorption. |

### Interactions with other substances:
- None reported.

VITAMIN/MINERAL

# Potassium

**Definition and description:** Major electrolyte inside cells. It is the third-most-common element in the body. Stimulates muscle contraction. It is also a co-factor for several enzymes and involved in insulin synthesis.

**Other names:** Potassium chloride, potassium bicarbonate, potassium citrate, potassium acetate, potassium gluconate. Also see brand-name list, page 390.

 ## Dosage

**Requirement:**
• Not established.

**Safe dosage:**
• Estimated safe and adequate intake— 1.88 to 5.62g.

**Toxic dosage:**
• Toxicity is unusual because the kidney excretes excess potassium. Toxicity can occur when kidneys are damaged or when there is a sudden, large increase in dietary potassium of 2 to 4g in excess of current intake.
• Overdose may be fatal.

 ## Possible benefits

**Benefits before pregnancy:**
• See *Deficiency before pregnancy.*

**Benefits to mother:**
• See *Deficiency in mother.*

**Benefits to fetus:**
• None reported.

**Benefits to newborn:**
• None reported.

**Benefits during lactation:**
• See *Deficiency during lactation.*

 ## Possible effects of deficiency

**Deficiency before pregnancy:**
• Excess potassium losses cause muscle weakness; heart arrythmias* can occur.
• Excess potassium loss occurs with vomiting, diarrhea or use of laxatives or diuretics.
• Additional potassium intake prevents problems.

**Deficiency in mother:**
• Blood levels of potassium fall as a normal occurrence of pregnancy. Supplementation is neither beneficial nor necessary.

**Deficiency in fetus:**
• None reported.

**Deficiency in newborn:**
• None reported.

**Deficiency during lactation:**
• Dietary potassium may increase or decrease breast-milk potassium levels.

 ## Possible adverse effects

**Effects before pregnancy:**
• Adverse effects are extremely rare because the kidney adapts to large changes in potassium intake.
• Toxicity usually causes vomiting, but it can also cause heartbeat irregularities and breathing-muscle paralysis.
• Liquid potassium chloride can cause gastric irritation and ulceration.

**Effects on mother:**
• See *Effects before pregnancy.*

**Effects on fetus:**
• None reported.

**Effects on newborn:**
• None reported.

**Effects during lactation:**
• No specific effects reported on lactation or breast milk.

- Adverse effects are extremely rare because the kidney adapts to large changes in potassium intake.
- Toxicity in the mother usually causes vomiting, but it can also cause heartbeat irregularities and breathing-muscle paralysis.
- Liquid potassium chloride can cause gastric irritation and ulceration.

 ## Additional information

- Sodium intake, in part, determines the amount of potassium lost in the urine.
- Sodium-to-potassium ratio should not exceed 1:1.
- The greater the sodium intake, the greater the potassium requirement.

 ## Recommendations for use

### Women considering pregnancy:
- Eat a well-balanced diet.
- Take potassium supplements only under your doctor's supervision.
- If you have kidney disease or heart disease, consult your doctor.

### Recommendations during pregnancy:
- Eat a well-balanced diet.
- Take potassium supplements only under your doctor's supervision.
- If you have kidney disease or heart disease, consult your doctor.

### Recommendations during lactation:
- Eat a well-balanced diet.
- Take potassium supplements only under your doctor's supervision.
- If you have kidney disease or heart disease, consult your doctor.

 ## Interactions

### Interactions with medications, vitamins and minerals:

| Interacts with | Combined effect |
| --- | --- |
| Amiloride | Increases potassium reabsorption in kidney. |
| Captopril | Increases potassium reabsorption in kidney. |
| Lasix | Increases potassium loss in urine. |
| Osmotic laxatives | Increases potassium loss. |
| Sodium | High sodium intake may increase potassium loss in kidney. Decreases sodium retention with excessive intake of potassium. |
| Spironolactone | Increases potassium reabsorption in kidney. |
| Triamterene | Increases potassium reabsorption in kidney. |
| Thiazide diuretics | Increases potassium loss in urine. |

### Interactions with other substances:
- High intake of salt may increase potassium loss in kidney.
- Alcohol intake increases potassium loss.

*See Glossary.

VITAMIN/MINERAL

# Prenatal multivitamin/mineral supplement

**Definition and description:** A multivitamin/mineral supplement especially formulated for women during pregnancy and lactation. Prenatal multivitamin/mineral supplements usually contain RDA amounts of vitamins and minerals for pregnant women. These supplements differ most from regular multivitamin/mineral supplements in their iron and folate contents. Some prenatal supplements also contain stool softeners or bulk-forming laxatives.

**Other names:** Multivitamin/mineral, therapeutic vitamin, perinatal vitamin. See *Additional information.*

 **Dosage**

- Note—Safe dosage has not been well-established for most nutrients. For nutrients whose requirements are not established, safe dosage is set by the Food and Nutrition Board. Safe dosage for remaining nutrients is the highest level, with no known side-effects or toxicities.

| Requirement while Pregnant/Lactating | | Safe Dosage | Toxic Dosage |
|---|---|---|---|
| • Vitamin A | 1,000/1,200mcg R.E. 5,000/6,000 I.U. | 8,000 I.U. | 25,000 I.U. |
| • Vitamin D | 10/10mcg, 400 I.U. | 15mcg/600 I.U. | 50mcg/2,000 I.U. |
| • Vitamin E | 10/11mg | 400mg | 1,000mg |
| • Vitamin C | 80/100mg | 400mg | 1g |
| • Thiamine | 1.4/1.5mg | 5g | 10g |
| • Riboflavin | 1.5/1.7mg | Very safe | Not reported |
| • Niacin | 15/18mg | 300mg | More than 300mg |
| • Vitamin B$_6$ | 2.6/2.5mg | 50mg | 500mg |
| • Folate | 800/500mcg | 1mg | 15mg |
| • Vitamin B$_{12}$ | 4/4mcg | Very safe | Not reported |
| • Pantothenic acid | Not established | 4-7mg | 20mg |
| • Vitamin K | Not established | 70-140mcg | 20mg |
| • Biotin | Not established | 100-200mcg | Not reported |
| • Calcium | 1,200/1,200mg | 1.6g | 3g |
| • Phosphorus | 1,200/1,200mg | 1.6g | 1g/kg |
| • Magnesium | 450/450mg | 1.7g | 1.7g |
| • Iron | 30-60/18mg | 190mg | 2g |
| • Zinc | 20/25mg | 25mg | 1.8g |
| • Iodine | 175/0.2mg | 0.3mg | 2mg |
| • Chromium | Not established | 0.05-0.2mg | Not reported |
| • Fluoride | Not established | 1.5-4mg | 20mg |
| • Manganese | Not established | 2.5-5mg | Not reported |
| • Selenium | Not established | 0.05-0.2mg | 1mg |
| • Sodium | Not established | 1.1-3.3g | 35g |
| • Potassium | Not established | 1.88-5.62g | 18g |
| • Copper | Not established | 2-3mg | 15mg |
| • Molybdenum | Not established | 0.1-0.5mg | 10-15mg |

# Prenatal multivitamin/mineral supplement, continued

 **Possible benefits**

### Benefits before pregnancy:

- Prenatal multivitamin/mineral supplement is usually not indicated before pregnancy.
- Sometimes prenatal vitamin/mineral supplements are prescribed for women who have anemia* caused by folate deficiency and iron deficiency.
- May be beneficial for women who have closely spaced pregnancies.
- Studies from Great Britain suggest supplementation with multivitamins, especially folate, before conception may be helpful in decreasing neural-tube defects* in infants born to mothers who have a high risk.

### Benefits to mother:

- Prenatal vitamins supply vitamins and minerals that are required during pregnancy. These levels may be difficult to obtain through dietary intake.

### Benefits to fetus:

- Prenatal multivitamin/mineral supplements assure adequate intake of nutrients during pregnancy, which helps produce a healthy baby.

### Benefits to newborn:

- See *Benefits to fetus*.

### Benefits during lactation:

- Prenatal vitamins supply vitamins and minerals that are required during lactation. These levels may be difficult to obtain through dietary intake.
- Prenatal multivitamin/mineral supplements are usually prescribed during lactation to replenish the mother's vitamin/mineral stores that may be depleted in pregnancy.

 **Possible effects of deficiency**

### Deficiency before pregnancy:

- Failure to take a prenatal vitamin, if prescribed for anemia*, may result in worsening or continuation of anemia*.

### Deficiency in mother:

- Failure to take prenatal vitamin supplement may result in nutritional deficiencies, especially iron and folate. See Folate, page 294, and Iron, page 299.

### Deficiency in fetus:

- Failure to take prenatal vitamin supplement may result in nutritional deficiencies, especially iron and folate. See Folate, page 294, and Iron, page 299.

### Deficiency in newborn:

- Failure to take prenatal vitamin supplement may result in nutritional deficiencies, especially iron and folate. See Folate, page 294, and Iron, page 299.

### Deficiency during lactation:

- Failure to take prenatal vitamin supplement may result in nutritional deficiencies, especially iron and folate. See Folate, page 294, and Iron, page 298.

 **Possible adverse effects**

### Effects before pregnancy:

- Some women do not tolerate multivitamin/mineral supplements.
- Taking a prenatal vitamin with meals usually increases tolerance.

➤➤→

# Prenatal multivitamin/mineral supplement, continued

## Effects on mother:
- Some women do not tolerate multivitamin/mineral supplements, especially during the first trimester.
- Taking a prenatal vitamin with meals usually increases tolerance.
- Prenatal vitamins that contain high levels of calcium and magnesium may reduce the amount of iron absorbed.
- Supplements should *not* contain any components above 100% of the RDA, especially vitamin A or vitamin D.
- High levels of iron in a prenatal supplement may contribute to constipation. Some prenatal supplements contain stool softeners or bulking agents. These products are listed under *Additional information*.

## Effects on fetus:
- None reported if the supplement does not contain any components above 100% of the RDA, especially vitamin A and vitamin D.

## Effects on newborn:
- See *Effects on fetus*.

## Effects during lactation:
- See *Effects before pregnancy* and *Effects on fetus*.

## Additional information:
- Filibon O.T. Prenatals® contain stool softeners.
- Prenatal supplements that contain bulking agents include Chromagen®, Filibon F.A.®, Filibon Forte®, Materna®, Natalins®, Natalins Rx® and Niferex PN®.

## Recommendations for use

### Women considering pregnancy:
- Take a prenatal multivitamin/mineral supplement only on your doctor's advice.
- If you have a family or personal history of neural-tube defects*, consult your doctor about supplementation before pregnancy.

- If you take anticonvulsant medications, consult your doctor about supplementation before pregnancy.

## Recommendations during pregnancy:
- Take a prenatal multivitamin/mineral supplement if your doctor prescribes one.
- If you are unable to tolerate the supplement, you may have to wait until later in your pregnancy to take the supplement. Most women are able to tolerate the supplement in their second and third trimester.
- If you start pregnancy in a nutrient-depleted state, it is important to take supplements throughout pregnancy.

## Recommendations during lactation:
- Take a prenatal multivitamin/mineral supplement if your doctor recommends one.
- A multivitamin/mineral supplement may be adequate during lactation.

## Interactions

### Interactions with medications, vitamins and minerals:

| Interacts with | Combined effect |
| --- | --- |
| Calcium | Calcium levels above 200mg may interfere with iron absorption. |
| Magnesium | Magnesium levels above 100mg may interfere with iron absorption. |
| Other vitamins and minerals | The level contained in prenatal vitamins is usually not high enough to interfere with other nutrients or medications. |

### Interactions with other substances:
- Fiber may interfere with absorption of minerals if eaten at the same time as the supplement.
- Orange juice increases iron absorption.

*See Glossary.

Note: This page purposely left blank.

# Pyridoxine

### Definition and description:
Pyridoxine is a coenzyme mainly for metabolizing protein. It is involved in converting tryptophan to the brain chemical serotonin. Involved in making *heme*\*, an important part of blood cells.

**Other names:** Vitamin B$_6$, pyridoxal, pyridoxamine.

 **Dosage**

### Requirement:
* Non-pregnant woman—2mg.
* Pregnant woman—2.6mg.
* Lactating woman—2.5mg.

### Safe dosage:
* Up to 50mg. Safe dose has not been established in pregnancy.

### Toxic dosage:
* 200mg.

 **Possible benefits**

### Benefits before pregnancy:
* See *Deficiency before pregnancy.*

### Benefits to mother:
* Pyridoxine supplementation in mothers, especially by lozenge, may reduce dental disease in mother during pregnancy.
* Pyridoxine supplementation may decrease the incidence of severe morning sickness.

### Benefits to fetus:
* See *Deficiency in fetus.*

### Benefits to newborn:
* See *Deficiency in newborn.*

### Benefits during lactation:
* See *Deficiency during lactation.*

 **Possible effects of deficiency**

### Deficiency before pregnancy:
* Oral-contraceptive users, especially those on combined estrogen-progestogen pills, may have pyridoxine deficiency. Symptoms include depression, high blood fat, lethargy, impaired sugar tolerance, personality changes, irritability, mouth and tongue sores, and rash on the forehead.

### Deficiency in mother:
* Pyridoxine deficiency is associated with the development of pregnancy-induced hypertension\*.
* Women with pyridoxine deficiency and gestational diabetes mellitus\* have shown improvement of gestational diabetes mellitus\* with pyridoxine supplements.

### Deficiency in fetus:
* Women with a pyridoxine deficiency during pregnancy may give birth to infants with lower Apgar scores\*.

### Deficiency in newborn:
* Seizures have been reported in newborns on a pyridoxine-deficient diet. Supplementation during pregnancy helps prevent this.

### Deficiency during lactation:
* Breast-milk pyridoxine content varies proportionately with the amount of pyridoxine in the mother's diet.
* Seizures may occur in infants whose mother's breast milk has low levels of pyridoxine. Pyridoxine supplementation prevents this type of seizure.
* Use of oral contraceptives may decrease pyridoxine levels in breast milk.
* Many lactating women consume less than the RDA for pyridoxine and their milk may have inadequate levels of pyridoxine. Supplementation to RDA levels is beneficial.

 **Possible adverse effects**

### Effects before pregnancy:
* Large doses of pyridoxine have been consumed for the treatment of premenstrual syndrome (PMS). This treatment has not been established as effective; at doses above 500mg/day it can cause dizziness, nausea, vomiting, rapid heartbeat, skin rash, weight gain and nerve damage.

### Effects on mother:
• See *Effects before pregnancy.*

### Effects on fetus:
• High doses of pyridoxine may increase the risk of birth defects and lower fetal weight.
• Chronic use by mother of doses over 50mg is associated with abnormal nerve development.

### Effects on newborn:
• Seizures have been seen in infants whose mothers took large amounts of pyridoxine during pregnancy. These infants may have inherited a pyridoxine-metabolism disorder. The infants improved when they were given pyridoxine supplements.

### Effects during lactation:
• Oral doses of 600mg/day of pyridoxine can inhibit lactation.

 ## Recommendations for use

### Women considering pregnancy:
• Eat a well-balanced diet. See Appendix 1, page 375, for a list of foods that contain high amounts of pyridoxine.
• If you use oral contraceptives, especially combined estrogen and progestogen, you may want to supplement to RDA levels.
• Consult your doctor regarding treatment for premenstrual syndrome (PMS).

### Recommendations during pregnancy:
• Eat a well-balanced diet. See Appendix 1, page 375, for a list of foods that contain high amounts of pyridoxine.
• Pyridoxine deficiency is common during pregnancy, so most prenatal vitamins contain pyridoxine. Take your prenatal vitamins.

### Recommendations during lactation:
• Eat a well-balanced diet. See Appendix 1, page 375, for a list of foods that contain high amounts of pyridoxine.
• Supplement with additional pyridoxine if your intake is less than the RDA of 2.3 to 2.5mg.

• If you take oral contraceptives, supplement with 2 to 10mg of pyridoxine.

 ## Interactions

### Interactions with medications, vitamins and minerals:

| Interacts with | Combined effect |
| --- | --- |
| Adrenal corticosteroids | Increases need for pyridoxine. |
| Ethosuxamide | Decreases blood-pyridoxine levels. |
| Hydralazine | Causes pyridoxine depletion. |
| Isoniazid (INH) | Increases urinary loss of pyridoxine, causing pyridoxine depletion. |
| Niacin | High doses of niacin interfere with pyridoxine metabolism and increase pyridoxine requirement. Pyridoxine deficiency may increase niacin requirement. |
| Oral contraceptives | May increase need for pyridoxine. |
| Phenobarbital | Decreases levels of pyridoxine. Pyridoxine can also decrease effectiveness of phenobarbital. |
| Phenytoin | Decreases blood pyridoxine levels. |
| Riboflavin | Large doses of pyridoxine interfere with the utilization of riboflavin. |

### Interactions with other substances:
• Alcohol decreases absorption and interferes with the activation of pyridoxine.

*See Glossary.

# Riboflavin

**Definition and description:** Part of a group of coenzymes called *flavoproteins* involved with the process of metabolizing protein, fat and carbohydrates for energy. It is important for maintenance of the skin, the mucous membranes, the cornea of the eye and the nervous system.

**Other names:** Vitamin B$_2$.

 ## Dosage

**Requirement:**
- Non-pregnant woman (15 to 22 years)—1.3mg.
- Non-pregnant woman (23 to 50+ years)—1.2mg.
- Pregnant woman—1.5 to 1.6mg.
- Lactating woman—1.7 to 1.8mg.

**Safe dosage:**
- Riboflavin is very safe.

**Toxic dosage:**
- None reported.

 ## Possible benefits

**Benefits before pregnancy:**
- See *Deficiency before pregnancy.*

**Benefits to mother:**
- See *Deficiency in mother.*

**Benefits to fetus:**
- See *Deficiency in fetus.*

**Benefits to newborn:**
- See *Deficiency in newborn.*

**Benefits during lactation:**
- See *Deficiency during lactation.*

 ## Possible effects of deficiency

**Deficiency before pregnancy:**
- Deficiency of riboflavin causes cracks in lips, changes in the tongue, skin changes around the nose, and eye problems.

**Deficiency in mother:**
- There is an increased incidence of excessive vomiting in the second trimester with riboflavin deficiency.

**Deficiency in fetus:**
- There is an increased incidence of premature births with riboflavin deficiency.

**Deficiency in newborn:**
- Riboflavin deficiency can occur in infants whose mothers are deficient in riboflavin. It is characterized by retarded growth, cracks in the lips and a purple-red, swollen tongue. Other symptoms may include eye infections and sensitivity to sunburn.
- Premature infants may be deficient in riboflavin and require riboflavin supplementation to prevent deficiency symptoms.

**Deficiency during lactation:**
- There is an increased incidence of unsuccessful lactation with riboflavin deficiency.
- Breast-milk riboflavin levels are affected by the mother's body riboflavin stores and dietary intake. Adequate riboflavin intake assures adequate riboflavin in breast milk.

 ## Possible adverse effects

- None reported.

**Additional information**

- High doses of riboflavin make the urine very yellow.

 **Recommendations for use**

**Women considering pregnancy:**
- Drink milk and eat egg whites, leafy-green vegetables, fish, meat and poultry to ensure adequate intake.
- Women who exercise 30 to 50 minutes a day or more may need additional riboflavin.

**Recommendations during pregnancy:**
- Drink milk and eat egg whites, leafy-green vegetables, fish, meat and poultry to ensure adequate intake.
- Women who exercise 30 to 50 minutes a day or more may need additional riboflavin.
- If you have anemia*, supplementation with riboflavin is suggested.

**Recommendations during lactation:**
- Drink milk and eat egg whites, leafy-green vegetables, fish, meat and poultry to ensure adequate intake.
- Women who exercise 30 to 50 minutes a day or more may need additional riboflavin.
- If you have anemia*, supplementation with riboflavin is suggested.

 **Interactions**

**Interactions with medications, vitamins and minerals:**

| Interacts with | Combined effect |
| --- | --- |
| Amitriptylene | Interferes with ribo-flavin metabolism. |
| Chlorpromazine | Interferes with ribo-flavin metabolism. |
| Erythromycin | Decreases riboflavin absorption. |
| Folate | Decreases maternal and fetal riboflavin blood levels. |
| Imipramine | Interferes with ribo-flavin metabolism. |
| Iron | Decreases maternal and fetal blood ribo-flavin levels. |
| Phenothiazines | Decreases riboflavin effect. |
| Oral contraceptives | May increase ribo-flavin utilization. |
| Probenecid | Decreases riboflavin effect. |
| Pyridoxine | Large doses of pyri-doxine interfere with the utilization of riboflavin. |
| Streptomycin | Decreases riboflavin absorption. |
| Tetracycline | Decreases riboflavin absorption. |
| Tricyclic anti-depressants | Decreases riboflavin effect. |

**Interactions with other substances:**
- Tobacco decreases riboflavin absorption.
- Excessive intake of riboflavin may prevent accurate readings of urine tests for catecholamines and urobilin.

*See Glossary.

VITAMIN/MINERAL

# Selenium

**Definition and description:** An essential trace element active in enzyme systems that functions as an antioxidant* to protect tissue from damage. Combines with heavy metals to prevent heavy-metal poisoning. It also plays a role in energy metabolism.

**Other names:** Kelp-bound selenium, yeast-selenium and selenite.

 **Dosage**

**Requirement:**
• Not established.

**Safe dosage:**
• Estimated safe and adequate intake— 0.05 to 0.2mg.

**Toxic dosage:**
• Greater than 1mg/day over an extended period.
• Overdose may be fatal.

 **Possible benefits**

**Benefits before pregnancy:**
• May be helpful at any age in preventing cell damage leading to cancer.

**Benefits to mother:**
• See *Benefits before pregnancy.*

**Benefits to fetus:**
• None reported.

**Benefits to newborn:**
• None reported.

**Benefits during lactation:**
• See *Deficiency during lactation.*

 **Possible effects of deficiency**

**Deficiency before pregnancy:**
• None reported.

**Deficiency in mother:**
• None reported.

**Deficiency in fetus:**
• None reported.

**Deficiency in newborn:**
• None reported.

**Deficiency during lactation:**
• No specific effects reported on lactation.
• Increase in selenium intake can increase the selenium content of breast milk.

 **Possible adverse effects**

**Effects before pregnancy:**
• Toxic doses of selenium may cause liver damage, kidney damage, irritability, indigestion, increase in dental cavities, streaked fingernails, garlic breath, red skin lesions, hives*, brittle dry hair, lethargy, weakness or paralysis.

**Effects on mother:**
• See *Effects before pregnancy.*

**Effects on fetus:**
• Women working with sodium-selenite powder, an industrial form of selenium not used in food or supplements, may have a higher rate of miscarriages.

**Effects on newborn:**
• None reported.

**Effects during lactation:**
• No specific effects reported on lactation or breast milk.
• See *Effects before pregnancy.*

 **Additional information**

• Selenium sulfide is also used in shampoos and ointments. Don't use shampoo or ointment with selenium if your skin is inflamed.
• Typical diet contains about 0.15mg of selenium.

## Recommendations for use

### Women considering pregnancy:
- Eat a diet containing seafood, kidney, liver and meat to ensure an adequate intake of selenium.

### Recommendations during pregnancy:
- Eat a diet containing seafood, kidney, liver and meat to ensure an adequate intake of selenium.
- Supplements are not recommended.

### Recommendations during lactation:
- Eat a diet containing seafood, kidney, liver and meat to ensure an adequate intake of selenium.
- Supplements are not recommended.

 ## Interactions

### Interactions with medications, vitamins and minerals:

| Interacts with | Combined effect |
| --- | --- |
| Vitamin C | Blood levels of vitamin C may decrease with selenium supplementation. |

### Interactions with other substances:
- None reported.

*See Glossary.

# Sodium

**Definition and description:** A major electrolyte in body fluids that is involved mainly in controlling water volume and pressure.

**Other names:** Sodium chloride (table salt), sodium citrate, sodium fluoride, sodium bicarbonate, electrolyte solution.

 **Dosage**

**Requirement:**
- Not established.

**Safe dosage:**
- Estimated safe and adequate intake—1.1g to 3.3g.

**Toxic dosage:**
- Acute* toxicity at 35 to 40g.
- Chronic* toxicity occurs at much lower levels. Toxicity is dependent on potassium and chloride ratios.

 **Possible benefits**

**Benefits before pregnancy:**
- See *Deficiency before pregnancy.*

**Benefits to mother:**
- See *Deficiency in mother.*

**Benefits to fetus:**
- None reported.

**Benefits to newborn:**
- See *Deficiency in newborn.*

**Benefits during lactation:**
- See *Deficiency during lactation.*

 **Possible effects of deficiency**

**Deficiency before pregnancy:**
- Deficiency is very rare under normal conditions.
- Excessive perspiration and loss of body fluid may decrease fluid volume and eventually the amount of sodium in the body. Additional sodium intake of 1.2g to 7g/liter of fluid lost will replace sodium.

- Symptoms of sodium deficiency include weakness and convulsions.

**Deficiency in mother:**
- Adequate sodium intake promotes necessary volume expansion. Sodium restriction may cause fluid and weight loss.
- See *Deficiency before pregnancy.*

**Deficiency in fetus:**
- None reported.

**Deficiency in newborn:**
- Sodium deficiency has been reported in infants of mothers who vigorously restricted sodium during pregnancy.
- Low blood-sodium levels are dangerous for the infant if left untreated. This may cause convulsions in infants.

**Deficiency during lactation:**
- Sodium content of breast milk is unaffected by changes in dietary sodium intake.

 **Possible adverse effects**

**Effects before pregnancy:**
- Many studies indicate increased sodium intake may increase the risk of developing high blood pressure.
- Potassium intake may have a protective effect on high sodium intake.

**Effects on mother:**
- Sodium restriction does not prevent pre-eclampsia* or eclampsia* of pregnancy and is not effective in its treatment.
- Changes in sodium intake cause little or no change in blood pressure of pregnant women with normal blood pressure.
- Excessive sodium intake may cause swelling.
- Sodium bicarbonate may cause swelling, heart failure and alkalosis*.

**Effects on fetus:**
- None reported.

### Effects on newborn:
- Sodium bicarbonate is associated with bleeding in the brain of some newborns treated with high doses by injection.

### Effects during lactation:
- None reported.

 ## Additional information

- Sodium bicarbonate contains a significant amount of sodium.
- Many medications contain sodium.
- Check with your doctor or pharmacist if you are concerned about sodium content.

 ## Recommendations for use

### Women considering pregnancy:
- Although still controversial, most dietitians recommend a sodium intake of 3 to 5g/day.
- If you take lithium, don't change your sodium intake without your doctor's supervision. See Lithium, page 162.

### Recommendations during pregnancy:
- Although still controversial, most dietitians recommend a sodium intake of 3 to 5g/day.
- Sodium restriction below 1g is not recommended during pregnancy.
- Inform your doctor if you are restricting sodium.
- Do not use sodium-containing antacids, such as sodium bicarbonate, during pregnancy.
- If you take lithium, don't change your sodium intake without your doctor's supervision. See Lithium, page 162.

### Recommendations during lactation:
- Although still controversial, most dietitians recommend a sodium intake of 3 to 5g/day.
- If you take lithium, don't change your sodium intake without your doctor's supervision. See Lithium, page 162.

 ## Interactions

### Interactions with medications, vitamins and minerals:

| Interacts with | Combined effect |
| --- | --- |
| Lithium | Changes in sodium intake alter lithium excretion. |
| Potassium | Sodium-to-potassium ratio should not exceed 1:1. |

### Interactions with other substances:
- None reported.

*See Glossary.

VITAMIN/MINERAL

# Thiamine

**Definition and description:** Functions as a coenzyme in energy metabolism. Keeps your appetite, digestive tract and nervous system healthy.

**Other names:** Thiamine pyrophosphate, vitamin $B_1$.

 ## Dosage

### Requirement:
- Non-pregnant woman (15 to 22 years)—1.1mg.
- Non-pregnant woman (23 to 50 years)—1mg.
- Pregnant woman—1.5 to 1.6mg.
- Lactating woman—1.6 to 1.7mg.

### Safe dosage:
- Up to 5g.

### Toxic dosage:
- 10g.

 ## Possible benefits

### Benefits before pregnancy:
- See *Deficiency before pregnancy.*

### Benefits to mother:
- See *Deficiency in mother.*

### Benefits to fetus:
- See *Deficiency in fetus.*

### Benefits to newborn:
- See *Deficiency in newborn.*

### Benefits during lactation:
- See *Deficiency during lactation.*

 ## Possible effects of deficiency

### Deficiency before pregnancy:
- Deficiency of thiamine causes beriberi* and Wernicke-Korsakoff syndrome*. The symptoms most frequently observed are mental confusion, loss of appetite, muscle weakness, loss of balance, swelling and enlarged heart.

### Deficiency in mother:
- Wernicke's encephalopathy* has been reported in women with excessive vomiting. Permanent damage can occur if supplementation with thiamine is not initiated.

### Deficiency in fetus:
- If a mother is severely thiamine deficient, the child can be born with thiamine deficiency.

### Deficiency in newborn:
- Thiamine deficiency in infants can cause cardiac failure and death.

### Deficiency during lactation:
- Levels of thiamine in breast milk are affected by the mother's thiamine stores and dietary intake.
- Infantile beriberi* has been seen in seemingly well-nourished mothers with thiamine-deficient diets.

 ## Possible adverse effects

### Effects before pregnancy:
- Adverse effects of headache, irritability, rapid pulse, trembling and weakness occur with high doses.

### Effects on mother:
- See *Effects before pregnancy.*

### Effects on fetus:
- None reported.

### Effects on newborn:
- None reported.

### Effects during lactation:
- None reported.

 ## Additional information

- Reports of adverse effects are more common with thiamine injections than oral dosages of thiamine.

## Recommendations for use

### Women considering pregnancy:
- Eat a well-balanced diet containing enriched and whole grains, fortified cereal, pork, soybeans, black-eyed peas, pasta, almonds, dried peas and beans.
- Thiamine supplementation is generally not necessary.

### Recommendations during pregnancy:
- Eat a well-balanced diet containing enriched and whole grains, fortified cereal, pork, soybeans, black-eyed peas, pasta, almonds, dried peas and beans.
- Thiamine supplementation is generally not necessary during pregnancy.
- If you have excessive vomiting, thiamine supplementation is indicated.

### Recommendations during lactation:
- Eat a well-balanced diet containing enriched and whole grains, fortified cereal, pork, soybeans, black-eyed peas, pasta, almonds, dried peas and beans.
- Thiamine supplementation is generally not necessary during lactation.

 ## Interactions

### Interactions with medications, vitamins and minerals:

| Interacts with | Combined effect |
| --- | --- |
| Pyridoxine | Massive doses of thiamine increase the need for pyridoxine. |
| Riboflavin | Massive doses of thiamine increase the need for riboflavin. |

### Interactions with other substances:
- Raw fish contains an enzyme that breaks down thiamine. Thiamine is then inactive in your body.
- Large amounts of tea can interfere with thiamine absorption.
- Alcohol decreases thiamine absorption and increases metabolism of thiamine.

*See Glossary.

VITAMIN/MINERAL

# Vitamin A

**Definition and description:** Maintains mucous membranes. Helps you see in dim light and prevents xerophthalmia\*. Essential to the tissues lining lungs, digestive organs and genitourinary tract. Helps bones grow normally. Maintains membranes of body cells. Important for reproduction.

**Other names:** There are two forms of vitamin A (preformed or retinol) and a precursor form called *carotene.* Carotene is converted to vitamin A in your liver. Retinol, retinoic acid, carotenoids, carotene, beta-carotene, vitamin-A palmitate, vitamin-A acetate. Vitamin-A analogs include isotretinoin (Accutane®), tretinoin (Retin-A®), 13-cis-retinoic acid. See Isotretinoin, page 154.

 ## Dosage

**Requirement:**
- Non-pregnant woman—800mcg retinol equivalents (R.E.) or 4,000 International units (I.U.).
- Pregnant woman—1,000mcg R.E. or 5,000 I.U.
- Lactating woman—1,200mcg R.E. or 6,000 I.U.

**Safe dosage:**
- Up to 8,000 I.U. of retinol.
- Excessive carotene intake is not harmful but can cause yellow coloration of the skin. This disappears when dose is reduced.

**Toxic dosage:**
- 25,000 I.U.

 ## Possible benefits

**Benefits before pregnancy:**
- Vitamin A and beta-carotene may be beneficial for reducing and treating cancer.

**Benefits to mother:**
- See *Benefits before pregnancy.*

**Benefits to fetus:**
- See *Deficiency in fetus.*

**Benefits to newborn:**
- See *Deficiency in newborn.*

**Benefits during lactation:**
- See *Benefits before pregnancy.*

 ## Possible effects of deficiency

**Deficiency before pregnancy:**
- Vitamin-A deficiency causes night blindness and reduced ability to resist infections.

**Deficiency in mother:**
- Vitamin-A deficiency may increase the risk of abruptio placenta\*.

**Deficiency in fetus:**
- Vitamin-A deficiency produces congenital malformations, including small brains, blindness, cleft lips\*, xerophthalmia\*, anophthalmia\*, mental retardation, skeletal defects, abnormal tooth development and eye defects.
- Vitamin-A deficiency may be associated with a higher prevalence of premature births and prenatal growth retardation.

**Deficiency in newborn:**
- Vitamin-A deficiency causes xerophthalmia\* and, if not treated, blindness.

**Deficiency during lactation:**
- Breast milk is affected by the level of vitamin-A stores and the vitamin-A content of the mother's diet.
- Supplemental vitamin A increases a mother's level of vitamin A and the vitamin-A content of her breast milk.
- See *Deficiency before pregnancy.*

## Possible adverse effects

### Effects before pregnancy:
- The most-frequently observed symptoms of vitamin-A toxicity are increased brain- and spinal-fluid pressure causing bulging forehead in infants and children, headache in adults, lack of appetite, nausea, vomiting and skin breakdown.

### Effects on mother:
- See *Effects before pregnancy.*

### Effects on fetus:
- Excessive vitamin A may cause malformed fetuses and kidney abnormalities.
- Isotretinoin (Accutane®)—a vitamin-A synthetic or analog) taken early in pregnancy leads to a high risk of miscarriage and congenital malformations, including small, malformed or absent ears, cleft palate*, cortical blindness*, abnormalities of blood vessels and water on the brain. See Isotretinoin, page 154.

### Effects on newborn:
- See *Effects on fetus.*

### Effects during lactation:
- See *Effects before pregnancy.*

 ## Additional information

- Vitamin-A analogs or synthetics—isotretinoin (Accutane®), page 154, and tretinoin (Retin-A®)—are used as medications. There is adequate evidence Accutane® is associated with problems in pregnancy, but there is only speculative evidence that Retin-A is associated with problems in pregnancy. However, at this time the benefits of consuming Retin-A do not outweigh the possible risks.
- There is twice as much vitamin A in colostrum (early milk) as in mature milk.
- Vitamin-A deficiency in infants and young children is a major cause of blindness.

 ## Recommendations for use

### Women considering pregnancy:
- Eat a well-balanced diet. See Appendix 1, page 375, for a list of foods that contain high amounts of vitamin A.
- Discontinue use of isotretinoin (Accutane®) and tretinoin (Retin-A®) for 3 months before attempting pregnancy.
- Levels of vitamin A above 25,000 I.U. are not recommended.
- Consult your doctor if you take vitamin A above recommended daily allowances.

### Recommendations during pregnancy:
- Eat a well-balanced diet. See Appendix 1, page 375, for a list of foods that contain high amounts of vitamin A.
- Discontinue use of isotretinoin (Accutane®) and tretinoin (Retin-A®) immediately!
- Consult your doctor if you were taking isotretinoin when you conceived.
- Levels of vitamin A above 8,000 I.U. are not recommended.
- Consult your doctor if you take vitamin A above recommended daily allowances.

### Recommendations during lactation:
- Eat a well-balanced diet. See Appendix 1, page 375, for a list of foods that contain high amounts of vitamin A.
- Discontinue use of isotretinoin (Accutane®) and tretinoin (Retin-A®).
- Levels of vitamin A above 25,000 I.U. are not recommended.
- Consult your doctor if you take vitamin A above recommended daily allowances.

VITAMIN/MINERAL

# Vitamin A, continued

 **Interactions**

**Interactions with medications, vitamins and minerals:**

| Interacts with | Combined effect |
|---|---|
| **Cholestyramine** | Decreases vitamin-A absorption. |
| **Colestipol** | Can lower blood-vitamin-A levels. |
| **Mineral oil** | Decreases vitamin-A absorption. |

| | |
|---|---|
| **Oral contraceptives** | Increases blood vitamin-A levels. |
| **Vitamin C** | Large doses of vitamin A may cause deficiency. |
| **Vitamin E** | Large doses of vitamin A may cause deficiency. |
| **Vitamin K** | Large doses of vitamin A may cause deficiency. |

**Interactions with other substances:**

• Cigarette smoking reduces blood-vitamin-A levels.

*See Glossary.

**Definition and description:** Vitamin B12 is a group of cobalt-containing enzymes involved as a coenzyme in many reactions, including the breakdown of certain amino acids and the utilization of folate. Helps metabolize carbohydrates and fats. Also helps produce blood cells, body cells and the covering of nerve fibers. Vitamin B12 is broken down into cobalamin, which combines with a special protein called *intrinsic factor*. It cannot be absorbed into the body until it is combined with an intrinsic factor.

**Other names:** Cobalamin, methylcobalamin, adenosylcobalamin, hydroxycobalamin, cyanocobalamin.

 ## Dosage

**Requirement:**
- Non-pregnant woman—3mcg.
- Pregnant woman—4mcg.
- Lactating woman—4mcg.

**Safe dosage:**
- Appears safe at levels 10,000 times above requirement.

**Toxic dosage:**
- None reported.

 ## Possible benefits

**Benefits before pregnancy:**
- See *Deficiency before pregnancy.*

**Benefits to mother:**
- See *Deficiency in mother.*

**Benefits to fetus:**
- See *Deficiency in fetus.*

**Benefits to newborn:**
- None reported.

**Benefits during lactation:**
- See *Deficiency during lactation.*

 ## Possible effects of deficiency

**Deficiency before pregnancy:**
- Vitamin-B12 deficiency may cause infertility.
- Deficiency causes weakness, fatigue, sore tongue, poor appetite, weight loss and changes in the way foods taste.

**Deficiency in mother:**
- See *Deficiency before pregnancy.*

**Deficiency in fetus:**
- Fetal death increases in mothers with a vitamin-B12 deficiency.

**Deficiency in newborn:**
- None reported in humans.
- Deficiency of vitamin B12 can cause low birth weight and an increase in stillbirths in rats.

**Deficiency during lactation:**
- Breast-milk vitamin B12 content varies proportionately with stores and dietary intake of the mother.
- Megaloblastic anemia* can occur if the mother is B12-deficient. Vitamin B12 supplementation can prevent megaloblastic anemia*, which is fatal if untreated.
- Vegetarian mothers are at risk to develop B12 deficiency and megaloblastic anemia*.

 ## Possible adverse effects

**Effects before pregnancy:**
- None reported.

**Effects on mother:**
- None reported.

**Effects on fetus:**
- None reported in humans.
- Large doses of vitamin A (retinol) can produce cleft palate* and other facial changes in animals.

# Vitamin B₁₂, continued

## Effects on newborn:
• None reported.

## Effects during lactation:
• None reported.

## Recommendations for use

### Women considering pregnancy:
• Eat a diet containing meat, poultry, fish, eggs and dairy products. Vitamin B₁₂ is only contained in animal foods or foods fortified with vitamin B₁₂.
• Supplement if you have a defect in B₁₂ absorption or are a strict vegetarian.
• Supplements are given as an injection if you have a defect in B₁₂ absorption.

### Recommendations during pregnancy:
• Eat a diet containing meat, poultry, fish, eggs and dairy products. Vitamin B₁₂ is only contained in animal foods or foods fortified with vitamin B₁₂.
• Supplement if you have a defect in B₁₂ absorption or are a strict vegetarian.
• Supplements are given as an injection if you have a defect in B₁₂ absorption.

### Recommendations during lactation:
• Eat a diet containing meat, poultry, fish, eggs and dairy products. Vitamin B₁₂ is only contained in animal foods or foods fortified with vitamin B₁₂.
• Supplement if you have a defect in B₁₂ absorption or are a strict vegetarian.
• Supplements are given as an injection if you have a defect in B₁₂ absorption.

## Interactions

### Interactions with medications, vitamins and minerals:

| Interacts with | Combined effect |
| --- | --- |
| Barbituates | Decreases blood B₁₂ levels. |
| Cholestyramine | Can decrease absorption of B₁₂ and decrease blood B₁₂ levels. |
| Methotrexate | Decreases absorption and blood B₁₂ levels. |
| Neomycin | Decreases blood B₁₂ levels. |
| Oral contraceptives | Decreases blood B₁₂ levels. |
| Phenobarbital | Decreases blood and central-spinal-fluid levels of B₁₂. |
| Phenytoin | Decreases blood and central-spinal-fluid levels of B₁₂. |
| Vitamin C | Vitamin C supplementation greater than 500mg may cause depletion of vitamin B₁₂. |

### Interactions with other substances:
• Cigarette smokers have lower levels of vitamin B₁₂ than non-smokers.
• Heavy use of alcohol decreases B₁₂ absorption.

*See Glossary.

**Definition and description:** The role of vitamin C in the body has not been well-defined. It is implicated in the formation of connective tissue, formulation of brain chemicals, synthesis of steroid hormones, maintenance of white blood cells, metabolism of folate and breakdown of proteins. May be important in wound healing. Plays a part in medication metabolism.

**Other names:** Ascorbic acid, dehydroascorbic acid.

 ## Dosage

**Requirement:**
- Non-pregnant woman—60mg.
- Pregnant woman—80mg.
- Lactating woman—100mg.

**Safe dosage:**
- Up to 400mg.

**Toxic dosage:**
- 1g.

 ## Possible benefits

**Benefits before pregnancy:**
- Vitamin-C supplementation may slightly decrease the duration of the common cold.

**Benefits to mother:**
- See *Benefits before pregnancy.*

**Benefits to fetus:**
- See *Deficiency in fetus.*

**Benefits to newborn:**
- See *Deficiency in fetus.*

**Benefits during lactation:**
- See *Deficiency during lactation.*

 ## Possible effects of deficiency

**Deficiency before pregnancy:**
- Vitamin-C deficiency causes scurvy*, a potentially fatal disease characterized by weakening of connective tissues, resulting in small-blood-vessel hemorrhaging.

**Deficiency in mother:**
- See *Deficiency before pregnancy.*

**Deficiency in fetus:**
- Adequate vitamin C intake and stores during pregnancy are important for the prevention of premature births and possibly miscarriages.

**Deficiency in newborn:**
- None reported.

**Deficiency during lactation:**
- Vitamin-C content of breast milk varies with dietary intake. Breast milk is able to adjust to lower vitamin-C content.
- Vitamin-C supplementation can increase the amount of vitamin C in breast milk.

 ## Possible adverse effects

**Effects before pregnancy:**
- Kidney stones, diarrhea and iron overload may occur at 1g or higher.
- Impaired ability to fight bacterial infections and withdrawal symptoms may occur at 2g.
- Reduced resistance to high altitudes may occur at 3g or higher.

**Effects on mother:**
- See *Effects before pregnancy.*

**Effects on fetus:**
- Very high intakes early in pregnancy may result in an increase in miscarriages.
- Excessive vitamin-C intake may increase fetal abnormalities.

# Vitamin C, continued

## Effects on newborn:
- Large doses of vitamin C in pregnancy increase the need for vitamin C in the newborn. Some infants have developed scurvy* after birth. Their enzymes for metabolizing vitamin C are activated because of the high levels of vitamin C in the mother's blood. After birth these enzymes continue to metabolize vitamin C at an accelerated rate.

## Effects during lactation:
- Vitamin-C supplementation to 1g in the mother does not increase breast-milk vitamin-C levels.
- No reports of the effect of higher levels of supplementation.

 **Recommendations for use**

### Women considering pregnancy:
- Eat a well-balanced diet. See Appendix 1, page 375, for a list of foods that contain high amounts of vitamin C.

### Recommendations during pregnancy:
- Eat a well-balanced diet. See Appendix 1, page 375, for a list of foods that contain high amounts of vitamin C.
- Avoid consuming more than 400mg of vitamin C a day, especially during the third trimester.
- If you take extra vitamin C, tell your baby's doctor so your baby can be observed for signs of vitamin-C deficiency.

### Recommendations during lactation:
- Eat a well-balanced diet. See Appendix 1, page 375, for a list of foods that contain high amounts of vitamin C.

 **Interactions**

### Interactions with medications, vitamins and minerals:

| Interacts with | Combined effect |
| --- | --- |
| Adrenal corticosteroids | Increases need for vitamin C. |
| Amphetamines | Excess vitamin C decreases amphetamine absorption. |
| Barbiturates | Increases amount of vitamin C lost in urine. |
| Copper | Vitamin-C intake above 1.5g reduces blood copper levels. |
| Iron | Increases the absorption of iron if the meal contains 25 to 75mg of vitamin C. |
| Oral contraceptives | Decreases blood-vitamin-C levels. |
| Salicylates | Decreases blood-vitamin-C levels. |
| Selenium | Decreases blood-vitamin-C levels. |
| Vitamin A | Large doses of vitamin A may cause a vitamin-C deficiency |
| Vitamin B$_{12}$ | Excess vitamin C destroys B$_{12}$. |

### Interactions with other substances:
- Excess vitamin C makes sugar-urine tests inaccurate.
- Cigarette smoking decreases blood-vitamin-C levels.

*See Glossary.

**Definition and description:** Promotes intestinal absorption of calcium and phosphate. May also influence the process of bone mineralization. Vitamin D is essential for normal bone growth and development.

**Other names:** Vitamin D2 (ergocalciferol), vitamin D3 (cholecalciferol), 1,25-dihydroxyergocalciferol, 1,25-dihydroxyvitamin D3 (calcitriol), synthetic vitamin-D analogue, dihydrotachysterol, calcifediol.

 ## Dosage

**Requirement:**
- Non-pregnant (15 to 18 years)—l0mcg.
- Non-pregnant (19 to 22 years)—7.5mcg.
- Non-pregnant (23 to 50 years)—5mcg.
- Pregnant woman—10 to 15mcg.
- Lactating woman—l0 to 15mcg.

**Safe dosage:**
- Up to 15mcg (up to 600 I.U.).

**Toxic dosage:**
- 50mcg (2,000 I.U.).

 ## Possible benefits

**Benefits before pregnancy:**
- See *Deficiency before pregnancy.*

**Benefits to mother:**
- See *Deficiency in mother.*

**Benefits to fetus:**
- See *Deficiency in fetus.*

**Benefits to newborn:**
- See *Deficiency in newborn.*

**Benefits during lactation:**
- See *Deficiency during lactation.*

 ## Possible effects of deficiency

**Deficiency before pregnancy:**
- In the absence of vitamin D, deposits of calcium and phosphate into bones is impaired. The result is rickets* in children and osteomalacia* in adults. These diseases are still common in third-world countries.

**Deficiency in mother:**
- Vitamin-D deficiency can cause decreased weight gain and pelvic deformities that prevent normal vaginal delivery.

**Deficiency in fetus:**
- Vitamin-D deficiency in the mother can cause low calcium levels and rickets* in the fetus and newborn.
- Low calcium level is associated with convulsions.
- Abnormal tooth development has been seen in infants whose mothers had inadequate intake of vitamin A, D, protein and calories during pregnancy.

**Deficiency in newborn:**
- Babies with rickets* can have convulsions and growth failure.
- Vitamin-D deficiency in the mother can cause low calcium levels and rickets* in the fetus and newborn.
- Abnormal tooth development has been seen in infants whose mothers had inadequate intake of vitamin A, D, protein and calories during pregnancy.

**Deficiency during lactation:**
- Low vitamin-D intake decreases the amount of vitamin D in breast milk.
- Dark-skinned infants or infants in climates where sunlight is minimal may be at significant risk for rickets*. These infants may need vitamin-D supplementation in addition to breast milk.
- Vitamin-D supplementation is very important when a baby is born with rickets*.

# Vitamin D, continued

## Possible adverse effects

### Effects before pregnancy:
- Vitamin D is the most toxic vitamin. Symptoms of toxicity include loss of appetite, nausea, vomiting, abdominal pain, excessive urination, excessive thirst and headache.
- At high levels, confusion, loss of consciousness and death can occur.

### Effects on mother:
- See *Effects before pregnancy.*

### Effects on fetus:
- Excessive vitamin-D intake by the mother may be associated with high calcium levels in the infant, head-bone abnormalities, heart abnormalities, lung abnormalities, high blood pressure, mental retardation, hernia*, abnormal sex characteristics and high levels of calcium in the kidney.

### Effects on newborn:
- Vitamin D above the RDA may cause slowing of growth, failure to thrive, kidney malfunction and severe mental retardation.

### Effects during lactation:
- Large doses of vitamin D taken by the mother may lead to greater-than-normal vitamin-D levels in breast milk and high calcium levels in the infant. Symptoms of high calcium levels include loss of appetite, vomiting, excessive thirst, weight loss and failure to thrive.

## Additional information

- 10mcg of vitamin D (cholecalciferol) is equal to 400 I.U. of vitamin D.
- Vitamin D requirements depend on sun exposure and skin color. Light skin and more sun exposure provide increased vitamin D.

## Recommendations for use

### Women considering pregnancy:
- Eat a diet that includes salmon, sardines, herring and mackerel. Drink vitamin-D-fortified milk.
- If you are dark-skinned and live in a climate with limited sunlight or if you have very limited exposure to the sun, a vitamin-D supplement with no more than 10mcg or 400 I.U. is recommended.
- If you have abnormal parathyroid hormones or take heparin, consult your doctor about vitamin-D supplements.

### Recommendations during pregnancy:
- Eat a diet that includes salmon, sardines, herring, tuna, egg yolks and mackerel. Drink vitamin-D-fortified milk.
- If you are dark-skinned and live in a climate with limited sunlight, a vitamin-D supplement with no more than 15mcg or 600 I.U. is recommended.
- If you have abnormal parathyroid hormones or take heparin, consult your doctor about vitamin-D supplements.

### Recommendations during lactation:
- The Committee on Nutrition of the American Academy of Pediatrics recommends vitamin-D supplements for breast-fed infants if the mother's vitamin D intake is inadequate or if the infant lacks sufficient exposure to sunlight.
- If you have abnormal parathyroid hormones or take heparin, consult your doctor about vitamin-D supplements and the safety of breast-feeding.
- If you take doses of vitamin D above the RDA, inform your baby's doctor, and watch for signs and symptoms of vitamin-D toxicity.

**Interactions**

## Interactions with medications, vitamins and minerals:

| Interacts with | Combined effect |
|---|---|
| Adrenal corti-costeroids | Increases need for vitamin D. |
| Barbiturates | Increases need for vitamin D. |
| Cholestyramine | May decrease vitamin-D absorption. |
| Heparin | May inhibit kidney conversion of vitamin D. Increases need for vitamin-D supplementation. |
| Magnesium | Vitamin D increases magnesium absorption. |
| Mineral oil | Decreases vitamin-D absorption. |
| Phenolphthalein | Decreases vitamin-D absorption. |
| Phenytoin | Increases need for vitamin D. Decreases blood-vitamin-D levels. Increases utilization of vitamin D. |
| Vitamin-A overdose | Increases the toxicity of vitamin-D overdose. |

## Interactions with other substances:

- Vitamin D may increase the calcium around damaged joints in persons with gout* and rheumatoid arthritis*.
- Alcohol interferes with vitamin-D metabolism.

*See Glossary.

VITAMIN/MINERAL

# Vitamin E

**Definition and description:** Helps prevent oxidation, a process that allows certain chemicals in the body to become harmful. Plays a role in the metabolism of polyunsaturated fats, muscle integrity and red-blood-cell integrity.

**Other names:** D1-alpha-tocopherol acetate (most common form in supplements), synthetic free d1-alpha-tocopherol, alpha-tocopherol, d-alpha-tocopherol, tocotrienols.

 **Dosage**

**Requirement:**
- Non-pregnant woman—8mg alpha-tocopherol equivalents.
- Pregnant woman—10mg alpha-tocopherol equivalents.
- Lactating woman—11mg alpha-tocopherol equivalents.

**Safe dosage:**
- Up to 400mg alpha-tocopherol equivalents.

**Toxic dosage:**
- 1,000mg alpha-tocopherol equivalents.

 **Possible benefits**

**Benefits before pregnancy:**
- See *Deficiency before pregnancy.*

**Benefits to mother:**
- Vitamin-E cream or oil may reduce stretch marks.

**Benefits to fetus:**
- None reported.

**Benefits to newborn:**
- Vitamin E has been used in premature infants to prevent eye damage caused by oxygen therapy.

**Benefits during lactation:**
- Vitamin-E cream may reduce breast and nipple soreness. Clean breasts before nursing.

 **Possible effects of deficiency**

**Deficiency before pregnancy:**
- None reported in humans.
- Deficiency of vitamin E can cause sterility in rats.

**Deficiency in mother:**
- None reported in humans.
- In rats, deficiency of vitamin E can increase lethargy, difficulty breathing, vaginal bleeding and death after delivery.

**Deficiency in fetus:**
- None reported in humans.
- In rats, a deficiency of vitamin E can cause an increase in miscarriages, stillbirths and congenital malformations, including no brain, hernia*, club foot*, cleft lip*, webs between fingers and scoliosis*.

**Deficiency in newborn:**
- Vitamin-E deficiency may cause anemia* and bleeding. Risk for deficiency is greater in premature infants.

**Deficiency during lactation:**
- None reported.

 **Possible adverse effects**

**Effects before pregnancy:**
- Excessive doses of vitamin E may cause nausea, gastric distress, diarrhea, chapped lips, hives*, thrombophlebitis*, fatique, breast enlargement, elevation in blood triglycerides (fats) and high blood pressure.

**Effects on mother:**
- See *Effects before pregnancy.*

### Effects on fetus:
- None reported in humans.
- In rats, large doses of vitamin E can cause eye abnormalities.

### Effects on newborn:
- None reported.

### Effects during lactation:
- Excessive vitamin E increases vitamin E in breast milk.
- Vitamin-E cream applied to breasts can raise the blood-vitamin-E levels of infants. This is *not* recommended.

 **Additional information**

- 1mg d1-alpha-tocopherol acetate equals 1 I.U.
- 1mg synthetic free d1-alpha-tocopherol has 1.1 I.U.
- 1mg alpha-tocopherol and d-alpha-tocopherol have 1.49 I.U.

 **Recommendations for use**

### Women considering pregnancy:
- Eat a well-balanced diet. Good sources of vitamin E include vegetable oils, wheat germ, spinach, collards, nuts and dried beans.
- Supplementation is not necessary.

### Recommendations during pregnancy:
- Eat a well-balanced diet. Good sources of vitamin E include vegetable oils, wheat germ, spinach, collards, nuts and dried beans.
- Supplementation is not necessary.

### Recommendations during lactation:
- Eat a well-balanced diet. Good sources of vitamin E include vegetable oils, wheat germ, spinach, collards, nuts and dried beans.
- Supplementation is not necessary for full-term babies.
- Consult your baby's doctor about supplementation if your baby is born prematurely.

 **Interactions**

**Interactions with medications, vitamins and minerals:**

| Interacts with | Combined effect |
| --- | --- |
| Coumadin | Excessive vitamin E may increase effects of coumadin. |
| Iron | Vitamin-E requirements may increase in women taking high amounts of iron. |
| Mineral oil | May decrease amount of vitamin E absorbed. |
| Vitamin A | Large doses of vitamin A may cause vitamin-E deficiency. |
| Vitamin D | High doses of vitamin E may increase vitamin-D requirements. |
| Vitamin K | Vitamin E may increase the effects of vitamin-K deficiency by increasing the amount of time it takes for blood to clot. |

**Interactions with other substances:**
- An increase in linoleic acid (a polyunsaturated fat) increases vitamin-E requirement. This is rarely a problem because most sources of linoleic acid also contain vitamin E.

*See Glossary.

VITAMIN/MINERAL

# Vitamin K

**Definition and description:** Involved in manufacturing of blood-clotting factors in the liver. Vitamin K is produced in the large intestine.

**Other names:** Vitamin K$_1$ (phylloquinone), vitamin K$_2$ (menaquinones), synthetic vitamin K (phytonadione), vitamin K$_3$ (menadione), vitamin K$_4$ (menadial).

 ## Dosage

### Requirement:
- About half of the vitamin K is made in the intestine.
- No specific requirement because of intestine's role in manufacturing vitamin K.

### Safe dosage:
- Estimated safe and adequate intake 70 to 140mcg.

### Toxic dosage:
- 20mg.

 ## Possible benefits

### Benefits before pregnancy:
- See *Deficiency before pregnancy.*

### Benefits to mother:
- See *Deficiency before pregnancy.*

### Benefits to fetus:
- Oral doses of vitamin K given to the mother during the last few weeks of pregnancy helps prevent hemorrhagic disease* of the newborn.

### Benefits to newborn:
- Newborns in the United States and Canada receive injections of vitamin K at birth to prevent hemmorrhagic disease* of the newborn.

### Benefits during lactation:
- See *Deficiency during lactation.*

 ## Possible effects of deficiency

### Deficiency before pregnancy:
- Vitamin-K deficiency is very rare because the body produces vitamin K in the large intestine. Deficiencies are seen when there are conditions that cause malabsorption, damage to the intestine or medications that interfere with vitamin-K's function. In any of these cases, excessive bleeding can occur, and vitamin-K functions should be closely monitored.

### Deficiency in mother:
- See *Deficiency before pregnancy.*

### Deficiency in fetus:
- None reported.

### Deficiency in newborn:
- The newborn's sterile intestine is unable to produce vitamin K. Hemmorrhagic disease* of the newborn may develop without supplementation.

### Deficiency during lactation:
- Vitamin-K content of breast milk is affected by the mother's dietary intake.
- Vitamin-K supplementation of the newborn is recommended, even when the mother supplements her diet with vitamin K.
- Breast-fed infants may be at greater risk for deficiency because their intestinal bacteria may produce less vitamin K.

 ## Possible adverse effects

### Effects before pregnancy:
- Vitamin K$_3$ (menadione) can cause anemia* and liver damage.

### Effects on mother:
- See *Effects before pregnancy.*

### Effects on fetus:
- Parenteral* doses of synthetic vitamin K3 (menadione) in the mother have been associated with hyperbilirubinemia* and kernicterus* of premature infants and severe hyperbilirubinemia* in full-term infants.

### Effects on newborn:
- See *Effects on fetus.*

### Effects during lactation:
- None reported.

 ## Additional information

- Cystic fibrosis* can cause malabsorption of vitamin K. Functioning levels should be closely monitored in these cases.

 ## Recommendations for use

### Women considering pregnancy:
- Eat a diet containing green, leafy vegetables.
- Take vitamin-K supplements only with your doctor's advice.

### Recommendations during pregnancy:
- Eat a diet containing green, leafy vegetables.
- Take vitamin-K supplements only with your doctor's advice.
- Vitamin-K supplements are unnecessary during pregnancy, except in women who are at risk for vitamin-K deficiency.
- Oral supplementation of vitamin K has been suggested for women on anticonvulsant therapy. But the effectiveness of this therapy has not been established. Consult your doctor.

### Recommendations during lactation:
- The American Academy of Pediatrics recommends all infants, especially breast-fed infants, receive 0.5 to 1.0mg of phytonadione at birth.
- Larger and/or repeat doses may be required for infants whose mothers take anticonvulsants or oral anticoagulants. Consult your baby's doctor.

 ## Interactions

### Interactions with medications, vitamins and minerals:

| Interacts with | Combined effect |
|---|---|
| Anticoagulants | Vitamin K may interfere with effectiveness of anticoagulants. Deficiency of vitamin K increases the effectiveness of anticoagulants. |
| Chloramphenicol | Changes the bacteria in the intestine. May decrease vitamin-K production. |
| Cholestyramine | Decreases vitamin-K absorption. |
| Metharbital | Can cause vitamin-K deficiency in infants born to mothers taking metharbital during pregnancy. |
| Mineral oil | Decreases vitamin-K absorption. |
| Neomycin | Decreases vitamin-K absorption. |
| Phenobarbital | Increases vitamin-K utilization. |
| Phenytoin | Increases vitamin-K utilization. |
| Primidone | Increases vitamin-K utilization. |
| Sulphonamides | Changes bacteria in the intestine. May decrease vitamin-K production. |
| Vitamin A | Large doses of vitamin A may cause a vitamin-K deficiency. |

### Interactions with other substances:
- None reported.

*See Glossary.

# Zinc

**Definition and description:** An essential trace element for humans. It is involved in many functions, such as protein production, bone building, making DNA and RNA (keepers of the body's genetic information), tasting, smelling and wound healing.

**Other names:** Zinc sulfate, zinc chloride, zinc acetate, zinc gluconate, chelated zinc, zinc oxide and pyrithione.

 ## Dosage

### Requirement:
- Non-pregnant woman—15mg.
- Pregnant woman—20mg.
- Lactating woman—25mg.

### Safe dosage:
- Up to 25mg/day of zinc.

### Toxic dosage:
- 33mg has been shown to cause toxic effects.
- Overdose can be fatal.

 ## Possible benefits

### Benefits before pregnancy:
- See *Deficiency before pregnancy.*

### Benefits to mother:
- See *Deficiency in mother.*

### Benefits to fetus:
- See *Deficiency in fetus.*

### Benefits to newborn:
- See *Deficiency in newborn.*

### Benefits during lactation:
- See *Deficiency during lactation.*

 ## Possible effects of deficiency

### Deficiency before pregnancy:
- Women of childbearing age eat an inadequate amount of zinc and may be marginally zinc-deficient. Marginal zinc deficiency may affect appetite, mood and senses of taste and smell. Other symptoms may include skin scaliness, delayed wound healing, depression, fatigue, hair loss, diarrhea and reduced resistance to infection.

### Deficiency in mother:
- The incidence of pregnancy-induced hypertension* may be higher in women with a low dietary intake of zinc. See *Deficiency before pregnancy.*

### Deficiency in fetus:
- Blood-zinc levels of women who miscarry may be lower than average.
- Severely zinc-deficient mothers may be more likely to have infants with birth defects.
- Infants born with fetal alcohol syndrome* (associated with high alcohol intake) have very low blood-zinc levels and more birth defects.

### Deficiency in newborn:
- Zinc deficiency may be a possible cause of dwarfism*, gonadal immaturity* and anemia* in young children. Adequate zinc intake might prevent these problems.
- Infants fed only breast milk for longer than 6 months may become zinc-deficient.

### Deficiency during lactation:
- The amount of zinc in breast milk is decreased in mothers with very low dietary zinc intakes. This effect is most apparent with longer periods of lactation.
- Infants fed only breast milk for longer than 6 months may become zinc-deficient.

 ## Possible adverse effects

### Effects before pregnancy:
- Toxic doses of zinc cause vomiting, diarrhea, restlessness, stomach irritation, depressed immune function and anemia*.

- Excessive zinc doses may decrease the level of HDL ("good") cholesterol and increase the risk for heart disease.

### Effects on mother:
- See *Effects before pregnancy*.

### Effects on fetus:
- Very high doses of zinc in the mother have been shown to cause fetal growth retardation and increased fetal death.

### Effects on newborn:
- None reported.

### Effects during lactation:
- Toxic doses do not appear to affect zinc levels in breast milk. See *Effects before pregnancy*.

 ## Additional information

- Zinc sulfate, zinc chloride, zinc acetate, zinc gluconate or chelated zinc for oral or topical treatment. Zinc oxide and pyrithione are available for topical use.

 ## Recommendations for use

### Women considering pregnancy:
- Eat a diet containing at least 15mg of zinc, or take a supplement.
- See Appendix 1, page 375, for a list of foods that contain high amounts of zinc.

### Recommendations during pregnancy:
- Eat a diet containing at least 20mg of zinc, or take a supplement.
- See Appendix 1, page 375, for a list of foods that contain high amounts of zinc.
- Doses above 25mg are not suggested during pregnancy.
- Take supplements only under your doctor's supervision.

### Recommendations during lactation:
- Eat a diet containing 25mg of zinc, or take a supplement.
- See Appendix 1, page 375, for a list of foods that contain high amounts of zinc.

 ## Interactions

**Interactions with medications, vitamins and minerals:**

| Interacts with | Combined effect |
| --- | --- |
| Calcium | At low calcium intakes, zinc may interfere with calcium absorption. |
| Copper | More than 50mg/day of zinc interferes with copper absorption. |
| Cortisone | May increase amount of zinc lost in urine. |
| Folate | High folate levels interfere with zinc absorption. Folate deficiency increases blood-zinc levels. |
| HDL cholesterol | May lower "good" HDL cholesterol at doses above 80mg. |
| Iron | Interferes with zinc absorption. Zinc may interfere with iron absorption. |
| Tetracycline | Decreases tetracycline absorption. |
| Valproic acid | Binds with zinc. May lower blood zinc levels. |

**Interactions with other substances:**
- Fiber in food interferes with zinc absorption.
- Fiber in unleavened bread interferes with zinc absorption more than leavened bread.
- Alcohol increases the amount of zinc lost in urine.
- Marijuana decreases concentration of zinc in fetal blood.
- Cigarette smoking reduces the amount of zinc in the placenta.

*See Glossary.

Note: This page purposely left blank.

# Other Substances

Some of the substances you may take during pregnancy and while breast-feeding are not covered under the previous sections. We include them here. Some products should be used with care because, in many cases, we do not have enough data to predict how they can affect you or your growing baby.

Other substances listed in this section should be avoided during pregnancy and lactation. Many negative consequences, such as birth defects and problems in the newborn, have been found among children born to women who used them during pregnancy.

If you have a problem with addiction to any of these substances, contact your doctor as soon as you think you might be pregnant. Your health and the health of your unborn baby may be affected if you continue to use these substances.

Be sure you check with your doctor about use of *any* products you are concerned about.

# Alcohol

**Definition and description:** A colorless, pungent liquid used as an intoxicating ingredient in fermented liquors.

**Other names:** Ethanol.

## Safe dosage:
• Safe-dosage level has not been determined.

## Toxic dosage:
• Exact toxic dose cannot be determined. Toxic level for fetus varies depending on many maternal factors, including presence and duration of alcoholism, dietary intake, cigarette and marijuana smoking, medications and caffeine ingestion.

 **Possible benefits**

## Benefits before pregnancy:
• None reported.

## Benefits to mother:
• None reported.

## Benefits to fetus:
• Alcohol can suppress the activity of the uterus and may suppress premature delivery. However, other medications are more effective. Your doctor should always assess the reasons for premature contractions or labor. Alcohol is usually not used for this purpose.

## Benefits to newborn:
• See *Effects on newborn.*

## Benefits during lactation:
• Small quantities of alcohol are reported to increase breast-milk production because of increased relaxation of the mother and increased letdown reflex*.

 **Possible adverse effects**

## Effects before pregnancy:
• Gynecological surgery, infertility, painful menstruation, heavy menstrual flow and premenstrual discomfort may be increased with the woman's drinking level, especially above 6 drinks a day at least once a week.
• Moderate drinking by the father (2 or more drinks a day) may cause a decrease in birth weight. Infants with lower birth weights have increased problems at birth.
• Over 1,000 or more alcoholic beverages contain a potent cancer-causing agent called *urethane.*

## Effects on mother:
• See *Effects before pregnancy.*

## Effects on fetus:
• Evidence indicates that consuming alcohol during pregnancy may cause birth defects.
• There is a common pattern of malformation in babies of alcoholic mothers called *fetal alcohol syndrome*.* Malformations include mental retardation, poor growth and characteristic facial features, such as small head circumference, small, short noses, indistinct groove between nose and mouth, and a thin upper lip. Other abnormalities may include poorly formed ears, cleft lip*, cleft palate*, small teeth with faulty enamel, benign skin tumors*, restriction in joint movement, poor nail growth, skeletal abnormalities and hernias* in the abdominal region. The percentage of infants having problems associated with fetal alcohol syndrome* is estimated to be 30 to 40% of all infants born to alcoholic mothers. The incidence of fetal alcohol syndrome* is directly related to the amount of alcohol consumed during pregnancy and the duration of the mother's alcoholism.

- The occurrence of congenital heart disease, kidney and genital defects, neural-tube defects* and club foot* may increase in babies born to women who drink.
- Moderate drinking by the father (2 or more drinks a day) may cause a decrease in birth weight.
- Amniotic fluid* appears to maintain alcohol long after alcohol disappears from the mother's blood. The fetus drinks amniotic fluid* and may be exposed to alcohol for much longer periods of time.

### Effects on newborn:

- Congenital heart disease may increase in babies born to women who drink.
- There is a common pattern of malformation in the babies of alcoholic mothers called *fetal alcohol syndrome*\*. See *Effects on fetus.*
- Children born to alcoholic mothers have been found to have significantly lower IQ test scores, excessive stubbornness, aggression, hyperactivity, sleep disorders and impaired sight.

### Effects during lactation:

- Heavy drinking causes mild sedation in infants. Infants are more susceptible to the effects of alcohol because the immature liver cannot metabolize it as rapidly as an adult's liver.
- Large doses of alcohol (greater than 5 ounces of 60-proof) can suppress lactation.
- Alcohol passes freely into breast milk. However, the toxic breakdown product of alcohol—acetaldehyde—apparently does not pass into milk.

 ## Additional information

- Studies have found mothers often reduce their alcohol intake in pregnancy but return to their prepregnancy levels by 1 year after delivery.

 ## Recommendations for use

### Women considering pregnancy:

- Abstinence from alcohol or a significant reduction in alcohol consumption is recommended for you and your baby's father if you are planning pregnancy.
- Adverse effects of alcohol can occur even before you know you are pregnant.

### Recommendations during pregnancy:

- Do not use alcohol during pregnancy.
- A safe alcohol-intake level has not been established.
- Inform your doctor if you drink heavily now or drank heavily before pregnancy.

### Recommendations during lactation:

- Do not use alcohol during lactation.

# Alcohol, continued

## Interactions

**Interactions with medications, vitamins and minerals:**

| Interacts with | Combined effect |
| --- | --- |
| Acetaminophen | Alcohol may increase risk of liver damagetoxicity. |
| Antihistamines | Increases drowsiness. |
| Antinauseants | Increases drowsiness. |
| Aspirin | Increases stomach irritation and blood loss. May also decrease blood clotting. |
| Barbiturates | Increases risk of malformations. Alcohol decreases effectiveness of barbiturates. Large amounts of alcohol may increase toxicity of barbiturates. Alcohol slows reaction time and increases drowsiness. Combined overdose may be very dangerous. |
| Benzodiazepines | Slows reaction time and increases drowsiness. Combined overdose may be very dangerous. |
| Cephalosporins | May produce facial flushing, difficulty breathing, fast heart rate, low blood pressure, nausea and vomiting. Life-threatening symptoms have rarely occurred. |
| Cimetidine | May decrease liver elimination of alcohol. |
| Disulfram | May produce facial flushing, difficulty breathing, fast heart rate, low blood pressure, nausea and vomiting. Life-threatening symptoms have occurred rarely. |
| Folate | Decreases absorption of folate. Decreases blood folate levels. May cause megaloblastic anemia*. |
| Indomethacin | Increases stomach irritation. Slows reaction time and increases drowsiness. |
| Insulin | Large amounts of alcohol may decrease blood sugar. |
| Iron | Increases iron absorption. Can cause iron overload. |
| Isoniazid (INH) | Increases risk of severe liver damage. Produces facial flushing, difficulty breathing, fast heart rate, low blood pressure, nausea and vomiting. Life-threatening symptoms have occurred rarely. |
| Magnesium | Increases magnesium loss. |
| Metronidazole | Increases risk of developing severe liver damage. Produces facial flushing, difficulty breathing, fast heart rate, low blood pressure, nausea and vomiting. Life-threatening symptoms have occurred rarely. |

| | |
|---|---|
| **Narcotics** | Slows reaction time and increases drowsiness. |
| **Non-acetylated salicylates (salsalates)** | May cause stomach irritation and blood loss. |
| **Oral antidiabetics** | Large amounts of alcohol may decrease blood sugar. Used together, there is an increased risk of malformations. Decreases effectiveness of oral anti-diabetics. May increase toxicity of antidiabetic agents. May produce facial flushing, difficulty breathing, fast heart rate, low blood pressure, nausea and vomiting. Life-threatening symptoms have occurred rarely. |
| **Phenothiazine** | Increases drowsiness. |
| **Phenytoin** | Alcohol decreases effectiveness of phenytoin. Used together, there is an increased risk of malformations. |
| **Potassium** | Increases potassium loss. |
| **Thiamine** | Decreases absorption of thiamine. |
| **Tricyclic anti-depressants** | Slows reaction time. Increases drowsiness. |
| **Vitamin B6** | Decreases absorption and interferes with the activation of vitamin $B_6$. |
| **Vitamin B12** | Decreases absorption of vitamin $B_{12}$. |
| **Vitamin D** | Interferes with the metabolism of vitamin D. |
| **Zinc** | Increases zinc loss. |

**Interactions with other substances:**
- Alcohol can decrease the absorption of fat and protein.
- Use with cigarette smoke causes more-deleterious effects on infant behavior and learning than is expected with either substance alone.
- Use with marijuana may cause more birth defects and fetal death than either substance alone.

*See Glossary.

SUBSTANCE

# Aspartame

**Definition and description:** Artificial sweetener used in drink mixes, gelatin desserts, soft drinks, yogurt-type products, flavored-milk beverages, frozen dairy and non-dairy desserts. It is a combination of two amino acids—*phenylalanine* and *aspartic acid*. When aspartame is metabolized, it breaks down to aspartate, methanol and phenylalanine. Aspartame is 40 times sweeter than the same amount of sugar.

**Other names:** Nutrasweet®, Equal®.

 ## Dosage

### Safe dosage:
- Consumption of 60 cans of aspartame-containing soda all at once did not raise blood levels of toxic substances. The FDA* has set 50mg/kg a day as the upper level of safe consumption.

### Toxic dosage:
- Exact toxic dose cannot be predicted.

 ## Possible benefits

### Benefits before pregnancy:
- May lower intake of calories. Women may not lose weight by lowering calories this way.
- Allows diabetics to lower sugar intake and enjoy foods that taste sweet.

### Benefits to mother:
- None reported.

### Benefits to fetus:
- None reported.

### Benefits to newborn:
- None reported.

### Benefits during lactation:
- None reported.

 ## Possible adverse effects

### Effects before pregnancy:
- People who have phenylketonuria* should not use aspartame. Phenylalanine is one of the breakdown products of aspartame.
- No problems are indicated for other individuals unless they are allergic to aspartame.
- Methanol, one of the breakdown products, is toxic. However, accumulation of high amounts of methanol does not occur, even with an intake of 60 cans of aspartame-containing soda all at once.

### Effects on mother:
- See *Effects before pregnancy*.

### Effects on fetus:
- No reports indicate adverse effects in healthy women. However, women who have phenylketonuria* must follow a low-phenylalanine diet or their babies may be born mentally retarded and show delayed development. Phenylalanine in aspartame contributes to phenylalanine in the diet.
- There are no reports specifically associating aspartame intake with adverse effects in the fetus or infant.
- Some people may carry unknown traits for phenylketonuria*. Excessive intake of aspartame is discouraged.

### Effects on newborn:
- See *Effects on fetus*.

### Effects during lactation:
- None reported.
- If a baby has phenylketonuria*, he or she will have to receive a special formula. Breast-feeding is not possible.

 ## Additional information

- Aspartame breaks down to phenylalanine, aspartic acid and methanol when heated. It no longer tastes sweet.
- Aspartame content in soda and other drinks is 500 to 600mg/liter.
- Aspartame content in foods may vary. If you desire information regarding aspartame content of any product, contact Searle Pharmaceuticals, Inc., Box 5110, Chicago, IL 60680.

## Recommendations for use

### Women considering pregnancy:
- Foods or drinks that contain aspartame do not appear to be hazardous and may be consumed in moderation.

### Recommendations during pregnancy:
- Foods or drinks that contain aspartame do not appear to be hazardous and may be consumed in moderation.
- If you have phenylketonuria* or carry a genetic trait, follow a low-phenylalanine diet. Consult your doctor.

### Recommendations during lactation:
- Foods or drinks that contain aspartame do not appear to be hazardous and may be consumed in moderation during lactation.
- If your baby has phenylketonuria*, consult your baby's doctor. Your baby will be placed on a special formula.

 ## Interactions

### Interactions with medications, vitamins and minerals:
- None reported.

### Interactions with other substances:
- A high-carbohydrate diet may increase the amount of phenylalanine transported to the brain.

*See Glossary.

SUBSTANCE

# Caffeine

**Definition and description:** This chemical, from the methyl-xanthine group, acts as a central-nervous-system stimulant. It may cause smooth-muscle relaxation, skeletal-muscle contraction and loss of body water.

**Other names:** Methyl xanthine.

 ## Dosage

### Safe dosage:
- Greater than 300mg/day (4 cups of coffee) by the mother has been associated with decreased birth weight and smaller head circumference in her baby.
- Drinkers of decaffeinated coffee may have the same effects as those who drink regular coffee.

### Toxic dosage:
- Exact toxic dose cannot be determined.
- Serious toxicity can occur after a single large dose or after frequent smaller doses.
- Toxic dose of caffeine can cause extreme irritability, abnormal heartbeat and confusion.
- Contact your doctor, poison-control center or emergency room if you think you have taken an overdose.

 ## Possible benefits

### Benefits before pregnancy:
- Acts as a stimulant.
- May have a role in in-vitro-fertilization* therapy, making sperm more successful in fertilizing eggs. This is still in the experimental stages.

### Benefits to mother:
- A change in caffeine consumption may temporarily increase the incidence of mild mental confusion and memory loss occurring in pregnancy.
- There may be a lower incidence of pregnancy-induced hypertension* in women who consume caffeine in moderation.

### Benefits to fetus:
- None reported.

### Benefits to newborn:
- Caffeine and theophylline are used to treat breathing problems in premature infants (apnea*).

### Benefits during lactation:
- None reported.

 ## Possible adverse effects

### Effects before pregnancy:
- 6 to 8 cups of coffee a day may be associated with decreased fertility.
- Fibrocystic breast disease* may be associated with caffeine consumption.

### Effects on mother:
- Adverse effects of caffeine, such as sleeplessness, jitteriness and irritability, may occur more quickly in pregnancy. The liver's ability to clear caffeine is greatly reduced during the last 6 months of pregnancy.
- Both coffee and decaffeinated-coffee drinkers have reduced calcium-absorption capabilities.

### Effects on fetus:
- Moderate-to-heavy caffeine use may increase the incidence of low birth weights, miscarriages, premature labor and fetal-breathing rate.

### Effects on newborn:
- Excessive caffeine consumption may increase newborn breathing problems.
- Infants born to mothers who are coffee and decaffeinated-coffee drinkers may have lower weight and lower iron stores.
- Coffee decreases the blood supply to the placenta*.

### Effects during lactation:
- The level of caffeine in breast milk is 1.5 to 3% of the amount of caffeine the mother ingests. If a mother drinks more than 6 to 8 cups of coffee a day, her baby can accumulate enough caffeine to display symptoms, such as irritability and sleeplessness.

- Some components of breast milk suppress or slow the maturation of liver enzymes, which are necessary for metabolizing caffeine. An infant metabolizes caffeine more slowly than an adult, so caffeine accumulates, even though only a small amount passes through breast milk.
- Excessive caffeine may interfere with the mother's milk letdown*.
- Breast milk of coffee and decaffeinated-coffee drinkers contains less calcium than that of non-coffee drinkers.

 **Additional information**

- Frequently used in combination products containing aspirin, phenacetin and codeine.
- Also found in beverages, such as coffee, teas and cola.
- Over 200 over-the-counter medications, foods and beverages contain caffeine.
- Chocolate contains a small amount of caffeine and much larger amounts of another methyl xanthine, theobromine. See Appendix 3, page 381.
- Aminophylline and theophylline are converted to caffeine in the baby's liver.

 **Recommendations for use**

### Women considering pregnancy:

- Due to possible effects on fertility, excessive caffeine intake (more than 600mg/day) is not recommended if you are trying to conceive. See Appendix 3, page 381.

### Recommendations during pregnancy:

- Caffeine consumption greater than 300mg/day is not recommended during pregnancy. Lesser amounts may change the blood supply to the placenta. Decaffeinated coffee may cause the same effects. See Appendix 3, page 381.
- Consult your doctor for recommendations.

### Recommendations during lactation:

- Excessive caffeine intake may cause wakeful, hyperactive infants. If you are concerned about your infant's sleeplessness, it may be beneficial to decrease or eliminate caffeine sources. Decaffeinated coffee may have the same effects. See Appendix 3, page 381.

 **Interactions**

**Interactions with medications, vitamins and minerals:**

| Interacts with | Combined effect |
|---|---|
| Calcium | May decrease calcium stores. |
| Phenylpropanolamine | Increases the stimulant effect. |

**Interactions with other substances:**

- Smoking may increase the stimulant effect of caffeine.

*See Glossary.

# Cigarettes (Smoke)

### Definition and description:
Cigarette smoke contains about 2,000 different compounds. The main pharmacological agents of cigarettes are nicotine, carbon monoxide and thiocyanates. *Nicotine* causes constriction of blood vessels and a change in the breathing in the fetus. *Carbon monoxide* causes a reduction in the amount of oxygen carried in blood.

**Other names:** Tobacco smoke.

 ## Dosage

### Safe dosage:
• No safe dosage.

### Toxic dosage:
• Toxic effects increase with the number of cigarettes you smoke.

 ## Possible benefits

### Benefits before pregnancy:
• None reported.

### Benefits to mother:
• None reported.

### Benefits to fetus:
• None reported.

### Benefits to newborn:
• None reported.

### Benefits during lactation:
• None reported.

 ## Possible adverse effects

### Effects before pregnancy:
• General health effects on women are well-known, including increase in the risks of lung cancer, heart disease and respiratory diseases. A less-dangerous but still undesirable effect is an increase in premature skin wrinkling.

### Effects on mother:
• There is an increased incidence of pregnancy complications among women who smoke, including bleeding after delivery, premature breaking of waters*, abruptio placenta*, placenta previa*, inflammation of the umbilical cord and amniotic-fluid* infections.

### Effects on fetus:
• There is an increased incidence of babies with no brains, congenital heart defects, cleft palate*, harelip*, urogenital abnormalites, increased fetal death rate, low birth weights and facial abnormalities in babies of mothers who smoked during pregnancy.
• Smoking increases the rate of miscarriage and pregnancy complications.
• Smoking late in pregnancy may decrease birth weight more than smoking early in pregnancy.
• Carboxyhemoglobin levels are increased in the blood. This decreases the amount of oxygen delivered to the fetus.
• Thiocyanate levels are increased in the blood. These compounds damage cells of the fetus.

### Effects on newborn·
• Infants born to smoking mothers have more respiratory oroblems, such as pneumonia* and bronchitis*.
• There may be an increased rate of Sudden infant death syndrome* (SIDS) in infants born to smoking mothers. It is unclear if this is due to exposure to cigarettes before birth or environmental exposure after birth or a combination of both.
• Infants born to smoking mothers show decreased growth rates throughout infancy and childhood.
• Hyperactivity may be more common among children born to mothers who smoke.
• Children whose mothers smoked during pregnancy may have slighly less-satisfactory neurological and intellectual maturation.

### Effects during lactation:
- Nicotine has been associated with a poor letdown reflex*, inhibition of lactation and a poor milk supply.
- The infant is exposed to high levels of environmental smoke (passive smoke) and the risk of burns from hot cigarette ashes if the mother smokes while breast-feeding.

 **Additional information**

- In addition to nicotine, cigarettes contain lead, cadmium and cyanide. These ingredients can be harmful to the fetus.
- Mothers who smoke choose bottle-feeding more frequently than non-smokers, and more discontinue breast-feeding by 6 weeks than those who do not smoke.
- There are reports of increased frequencies of upper-respiratory infection, pneumonia*, diminished, small airway function and heart pain in association with exposure to air contaminated with cigarette smoke. Findings suggest this may also occur in pregnancy but effects are not well-documented.
- Passive smoke inhaled from other individuals in the baby's environment may contribute to the effects of the mother's smoking.

 **Recommendations for use**

### Women considering pregnancy:
- Smoking is discouraged for everyone.

### Recommendations during pregnancy:
- Smoking is not recommended during pregnancy.

### Recommendations during lactation:
- Smoking is not recommended during lactation.

 **Interactions**

### Interactions with medications, vitamins and minerals:

| Interacts with | Combined effects |
|---|---|
| Aminophylline | Decreases aminophylline effect. |
| Beta carotene (vitamin A) | Reduces vitamin-A blood levels. |
| Oral contraceptives | Increases risk of stroke. |
| Theophylline | Decreases theophylline effect. |
| Vitamin B$_{12}$ | Reduces vitamin-B$_{12}$ blood levels. |
| Vitamin C | Reduces vitamin-C blood levels. |
| Zinc | Reduces the amount of zinc in the placenta, which may reduce the amount of zinc delivered to the fetus and may cause zinc deficiency. |

### Interactions with other substances:
- Use with caffeine may increase breathing problems in babies.
- Use with alcohol causes more deleterious effects on infant behavior and learning than would be expected with either substance alone.

*See Glossary.

SUBSTANCE

# Cocaine

**Definition and description:** Cocaine acts on the nervous system as a stimulant and reduces nerve impulses.

**Other names:** Coke, crack.

 ## Dosage

**Safe dosage:**
- No safe dose.

**Toxic dosage:**
- Any dose may have toxic effects.

 ## Possible benefits

**Benefits before pregnancy:**
- None reported.

**Benefits to mother:**
- None reported.

**Benefits to fetus:**
- None reported.

**Benefits during lactation:**
- None reported.

 ## Possible adverse effects

**Effects before pregnancy:**
- Increased heart rate, high blood pressure, heart attacks and strokes.
- Cocaine is an addictive substance.

**Effects on mother:**
- Intravenous* injection of cocaine may cause abruptio placenta*.
- See *Effects before pregnancy.*

**Effects on fetus:**
- Cocaine-using mothers have significantly higher rates of miscarriage, stillbirth, premature labor, malformations, low birth weight, short length, small head circumference, lower Apgar scores* and abruptio placenta* than women who do not use cocaine.

- Cocaine-using mothers have significantly higher rates of premature and rapid labor, abnormalities during labor and meconium staining* than women on methadone maintenance.

**Effects on newborn:**
- Babies of cocaine-using mothers have less interaction with caregivers and a poor response to environmental stimulation.
- Babies of cocaine-using mothers have a higher rate of sudden infant death syndrome* (SIDS) than infants of methadone-maintenance mothers.
- Babies of cocaine-using mothers may go through withdrawal.

**Effects during lactation:**
- Safety or risk has not been established.

 ## Recommendations for use

**Women considering pregnancy:**
- Cocaine use is not recommended.

**Recommendations during pregnancy:**
- Do not use cocaine during pregnancy.

**Recommendations during lactation:**
- Do not use cocaine during lactation.

 ## Interactions

**Interactions with medications, vitamins and minerals:**
- None reported.

**Interactions with other substances:**
- Use with methamphetamine will increase the rate of placental hemorrhage*.

*See Glossary.

**Definition and description:** Fiber is a component of plant cell walls. The body is unable to break down fiber by enzymes in the digestive tract. It moves through the intestinal tract without being absorbed and increases the water and cholesterol* content of the stool.

**Other names:** Dietary fiber, soluble fiber, insoluble fiber, bulk.

 ## Dosage

### Safe dosage:
• Increasing to more than 20g initially may interfere with the absorption of other nutrients. There is evidence humans adapt to very high fiber intakes over a period of time.

### Toxic dosage:
• Not established.

 ## Possible benefits

### Benefits before pregnancy:
• Fiber causes bulkier stools and decreases constipation.
• It helps control blood-sugar levels in diabetics and people with low blood sugar.
• Fiber absorbs cholesterol* and may decrease blood-cholesterol levels. This may decrease risk of developing heart disease.
• High-fiber diets may reduce the risk of developing colon cancer*.

### Benefits to mother:
• See *Benefits before pregnancy.*
• Hemorrhoids* can occur in pregnancy, especially the third trimester. Fiber, adequate fluid intake and exercise are effective for preventing or decreasing hemorrhoids*.
• May decrease "morning sickness."

### Benefits to fetus:
• None reported.

### Benefits to newborn:
• None reported.

### Benefits during lactation:
• See *Benefits before pregnancy.*
• Hemorrhoids* can occur after delivery. Fiber, adequate fluid intake and exercise are effective for preventing or decreasing hemorrhoids*.

 ## Possible adverse effects

### Effects before pregnancy:
• Greater than 20g of fiber a day (if consumed at the same time) may interfere with absorption of zinc, iron, calcium, magnesium and copper.
• If fiber intake is increased rapidly, it may cause bloating and gas.

### Effects on mother:
• See *Effects before pregnancy.*

### Effects on fetus:
• None reported, except in cases of excessive fiber consumption leading to deficiencies in zinc, iron, calcium, magnesium or copper. See specific charts for effects of deficiencies.

### Effects on newborn:
• See *Effects on fetus.*

### Effects during lactation:
• See *Effects before pregnancy.*

 ## Additional information

• If fiber is eaten separately from other foods, much higher levels of fiber can be tolerated.
• Increase fiber intake slowly.
• The National Cancer Institute recommends fiber intake of 25 to 30g/day.

≫→

# Fiber, continued

 **Recommendations for use**

### Women considering pregnancy:
- An increase in fiber intake is recommended for most individuals. Fiber is often in short supply in diets. See Appendix 1, page 375.
- Increase fiber intake slowly.
- The National Cancer Institute recommends fiber intake of 25 to 30g/day.

### Recommendations during pregnancy:
- An increase in fiber intake to 15g is recommended during pregnancy. See Appendix 1, page 375.
- Increase fiber intake slowly.

### Recommendations during lactation:
- An increase in fiber intake is recommended for most individuals. Fiber is often in short supply in diets. See Appendix 1, page 375.
- Increase fiber intake slowly.
- The National Cancer Institute recommends fiber intake of 25 to 30g/day.

 **Interactions**

**Interactions with medications, vitamins and minerals:**

| Interacts with | Combined effect |
| --- | --- |
| Calcium | Large amounts of fiber decrease absorption. |
| Copper | Large amounts of fiber decrease absorption. |
| Iron | Large amounts of fiber decrease absorption. |
| Magnesium | Large amounts of fiber decrease absorption. |
| Zinc | Large amounts of fiber decrease absorption. |

**Interactions with other substances:**
- None reported.

*See Glossary.

# Herbs

**Definition and description:** Any plant used as a medication.

| Various herbs | Reported effects |
|---|---|
| African yohimbe bark | Mild hallucinogen*. |
| Blessed thistle leaf | May induce menstruation. May stimulate mammary glands. |
| Blue or black cohosh | Antispasmodic*. Irritant. May induce menstruation or cause labor, cause low blood pressure and dizziness. Diuretic*. |
| Borage leaf | Diuretic*. Mood elevator. |
| Catnip | Mild hallucinogen*. |
| Cayenne | Relieves flatulence. Stimulant. Antispasmodic*. Astringent. |
| Chamomile flower | Antispasmodic*. |
| Cinnamon | Mild stimulant. |
| Coltsfoot | Diuretic*. |
| Comfrey leaf | Helps heal bones. Weak sedative. Astringent. |
| Coriander seed | Increases flow of saliva and stomach juice. |
| False unicorn | Diuretic*. Causes vomiting. Stimulant. Kills intestinal parasites. May induce menstruation. |
| Fennel seed | Weak diuretic*. Stimulant. |
| Horsetail | Astringent. Diuretic*. |
| Kava-kava | Mild hallucinogen*. |
| Kola nut; gotu kola | Stimulant. Diuretic*. |
| Lobelia | Mild mood elevator. |
| Mandrake | Hallucinogen*. |
| Mate | Stimulant. |
| Mistletoe | Stimulant. Causes contraction of smooth muscles. |
| Mormon tea | Stimulant. |
| Nutmeg | Hallucinogen*. |
| Oatstraw | Antispasmodic*. Stimulant. |
| Passion flower | Mild stimulant. |
| Pennyroyal | Stimulant. May induce menstruation, and sweating. Relieves flatulence. |
| Peppermint | Causes sweating. Stimulant. Antispasmodic*. Relieves flatulence. |
| Periwinkle | Hallucinogen*. |
| Red raspberry | Astringent. Antiseptic. Reduces vomiting. May stimulate uterine contractions. |
| Rue | May stimulate uterine contractions. Antispasmodic*. May decrease capillary fragility. |
| Sassafras | Decreases body temperature. |
| Scullcap | Antispasmodic*. |
| Senna | Laxative. |
| Shepherd's purse | Astringent. Diuretic*. Stimulant. |
| Snakeroot | Tranquilizer. |
| Spiknard | Stimulant. Causes sweating. |
| Squaw vine | Astringent. Diuretic*. |
| St. John's wort | Astringent. Diuretic*. Sedative. |
| Tansy | May stimulate uterine contractions. Stimulates appetite. Kills intestinal parasites. |
| Thorn apple | Strong hallucinogen*. |
| Valerian | Tranquilizer. |
| Wormwood | Addictive pain reliever. |
| Yarrow | Reduces blood-clotting time. |

SUBSTANCE

359

# Herbs, continued

 **Dosage**

- Not established for any herb. These natural products are unpredictable because one particular plant can contain more or less active ingredient than another of the same variety. Tea depends on how it is made. Potency can increases 10 times or more when it is steeped for 5 minutes.

**Safe dosage:**
- Not established.

**Toxic dosage:**
- Exact toxic dose cannot be predicted.

 **Possible benefits**

**Benefits before pregnancy:**
- Pennyroyal and blue or black cohosh are promoted for inducing menstruation. No studies support this promotion.

**Benefits to mother:**
- When combined with lobelia, false unicorn is promoted for preventing threatened miscarriages.
- Red raspberry is promoted to decrease premature labor pains and hemorrhoids, increase contractions and decrease bleeding after delivery.
- Scullcap is promoted for relieving cramps.
- St. John's wort, red raspberry, cayenne and shepherd's purse are promoted to decrease bleeding after delivery.
- Chamomile or comfrey sitz baths are promoted to increase vaginal-area healing.
- No studies support any of the above claims.

**Benefits to fetus:**
- None reported.

**Benefits to newborn:**
- Peppermint and chamomile are promoted for decreasing colic. No studies support this claim.

**Benefits during lactation:**
- Blessed thistle is promoted for stimulating the mammary glands to help increase milk supply. No studies support this claim.

 **Possible adverse effects**

**Effects before pregnancy:**
- See list under *Various herbs*.

**Effects on mother:**
- Any of the effects that occur when you are not pregnant continue and may increase because of the decreased ability of the kidneys and liver to metabolize and excrete herbs.
- Large doses of cayenne over long periods may cause abdominal pain and possible kidney inflammation.
- Large doses of valerian may cause nausea, diarrhea, increased urination, slowed heart rate, low blood pressure, melancholia* or hysteria*.
- Blue and black cohosh may cause low blood pressure or dizziness.
- Chamomile may cause a severe allergic reaction in individuals who are allergic to marigold, yarrow, asters, ragweed and chrysanthemums.
- Horsetail can irritate the kidney and cause acute nerve damage.
- Lobelia may be toxic in large amounts.
- Pennyroyal may cause miscarriage or premature labor.
- Periwinkle contains a substance that can damage blood cells, nerves and liver.
- Sassafras contains a potent carcinogen, safrole.
- Senna can cause severe diarrhea.

**Effects on fetus:**
- Safety or risk has not been established.

**Effects on newborn:**
- Safety or risk has not been established.

### Effects during lactation:
- Although effects vary depending on the herb, most herbs cross into breast milk. The concentration varies, depending on the herb.
- Toxic accumulation in the infant is possible because immature kidneys and liver have a decreased ability to metabolize and excrete the herbs.
- Toxic effects in the infant are similar to toxic effects in the mother. See list under *Various herbs* and *Effects on mother*.

 **Additional information**

- Herbs may interfere with or increase the action of other medication.

 **Recommendations for use**

### Women considering pregnancy:
- Inform your doctor if you take *any* herbs.
- Use caution when taking herbs because of the variation in strengths and potential medicinal properties.
- If you buy herbs, use a reputable source. Consult a reputable authority.

### Recommendations during pregnancy:
- Inform your doctor if you take *any* herbs.
- Use caution when taking herbs because of the variation in strengths and potential medicinal properties.
- If you buy herbs, use a reputable source. Consult a reputable authority.
- Do not take blessed thistle early in pregnancy.
- Do not take coltsfoot, mistletoe, yarrow or blue or black cohosh until the last 4 weeks of pregnancy.
- Do not take sassafras, pennyroyal, Senna, tansy or rue at *any time* during pregnancy.

### Recommendations during lactation:
- Use caution when taking herbs because of the variation in strengths and potential medicinal properties.
- If you buy herbs, use a reputable source. Consult a reputable authority.
- Inform your doctor and your baby's doctor if you take any herbs.

 **Interactions**

**Interactions with medications, vitamins and minerals:**

| Interacts with | Combined effect |
|---|---|
| **Catnip** | Decreases iron absorption. |
| **Cinnamon** | Decreases iron absorption. |
| **Cohosh, black** | Decreases iron absorption and absorption of other minerals. |
| **Coltsfoot** | Decreases iron absorption. |
| **Comfrey** | Decreases iron absorption. |
| **Red raspberry** | Decreases iron absorption. |
| **Rue** | Decreases iron absorption. |
| **St. John's wort** | Decreases iron absorption. |
| **Yarrow** | Decreases iron absorption. |

**Interactions with other substances:**
- None reported.

*See Glossary.

SUBSTANCE

# Marijuana

**Definition and description:** A preparation of leaves and flowering tops of the plant Cannibis sativa. It is usually made into cigarettes and inhaled as smoke for its mood-elevating effects.

**Other names:** Cannibis, pot, dope, Mary Jane, joints.

 ## Dosage

**Safe dosage:**
• No safe dosage.

**Toxic dosage:**
• Any dose may have toxic effects.

 ## Possible benefits

**Benefits before pregnancy:**
• The active substance THC has been isolated and used to treat nausea and vomiting in cancer patients.

**Benefits to mother:**
• None reported.

**Benefits to fetus and newborn:**
• None reported.

**Benefits during lactation:**
• None reported.

 ## Possible adverse effects

**Effects before pregnancy:**
• Altered mental states, mood elevation, altered time perception and increased appetite may occur with marijuana use.
• May decrease sperm and testosterone in long-time male smokers. This may cause infertility*.

**Effects on mother:**
• See *Effects before pregnancy.*

**Effects on fetus and newborn:**
• Abnormal eye spacing, abnormal eye formation, decreased birth weight and increased incidence of fetal-alcohol-syndrome*-like features have been found in children of mothers who were heavy users of marijuana.

• There may be an increase in premature births in heavy marijuana smokers.

**Effects during lactation:**
• If a mother smokes marijuana while nursing, the baby is exposed to the drug in breast milk and to the environmental marijuana. Brain-cell development in the infant occurs during the first months of life. Marijuana may alter brain cells. Any remote chance these cells could be altered should be cause for concern.

 ## Recommendations for use

**Women considering pregnancy:**
• No specific recommendations before pregnancy because studies are not reported. Considering the effects on fetal development, use moderation or abstain completely from marijuana use while attempting to conceive.

**Recommendations during pregnancy:**
• Do not use marijuana during pregnancy.

**Recommendations during lactation:**
• Do not use marijuana during lactation.

 ## Interactions

**Interactions with medications, vitamins and minerals:**

| Interacts with | Combined effect |
| --- | --- |
| Aminophylline | Smoking decreases effect of aminophylline. |
| Theophylline | Smoking decreases effect of theophylline. |
| Zinc | Zinc concentration in the infant is reduced at time of delivery. |

**Interactions with other substances:**
• Use with alcohol potentially causes more birth defects and fetal death than using either substance alone.

*See Glossary.

# Miscellaneous Food Items
## for Use in Pregnancy and Lactation

| Food | Effect | Recommendation |
|---|---|---|
| Bee pollen | May cause severe allergic reactions. No proven benefit. | Do not consume. |
| Broccoli, cauliflower, cabbage, Brussels sprouts (cruciferous vegetables) | May cause gas in nursing infant. No effect reported on baby during pregnancy. | If you notice increased irritability after eating, decrease intake and monitor. |
| Chocolate | Contains theobromine and caffeine, which may act as stimulants. See Appendix 3, page 381. No evidence chocolate causes problems during pregnancy or when nursing, unless specific allergies are present. | Consume in moderation. |
| Fish-oil pills (E.P.A.) | Promoted to decrease heart disease by decreasing blood-platelet stickiness, cholesterol and triglycerides. Can cause GI distress, diarrhea, nausea and gas. No studies have been done evaluating safety in pregnancy or lactation. | Pregnancy may not be the time to try to reduce risk of heart disease. If you take fish-oil pills, inform your doctor. |
| Garlic pills | Appear to have many medicinal properties, such as decreasing bacterial infections. May decrease atherosclerosis and lower blood pressure. No specific effects reported during pregnancy or lactation. See Appendix 3, page 381. | Consume as *fresh* garlic for medicinal effect. |
| Home-canned vegetables | Clostridium botulisum may be present. Symptoms are difficulty swallowing, double vision, labored breathing and death. Symptoms appear 1 to 2 days after eating. Very dangerous during pregnancy. | Properly heat home-canned vegetables. Avoid commercially canned food with leaky seals. |
| Hot dogs, contaminated cabbage, soft cheese | Listeriosis poisoning can occur. It can cause serious illness and death for the fetus and newborn. | Cook meat thoroughly. Wash cabbage thoroughly. Avoid unpasteurized dairy products. |

≫➔

| Food | Effect | Recommendation |
|------|--------|----------------|
| Licorice | The natural extract used in "natural" licorice candies may interfere with the action of diuretics and drugs to treat hypertension. May increase sodium retention and water retention. | Don't consume more than 2 twists per day of natural black licorice. |
| Lysine | Speculated to help protect against some sexually transmissible herpes viruses. No proven benefit. No studies have been done evaluating safety during pregnancy. | Eat a diet adequate in protein. Inform your doctor if you supplement with lysine. |
| Milk, dairy products, eggs, wheat, soy | In families with many allergies, nursing infants may be sensitive to certain foods. | If you notice increased irritability, congestion or GI upset in your baby, discuss with your baby's doctor. |
| Potatoes | Contain steroid alkaloids, which can be toxic to humans. Effects during pregnancy or on fetus are unknown. | Steroid alkaloids are especially present in British variety. Concentrated close to the skin. Moderate intake. Avoid green potatoes or potatoes with sprouts. Peel potatoes before eating. |
| Quinine water | Quinine, an ingredient found in quinine water, may not be safe during pregnancy. | Avoid consumption. |
| Raw eggs | Salmonella poisoning has been found in raw eggs. Symptoms include abdominal pain, chills, fever and frequent vomiting. Symptoms appear 7 to 72 hours after eating. Raw eggs with cracks are especially dangerous. No specific effects known during pregnancy or lactation. | Avoid raw eggs or soft-cooked eggs. |

| Food | Effect | Recommendation |
|------|--------|----------------|
| Raw fish; sushi | Cholera has been found in fish from water contaminated by human sewage. Effects can range from diarrhea to death. Scombrotoxism can result from eating raw tuna or mackerel. Other types of food poisoning or disease are possible but not as common. No specific effects known during pregnancy or lactation. | Eat only *cooked* fish. |
| Raw milk | Campylobacterosis has been found. Symptoms are diarrhea, abdominal cramps, fever and sometimes bloody stools. Tuberculosis has rarely been found in cows. No specific effects known during pregnancy or lactation. Listeriosis poisoning can occur. It can cause serious illness and death for the fetus and newborn. | Drink pasteruized milk. |
| Rotting foods | A compound that can be present in rotting food, Asperigillus flavus, can produce aflatoxin, which is a carcinogen. It has produced birth defects in animals. The effect in humans is unknown. | Store food in cool, dry environment. Don't eat questionable food. |
| Tryptophan | Speculated to help sleeplessness, decrease sensitivity to moderate pain, act as an anti-depressant and suppress appetite. No studies have been done evaluating safety during pregnancy. | Eat a diet adequate in protein. Inform your doctor if you supplement with tryptophan. |
| Uncooked chicken | Salmonella poisoning can occur. Symptoms include abdominal pain, chills, fever and frequent vomiting. Symptoms appear 7 to 72 hours after eating. No specific effects known during pregnancy or lactation. Listeriosis poisoning can occur. It can cause serious illness and death for the fetus and newborn. | Cook chicken thoroughly. |

FOOD ITEMS

365

# Selected Food Additives

There are no reports about the safety or dangers of these food additives in pregnancy or lactation. This table reviews common food additives and their safety levels in the modified opinion of the Center for Science in the Public Interest.

| Food Additive | Description | Safety Rating |
|---|---|---|
| Alginate, Propylene glycol | Thickening agent and foam stabilizer. Used in ice cream, cheese, candy, yogurt. Made from seaweed. | Safe |
| Alpha tocopherol | Vitamin E. Used as an anti-oxidant in vegetable oil. | Safe |
| Artificial flavoring | Used in soda pop, candy, breakfast cereals, gelatin, many other foods. | May be safe |
| Ascorbic acid | Antioxidant, nutrient, color stabilizer. | Safe |
| Aspartame | Artificial sweetener in drink mixes, gelatin, candy, other foods. | May be safe. See chart, page 350. |
| Beta-carotene | Coloring, nutrient in margarine, shortening, non-dairy whiteners, butter. Preformed vitamin A. | Safe |
| Blue No. 1 | Coloring in beverages, candy, baked goods. Small cancer risk. | May not be safe |
| Blue No. 2 | Coloring in pet food, beverages, candy. Small cancer risk in mice. | May not be safe |
| Brominated vegetable oil (BVO) | Emulsifier, clouding agent in soft drinks. | May not be safe |
| Butylated hydroxyanisole | Antioxidant in cereals, chewing gum, potato chips, oils, other foods. | May not be safe |
| Butylated hydroxytoluene (BHT) | Antioxidant in cereals, chewing gum, potato chips, oils, other foods. | May not be safe |
| Calcium propionate | Preservative in bakery goods. | Safe |
| Calcium stearyl lactylate | Dough conditioner. Whipping agent in bread dough, cake fillings, artificial whipping cream, processed egg whites. | Safe |
| Carrageenan | Thickening and stabilizing agent in ice cream, jelly, chocolate milk, infant formula. | May be safe |

| Food Additive | Description | Safety Rating |
|---|---|---|
| Casein, sodium caseinate | Thickening and whitening agent in ice cream, coffee creamers, sherbet. | Safe |
| Citric acid, sodium citrate | Acid, flavoring, chelating agent in ice cream, sherbet, fruit drink, candy, soda, instant potatoes. | Safe |
| Citrus red No. 2 | Coloring in skin of some Florida oranges. Dye does not leach through skin. | May be safe |
| Corn syrup | Sweetener, thickener in candy toppings, syrups, snack foods, imitation dairy products. | Safe |
| Dextrose (glucose, corn sugar) | Sweetener, coloring agent in bread, caramel, soda, cookies, other foods. | Safe |
| EDTA | Chelating agent in salad dressing, margarine, sandwich spreads, mayonnaise, processed fruits and vegetables, canned shellfish, soda. | Safe |
| Erythorbic acid | Antioxidant and color stabilizer in oily foods, cereals, soft drinks, cured meats. | Safe |
| Ferrous gluconate | Coloring, nutrient in black olives. | Safe |
| Fumaric acid | Tartness agent in powdered drinks, pudding, pie filling, gelatin. | Safe |
| Gelatin | Thickening and gelling agent in powdered drinks, pudding, pie filling, gelatin. | Safe |
| Glycerin (glycerol) | Maintains water content in marshmallows, candy, fudge, baked goods. | Safe |
| Green No. 3 | Coloring in candy, beverages. Small cancer risk. | May not be safe |
| Gums | Thickening agent and stabilizer in beverages, ice cream, frozen pudding, salad dressing, dough, cottage cheese, candy, drink mixes. | Safe |
| Heptyl paraben | Preservative in beer, non-carbonated soft drinks. | May be safe |
| Hydrogenated vegetable oil | Source of oil in margarine, many processed foods. | May be safe |

≫→

FOOD ADDITIVES

| Food Additive | Description | Safety Rating |
|---|---|---|
| Hydrolyzed vegetable protein (HVP) | Flavor enhancer in instant soups, frankfurters, sauce mixes, beef stew. | Safe |
| Invert sugar | Sweetener in candy, sodas, many other foods. | Safe |
| Lactic acid | Acidity regulator in Spanish olives, cheese, frozen desserts, carbonated beverages. | Safe |
| Lactose | Sweetener in whipped-topping mix, breakfast pastries. | Safe |
| Lecithin | Emulsifier, antioxidant in baked goods, margarine, chocolate, ice cream. | Safe |
| Mannitol | Sweetener in chewing gum, low-calorie foods. | Safe |
| Monoglycerides, diglycerides | Emulsifier in baked goods, margarine, candy, peanut butter. | Safe |
| Monosodium glutamate (MSG) | Flavor enhancer in soup, seafood, poultry, cheese, sauces, stews, other foods. | May be safe |
| Phosphoric acid | Acidifier, chelating agent in butter, emulsifier, nutrient-discoloration inhibitor in cheese, powdered foods, cured meat, soda, baked goods, breakfast cereals, dehydrated potatoes. | May be safe |
| Polysorbate 60 | Emulsifier in baked goods, frozen desserts, imitation dairy products. | Safe |
| Propyl gallate | Antioxidant in vegetable oil, meat products, potato sticks, chicken-soup base, chewing gum. | May be safe |
| Quinine | Flavoring in tonic water, quinine water, bitter lemon. | May not be safe. *Avoid in pregnancy.* |
| Red No. 3 | Coloring in cherries, candy, baked goods. Cancer risk. | May not be safe |
| Red No. 40 | Coloring in soda, candy, gelatin desserts, pastry, pet food, sausage. | May be safe |
| Saccharin | Synthetic sweetener in diet products. | May not be safe |

| Food Additive | Description | Safety Rating |
|---|---|---|
| Simplesse® | Synthetic fat made from protein to be introduced in 1989. Simplesse can be used in dairy products or oil-based foods. | May be safe. Some studies remain to be done. |
| Sodium benzoate | Preservative in fruit juice, carbonated drinks, pickles, preserves. | Safe |
| Sodium carboxyl-methylcellulose | Thickening and stabilizing agent in ice cream, beer, pie fillings, icings, diet foods, candy. | Safe |
| Sodium nitrite, nitrate | Preservative, coloring, flavoring used in bacon, ham, frankfurters, luncheon meats, smoked fish, corned beef. | May not be safe |
| Sorbic acid, potassium sorbate | Prevents growth of mold in cheese, syrup, jelly, cake, wine, dry fruits. | Safe |
| Sorbitan monostearate | Emulsifier in cakes, candy, frozen pudding, icings. | Safe |
| Sorbitol | Sweetener, thickening agent in dietetic drinks and foods, candy, shredded coconut, chewing gum. | Safe |
| Starch, modified | Thickening agent in soup, gravy, baby foods. | Safe |
| Sulfur dioxide, sodium bisulfite, sulfite | Preservative and bleach used in sliced fruit, wine, processed potatoes. May cause severe allergic reactions in certain people, especially asthmatics. | May not be safe. Avoid if you are allergic to sulfites. |
| Vanillin, ethyl vanillin | Substitute for vanilla in ice cream, baked goods, beverages, chocolate, candy, gelatin. | Safe |
| Yellow No. 5 | Coloring in gelatin, candy, pet food, baked goods. May cause allergic reactions. | May be safe |
| Yellow No. 6 | Coloring in beverages, sausage, baked goods, candy. Cancer risk. | May not be safe |

**Safe** = Testing indicates product is safe. There has been adequate testing.
**May be safe** = Testing indicates product is safe, but there has not been adequate testing.
**May not be safe** = Testing does not indicate safety or additive is unsafe in amounts consumed.

Reprinted from *Nutrition Action Healthletter,* available from Center for Science in the Public Interest, 1501 16th St., NW, Washington, DC, 20036, $19.95 for 10 issues, ©1989.

FOOD ADDITIVES

# Recommended Diet
# during Pregnancy and Lactation

$M$any factors are involved in a healthy baby's development. Your food intake is very important.

Below is a description of a healthy diet to follow during pregnancy and lactation. The description is divided into the three sources of calories—proteins, carbohydrates and fats. A 3-day menu plan follows the description.

The menu plan is provided as a guide for food selection. You have a personal eating style and habits and are not expected to follow a specific plan. Using this guide and Appendix 1, Food Sources of Nutrients, page 375, will help you obtain adequate nutrients.

There's no better time to start a healthy eating plan. Eating well will benefit you and your baby during pregnancy. Continuing this healthy plan will help maintain your well-being and encourage healthy, life-long eating patterns for your family.

## Energy Requirements and Weight Gain

The recommended diet during pregnancy is based on increased nutrient needs of you and your growing fetus. Your needs are increased to provide extra energy for tissue growth, body functions and fat deposits for nursing. The fetus needs energy to create and store protein, fat and carbohydrates. It also needs energy for body processes to function.

The total cost of these energy-using processes is 80,000 calories for your *total* pregnancy. This increase in energy averages 300 calories/day over 40 weeks of pregnancy. However, most fetal growth occurs in the second and third trimesters. Energy requirements resemble an inverted bowl, with the increase initially low, higher in midpregnancy and declining slightly at the end of pregnancy because of your decreased activity.

Healthy babies are born to many women who experience weight loss in the first trimester. Although weight loss is never recommended, it sometimes occurs with excessive nausea and vomiting. No harm usually occurs as long as adequate nutrients are supplied for the remainder of pregnancy.

Studies have shown if you follow a restricted-calorie diet during the second and especially third trimesters, your baby's weight can be decreased. In the last few weeks of pregnancy, your baby gains approximately 1 ounce/day.

In some cases, energy requirements differ from the usual recommendations. Teenagers who have been menstruating 2 years or less are usually still growing. They must supply calories for their normal growth and additional growth demands in pregnancy. Other instances of increased needs are mothers who are underweight at the beginning of pregnancy or those who have high-energy outputs. An example of high-energy output is an athlete who continues to train or a mother with a physically demanding job.

On the other end of the scale is the mother with a reduced-energy requirement or the women who needs to gain less weight for a healthy pregnancy. This includes mothers who are overweight at the beginning of pregnancy or those who are very inactive.

The table at right provides guidelines for calorie requirements during pregnancy and lactation. The best way to determine appropriateness of calorie intake is weight gain. The chart provides guidelines for suggested weight gain. The lines are labeled underweight, normal weight and overweight. This refers to your weight *before* pregnancy. The second table helps you determine if you were overweight, normal weight or underweight before pregnancy. A deviation from this pattern may not be cause for concern, but you may want to discuss your pattern with your doctor or nurse.

Increased energy needs during lactation are a direct result of the amount of energy in the milk and the amount of energy required to produce the milk. Milk production requires approximately 900 calories/day. The suggested calorie intake is an extra 500 calories a day above non-pregnancy levels. Some of the weight gained during pregnancy is used to provide fat stores and energy for the first few months of lactation.

## Suggested calorie intake during pregnancy and lactation

| Age | Non-pregnant | Pregnant | Lactating |
|---|---|---|---|
| 15-18 | 2,200 | 2,500 | 2,700 |
| 19-22 | 2,100 | 2,400 | 2,600 |
| 23-50 | 2,000 | 2,300 | 2,500 |

## Suggested desirable weights for heights in women

| Height (inches) | Weight (pounds) | Weight (kilograms) |
|---|---|---|
| 58 | 92-119 | 42-54 |
| 60 | 96-125 | 44-57 |
| 62 | 102-131 | 45-59 |
| 64 | 108-138 | 49-63 |
| 66 | 114-146 | 52-66 |
| 68 | 122-154 | 55-70 |
| 70 | 130-163 | 59-74 |
| 72 | 138-173 | 63-79 |

## Suggested Rate of Weight Gain

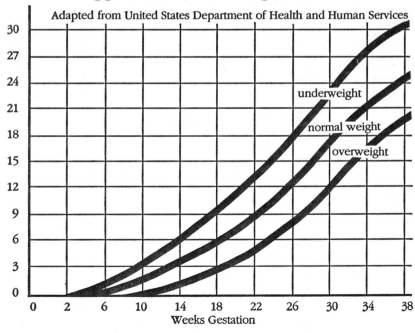

Adapted from United States Department of Health and Human Services

# Carbohydrate Requirements

There are no recommended dietary allowances (RDAs) for carbohydrate intake. Most nutrition experts recommend carbohydrate calories should constitute 50 to 55% of the total calories in your diet. Intake of carbohydrates should not fall below 100g/day. If this occurs, the level of ketone bodies in your blood may increase. Ketone bodies are starvation products. They accumulate when an inadequate carbohydrate level is provided in the diet and fat is broken down for energy. The effect of ketone bodies on the fetus is unknown. Eating carbohydrates that contain fiber helps prevent constipation and hemorrhoids during pregnancy. It also helps decreases nausea and vomiting. See Appendix 1, page 375, for fiber content of food.

The 3-day diet on the following page is an example of a diet that provides about 50% of the calories from carbohydrates.

# Fat Requirements

There are no RDAs for fat intake during pregnancy or lactation. Most nutrition experts recommend fat intake not exceed 30% of total calories when not pregnant. Fat carries fat-soluble vitamins and provides essential fatty acids. These needs can be met on a diet containing 15 to 25g of fat. This minimum amount represents less than 5% of total calories. The average North-American diet contains 37% calories as fat, so there is rarely a need for concern about fat deficiency. The concern is usually about fat *excess!*

Cholesterol intake and blood-cholesterol levels are health barometers that have recently become very important. High cholesterol levels are a risk factor for heart disease. The National Institute of Health has recommended all adults know their total cholesterol level.

Pregnancy and lactation are not times to evaluate your blood cholesterol. It is not unusual to see a 25% increase in blood-cholesterol levels due to the hormonal changes of pregnancy and lactation. Studies have not been done to determine the effect of treatment to lower cholesterol in pregnancy or lactation. This suggests it is unsafe and probably unnecessary to try to lower cholesterol levels at this time.

If you breast-feed, the type of fat you eat influences the fat content of your breast-milk. There are no specific guidelines for composition of the fat in lactating women's diets. A prudent recommendation is not more than 1/3 of your fat calories come from saturated fat, not more than 1/3 from polyunsaturated fat and at least 1/3 from monounsaturated fat. Saturated fat includes most fat from animal sources. Polyunsaturated fat includes vegetable oil and fish oil. Monounsaturated fat includes olive oil, canola oil (Puritan®) and parts of other oils.

# Protein Requirements

Protein requirements for pregnancy are based on the need to build tissue for the mother and baby. It is important to provide adequate calories from carbohydrates and fat so protein is used for building purposes rather than energy needs. The table below provides a guide for protein requirements during pregnancy and lactation. Appendix 1, page 375, provides protein levels in various food. Most diets are adequate in protein. Special diets, such as vegetarian diets, may be inadequate. If you are concerned about your protein intake, consult a registered dietitian.

| Age | Non-pregnant | Pregnant | Lactating |
|---|---|---|---|
| 15-18 years | 46 grams | 76 grams | 76 grams |
| 19-33 years | 46 | 76 | 76 |
| 23-50 years | 44 | 74 | 74 |

# 3-Day Diet for Pregnancy and Lactation

*Calories during pregnancy—2,300; calories during lactation—2,500*

## Day 1

| Food | Amount |
|---|---|
| **Breakfast** | |
| Fresh grapefruit | 1/2 medium |
| Pancakes, 5-inch | 3 |
| Maple syrup | 2T |
| Margarine | 1T |
| Peppermint herb tea | 1 cup |
| 1% milk | 1 cup |
| **Lunch** | |
| Split-pea soup with ham | 1 cup |
| French roll, hard | 1 medium |
| Apple butter | 1T |
| Margarine | 1t |
| 1% milk | 1 cup |
| **Dinner** | |
| Spinach salad with mushrooms | 1 cup |
| Poppy-seed dressing | 3T |
| Broiled halibut with | 4 oz. |
| parsley lemon butter | 2t |
| Noodles with Parmesan cheese | 3/4 cup |
| Asparagus with | 1 cup |
| Lemon butter | 1t |
| **Snacks** | |
| Popcorn | 2 cups |
| Apple | 1 medium |
| Ice cream | 3/4 cup |
| **For lactation add:** | |
| Whole-wheat bread | 1 slice |
| Peanut butter | 1T |

## Day 2

| Food | Amount |
|---|---|
| **Breakfast** | |
| Cantaloupe | 1/2 melon |
| Whole-grain cereal | 3/4 cup |
| Raisins and dates | 3T |
| 1% milk | 1 cup |
| **Lunch** | |
| Tomato bisque | 1 cup |
| Whole-wheat pita, stuffed with curried tuna | |
| Whole-wheat pita | |
| Waterpacked tuna | 2 oz. |
| Mayonnaise | 1T |
| Raisins | 2T |
| Curry powder | To taste |
| Tomato | 1/2 medium |
| Chutney | 2T |
| 1% milk | 1 cup |
| Banana | 1 medium |

## Dinner

| Food | Amount |
|---|---|
| Baked chicken almondine | 4 oz. |
| Cauliflower and red-pepper saute | 1-1/4 cup |
| Croissant | 1 medium |
| Frozen strawberry yogurt | 1 cup |
| **Snacks** | |
| Graham crackers | 4 squares |
| Peanut butter | 1T |
| Grapes | 1/2 cup |
| **For lactation add:** | |
| Fruit yogurt | 8 oz. |

## Day 3

| Food | Amount |
|---|---|
| **Breakfast** | |
| Grape juice | 1 cup |
| Raisin bagel | 1 medium |
| Ricotta cheese and cinnamon | 2 oz. |
| 1% milk | 1 cup |
| **Lunch** | |
| Pinto-bean burrito | |
| Flour tortilla | 1 medium |
| Rice | 1/2 cup |
| Green onion | 2T |
| Chopped tomato | 2T |
| Salsa | 2T |
| Pinto beans | 1/2 cup |
| Monterey jack cheese | 1 oz. |
| Pineapple chunks with | 1/2 cup |
| Vanilla yogurt | 3/4 cup |
| 1% milk | 1 cup |
| **Dinner** | |
| Egg rolls | 2 medium |
| Sliced beef tenderloin, marinated in red wine and tarragon | 3 oz. |
| Stir-fried mixed vegetables | 1 cup |
| Brown rice | 1 cup |
| Almond cookies | 2 medium |
| Tea | 1 cup |
| **Snacks** | |
| Raisins | 1/4 cup |
| Dried apricots | 3 medium |
| Orange juice | 3/4 cup |
| **For lactation add:** | |
| Sunflower seeds | 2T |
| Almonds | 2T |

DIET

# Nutrient Analysis for 3-Day Diet

| Nutrient | Average per Day | % Recommended Amount |
|---|---|---|
| Calories | 2,224 calories | 97 |
| Fat | 71.7g | |
| Fat (% of calories) | 29% | |
| Cholesterol | 104mg | |
| Carbohydrates | 294.5g | |
| Carbohydrates (% of cal.) | 53% | |
| Protein | 103g | 139 |
| Protein (% of cal.) | 18% | |
| Vitamin A | 12,968 I.U. | 259 |
| Vitamin C | 257mg | 322 |
| Thiamine | 1.78mg | 127 |
| Riboflavin | 2.5mg | 168 |
| Folate | 428mcg | 54 |
| Vitamin B$_{12}$ | 3.5mcg | 87 |
| Niacin | 25.8mg | 172 |
| Potassium | 4,401mg | 117 |
| Calcium | 1,424mg | 118 |
| Iron | 15.6mg | 87 |
| Zinc | 8.0mg | 40 |
| Pyridoxine | 1.8mg | 72 |

# Appendix 1
# Food Sources of Nutrients

T his Appendix provides a list of excellent food sources of calcium, fiber, folate, iron, magnesium, protein, pyridoxine (vitamin B6), vitamin A, vitamin C and zinc. Foods are listed with the highest-nutrient source first. These nutrient lists were obtained from the U.S.D.A. Handbook No. 8.

## Calcium
**Daily need in pregnancy and lactation—1,200mg**

| Food | Portion | Milligrams | Food | Portion | Milligrams |
|---|---|---|---|---|---|
| Sardines with bones | 3 oz. | 372 | American cheese | 1 oz. | 198 |
| Evaporated milk | 1/2 cup | 329 | Ice cream | 1 cup | 194 |
| Milk, 2%, 1%, skim | 1 cup | 300 | Cottage cheese, | | |
| Milk, whole | 1 cup | 288 | low-fat | 1 cup | 180 |
| Yogurt, low-fat | 1 cup | 274 | Canned salmon, | | |
| Soft-serve ice cream | 1 cup | 273 | with bones | 3 oz. | 167 |
| Swiss cheese | 1 oz. | 262 | Collard greens | 1/2 cup | 145 |
| Pudding | 1 cup | 250 | Spinach | 1/2 cup | 106 |
| Creamed soup | 1 cup | 240 | Mustard greens | 1/2 cup | 97 |
| Cottage cheese, | | | Corn muffin | 1 medium | 96 |
| creamed | 1 cup | 230 | Orange | 1 medium | 54 |
| Oysters | 1 cup | 226 | Broccoli | 1 stock | 49 |
| Ice milk | 1 cup | 204 | | | |
| Macaroni and cheese | 1 cup | 199 | | | |

## Fiber
**Daily need in pregnancy not established**

| Food | Portion | Grams | Food | Portion | Grams |
|---|---|---|---|---|---|
| Bran cereals | 1/2 cup | 8-13 | Zucchini | 1 cup | 3.6 |
| Baked beans, cooked | 1/2 cup | 8.8 | Apple | 1 medium | 3.5 |
| All-Bran® | 1/3 cup | 8.8 | Carrots | 1 cup | 3.1 |
| Bran Buds® | 1/3 cup | 7.9 | Strawberries | 1 cup | 3.0 |
| Kidney beans, | | | Popcorn | 3 cups | 3.0 |
| cooked | 1/2 cup | 7.3 | Grape Nuts® | 1/2 cup | 2.8 |
| Raspberries | 1 cup | 5.8 | Papayas | 1 medium | 2.8 |
| Green peas | 1/2 cup | 5.5 | Shredded Wheat® | 2/3 cup | 2.6 |
| Bran Chex® | 2/3 cup | 4.6 | Orange | 1 medium | 2.6 |
| Avocado, raw | 1 medium | 4.6 | Grapes | 1 cup | 2.6 |
| Lima beans, cooked | 1/2 cup | 4.5 | Bran muffin | 1 medium | 2.5 |
| Broccoli | 1 cup | 4.4 | Pineapple | 1 cup | 2.4 |
| Cracklin' Bran® | 1/2 cup | 4.3 | Bread, whole-grain | 1 slice | 2.0-6.0 |
| Spinach | 1 cup | 4.2 | Total® cereal | 1 cup | 2.0 |
| Wheat bran | 1/4 cup | 4.2 | Prunes | 2 medium | 2.0 |
| Pear, raw | 1 medium | 4.1 | Blueberries | 1/2 cup | 2.0 |
| Raisin bran cereal | 3/4 cup | 4.0-4.8 | Peach | 1 | 1.9 |
| Oat bran | 1/3 cup | 4.0 | Banana | 1 medium | 1.6 |
| Spaghetti, | | | Rye Krisps® | 2 crackers | 1.6 |
| whole-wheat | 1 cup | 3.9 | Apricots, raw | 3 medium | 1.4 |

# Folate
Daily need in pregnancy—800mcg; lactation—500mcg

| Food | Portion | Micrograms | Food | Portion | Micrograms |
|---|---|---|---|---|---|
| Brewer's yeast | 1T | 320 | Beets | 1 cup | 60 |
| Chicken liver | 4 oz. | 260 | Collards | 1 cup | 50 |
| Spinach | 1 cup | 200 | Orange | 1 medium | 45 |
| Chick peas | | | Avocado | 1/2 medium | 40 |
| (garbanzo beans) | 1 cup | 200 | Soybeans | 1 cup | 40 |
| Black-eyed peas | 1 cup | 140 | Broccoli | 1 cup | 40 |
| Melon, honeydew | | | Split peas | 1 cup | 40 |
| or cantaloupe | 1/4 melon | 100 | Lettuce | 1 cup | 30 |
| Orange juice | 1 cup | 87 | Cauliflower | 1 cup | 30 |
| Wheat germ | 1 oz. | 80 | | | |

# Iron
Daily need in pregnancy and lactation—18mg plus an oral supplement with 30-60mg

| Food | Portion | Milligrams | Food | Portion | Milligrams |
|---|---|---|---|---|---|
| Beef liver, fried | 3-1/2 oz. | 8.8 | Cube steak | 3-1/2 oz. | 3.5 |
| Oysters | 3-1/2 oz. | 8.1 | Prune juice | 1 cup | 3.3 |
| Kidney beans | 1 cup | 6.0 | Split peas | 1 cup | 3.0 |
| Peaches, dried | 10 halves | 5.3 | Green peas | 1 cup | 3.0 |
| Figs, dried | 10 | 4.2 | Lamb chop | 3-1/2 oz. | 3.0 |
| Clams | 1/2 cup | 4.1 | Leg of lamb | 3-1/2 oz. | 3.0 |
| Lima beans | 1 cup | 4.0 | Mixed fruit, dried | 3-1/2 oz. | 2.7 |
| Pork | 3-1/2 oz. | 4.0 | Blackstrap molasses | 1T | 2.3 |
| Flank steak | 3-1/2 oz. | 3.9 | Raisins | 2/3 cup | 2.1 |
| Rib steak | 3-1/2 oz. | 3.6 | Acorn squash | 1 cup | 2.0 |
| Pot roast | 3-1/2 oz. | 3.6 | Shrimp, cooked | 3-1/2 oz. | 2.0 |

# Magnesium
Daily need in pregnancy and lactation—450mg

| Food | Portion | Milligrams | Food | Portion | Milligrams |
|---|---|---|---|---|---|
| Spinach, boiled | 1/2 cup | 60 | Haddock, fried | 4 oz. | 20 |
| Oatmeal, cooked | 1 cup | 55 | Hamburger, broiled | 3 oz. | 20 |
| Potato | 1 large | 45 | Tomato | 1 medium | 20 |
| Milk | 1 cup | 40 | Broccoli, boiled | 1/2 cup | 14 |
| Banana | 1 medium | 35 | Lettuce, chopped | 1 cup | 10 |
| Red beans, canned | 1/2 cup | 35 | Rice, white, cooked | 2/3 cup | 10 |
| Walnut halves | 1/4 cup | 33 | Cheese, cheddar | 1 oz. | 8 |
| Chicken, white meat | 3-1/2 oz. | 29 | Egg | 1 large | 6 |
| Orange juice | 1 cup | 25 | Bread, white | 1 slice | 5 |
| Bread, whole-wheat | 1 slice | 25 | | | |

# Protein
Daily need in pregnancy and lactation—75g

| Food | Portion | Grams | Food | Portion | Grams |
|------|---------|-------|------|---------|-------|
| Chicken, no skin | 3 oz. | 28 | Ham | 3 oz. | 18 |
| Cottage cheese | 1 cup | 26 | Cheese | 3 oz. | 18 |
| Roast beef | 3 oz. | 25 | Sausage | 3 oz. | 17 |
| Pork chop, lean | 3 oz. | 25 | Beans, dried, cooked | 1 cup | 15 |
| Tuna | 3 oz. | 24 | Yogurt, low-fat | 1 cup | 12 |
| Steak, lean | 3 oz. | 24 | Peanuts | 1/4 cup | 9 |
| Cod, broiled | 3 oz. | 23 | Milk | 1 cup | 8 |
| Lamb, roast | 3 oz. | 23 | Egg | 1 medium | 6 |
| Shrimp | 3 oz. | 21 | Peanut butter | 1T | 4 |
| Hamburger, regular | 3 oz. | 21 | | | |

# Pyridoxine (Vitamin B6)
Daily need in pregnancy—2.6mg; lactation—2.5mg

| Food | Portion | Milligrams | Food | Portion | Milligrams |
|------|---------|------------|------|---------|------------|
| Brussels sprouts | 1 cup | 0.8 | Tomato juice | 1 cup | 0.4 |
| Kidney beans | 1 cup | 0.8 | Asparagus | 1 cup | 0.4 |
| Mackerel | 3-1/2 oz. | 0.7 | Avocado | 1/2 cup | 0.4 |
| Oysters | 1/2 cup | 0.6 | Hamburger | 3 oz. | 0.4 |
| Chicken breast | 3-1/2 oz. | 0.6 | Spinach | 1 cup | 0.4 |
| Black-eyed peas | 1 cup | 0.6 | Sunflower seeds | 1/4 cup | 0.4 |
| Banana | 1 medium | 0.6 | Beef, most cuts | 3 oz. | 0.3 |
| Bean soup | 1 cup | 0.5 | Fish | 3 oz. | 0.3 |
| Baked potato | 1 medium | 0.5 | Wheat germ | 1/4 cup | 0.3 |

# Vitamin A
Daily need in pregnancy and lactation—5,000 International Units (IU).

| Food | Portion | IU | Food | Portion | IU |
|------|---------|-----|------|---------|-----|
| Beef liver, cooked | 3 oz. | 45,420 | Beet greens | 1 cup | 7,400 |
| Carrots | 1 cup | 15,220 | Cantaloupe | 1/2 melon | 6,540 |
| Pumpkin, canned | 1 cup | 14,590 | Broccoli | 1 cup | 3,880 |
| Spinach, cooked | 1 cup | 14,580 | Papaya | 1 cup | 3,190 |
| Sweet potato | 1 medium | 11,610 | Apricots | 3 medium | 2,890 |
| Winter squash | 1 cup | 8,610 | Tomato juice | 1 cup | 1,940 |
| Turnip greens | 1 cup | 8,270 | Peach, raw | 1 medium | 1,320 |

# Vitamin C
## Daily need in pregnancy—80mg; lactation—100mg

| Food | Portion | Milligrams | Food | Portion | Milligrams |
|---|---|---|---|---|---|
| Turnip greens | 3-1/2 oz. | 139 | Strawberries | 1 cup | 85 |
| Pepper, green | 1 medium | 128 | Cauliflower | 1 cup | 78 |
| Kale | 3-1/2 oz. | 125 | Lime juice | 8 oz. | 72 |
| Orange juice | 8 oz. | 124 | Cantaloupe | 1 cup | 68 |
| Broccoli | 1 stalk | 113 | Red cabbage | 1 cup | 61 |
| Mustard greens | 3-1/2 oz. | 97 | Oysters | 4-6 medium | 60 |
| Collard greens | 3-1/2 oz. | 92 | Mango | 1 medium | 57 |
| Grapefruit juice | 8 oz. | 92 | Spinach | 3-1/2 oz. | 51 |
| Brussels sprouts | 6-8 medium | 87 | | | |

# Zinc
## Daily need in pregnancy—20mg; lactation—25mg

| Food | Portion | Milligrams | Food | Portion | Milligrams |
|---|---|---|---|---|---|
| Oysters, Atlantic | 3 oz. | 63.0 | Tuna, oil-packed, drained | 3 oz. | 0.9 |
| Oysters, Pacific | 3 oz. | 7.6 | Lima beans, cooked | 1/2 cup | 0.9 |
| Calves' liver, cooked | 3 oz. | 5.3 | Peas, green, cooked | 1/2 cup | 0.9 |
| Beef, lean, cooked | 3 oz. | 5.1 | Whitefish, broiled | 3 oz. | 0.9 |
| Lamb, lean, cooked | 3 oz. | 4.0 | Whole milk | 1 cup | 0.9 |
| Crabmeat | 1/2 cup | 3.4 | Macaroni, cooked | 1 cup | 0.7 |
| Black-eyed peas, cooked | 1/2 cup | 3.4 | Egg | 1 large | 0.5 |
| Pork loin, cooked | 3 oz. | 2.6 | Cottage cheese, creamed | 1/2 cup | 0.5 |
| Chicken | 3 oz. | 2.4 | Avocado | 1/2 medium | 0.5 |
| Shrimp | 1/2 cup | 1.4 | | | |
| Yogurt, plain | 1 cup | 1.1 | | | |
| Potato, baked with skin | 1 medium | 1.0 | | | |

# Appendix 2
# Calcium and Magnesium Content of Drugs or Supplements

This Appendix provides a list of the drug or supplement content of magnesium and calcium. Adapted from *The Right Dose* ©1987 by Patricia Hausman. Permission granted by Rodale Press, Inc. 33 E. Minor St; Emmaus, PA 18098.

## Calcium Content of Selected Supplements

| Brand Name | Milligrams | Brand Name | Milligrams |
|---|---|---|---|
| **Calcium Carbonate** | | **Calcium Phosphates:** | |
| Alka-2® | 200 | **Dibasic & Tribasic** | |
| Alka-2 Mints® | 340 | Di-Cal D Capsules® | 117 |
| Calciday-667® | 667 | Di-Cal D Wafers® | 232 |
| Calcitab® | 600 | Dicalcium Phosphate (Gray) | 112 |
| Calcium Carbonate—500mg | 200 | Dicalcium Phosphate | |
| Calcium Carbonate | 260 | (North American) | 89 |
| Calcium Complete® | 400 | Posture® (high-potency) | 600 |
| Calcium Gluconate | 63 | Posture® (moderate potency) | 300 |
| Calcium Junior—Chewable® | 300 | **Chelated Calcium** | |
| Calcium Lactate | 100 | Chelated Calcium (Arco) | 150 |
| Calcium Lactate—0.65mg | 85 | Chelated Calcium (Schiff) | 130 |
| Calcium Lactate—10 grains | 84 | Chelated Calcium (Thompson) | 200 |
| Calcium with Vitamin D—GNC® | 140 | **Miscellaneous Calcium** | |
| Calcium—600mg | 600 | Ca-Plus® | 280 |
| Caltrate 600® | 600 | Calcet® | 153 |
| Chewable Biocal®—250mg | 250 | Calcicaps Tablets® | 130 |
| Chooz® | 200 | Calcium Orotate® | 50 |
| New Biocal-500® | 500 | Calciwafers® | 165 |
| New Potent Calcium Plus® | 400 | FEMCAL Powder® | 317 |
| Os-Cal 250® | 250 | Neo-Calglucon Syrup® | 115 |
| Os-Cal 500® | 500 | | |
| Os-Cal Chewable® | 500 | | |
| Oyster Calcium® | 375 | | |
| Oyster Shell Calcium® | 250 | | |
| Oyster Shell Calcium®—500 | 500 | | |
| Oyster-Cal® | 375 | | |
| Rolaids® | 220 | | |
| Suplical® | 600 | | |
| Titralac® | 168 | | |
| Tums-EX® | 300 | | |
| Tums-Regular® | 190 | | |

# Magnesium Content of Selected Antacids

| Brand Name | Milligrams | Brand Name | Milligrams |
|---|---|---|---|
| Aludrox® | 43 | Maalox Plus Suspension® | 84 |
| Camalox Suspension® | 83 | Maalox Plus Tablets® | 84 |
| Camalox Tablets® | 83 | Maalox Suspension® | 84 |
| Delcid Suspension® | 302 | Milk of Magnesia® | 500 |
| Di-Gel Liquid® | 36 | Mylanta Liquid® | 84 |
| Di-Gel Tablets® | 50 | Mylanta Tablets ® | 84 |
| Gelusil Liquid® | 82 | Mylanta-II Liquid® | 167 |
| Gelusil-II Liquid® | 164 | Mylanta-II Tablets® | 167 |
| Gelusil-M Liquid® | 82 | Riopan Plus Chew® | 103 |
| Kolantyl Liquid® | 63 | Riopan Plus Suspension® | 103 |
| Kolantyl Tablets® | 167 | Riopan Suspension® | 93 |
| Kolantyl Wafers® | 71 | Riopan Tablets® | 93 |
| Maalox No. 1 Tablets® | 84 | Silain-Gel Liquid® | 119 |
| Maalox No. 2 Tablets® | 167 | Simeco Suspension® | 125 |

# Appendix 3
# Caffeine in Foods, Beverages and Drugs

This appendix provides a list of foods, beverages and medications that are sources of caffeine.

## Caffeine Content of
## Selected Foods and Medications

| Food | Portion | Milligrams | Range* |
|---|---|---|---|
| Baking chocolate | 1 oz. | 35 | |
| Cafe Amaretto® | 6 oz. | 60 | |
| Cafe Français® | 6 oz. | 52 | |
| Cafe Vienna® | 6 oz. | 57 | |
| Cherry Cola® | 12 oz. | 44 | |
| Chocolate cake | 1/16 of 9-inch cake | 14 | |
| Chocolate kisses | 6 pieces | 5 | |
| Cocoa mix | 1 packet | 4 | |
| Cocoa, dry, Hershey® | 1 oz. | 70 | |
| Coffee, decaffeinated | 5 oz. | 3 | 2-5 |
| Coffee, drip, automatic | 5 oz. | 137 | 110-164 |
| Coffee, instant | 5 oz. | 60 | 47-68 |
| Coffee, percolated, automatic | 5 oz. | 117 | 99-134 |
| Coca-Cola® | 12 oz. | 45 | |
| Diet Coca-Cola® | 12 oz. | 45 | |
| Dr Pepper® | 12 oz. | 40 | |
| Irish Mocha Mint® | 6 oz. | 27 | |
| Jolt Cola® | 12 oz. | 90 | |
| Kit-Kat® | 1-1/2 oz. bar | 5 | |
| Mountain Dew® | 12 oz. | 54 | |
| Orange Cappuccino® | 6 oz. | 74 | |
| Pepsi Cola® | 12 oz. | 38 | |
| Diet Pepsi Cola® | 12 oz. | 36 | |
| Semisweet chocolate chips | 1 oz. | 17 | |
| Shasta Cola® | 12 oz. | 44 | |
| Suisse Mocha® | 6 oz. | 40 | |
| Sweet German chocolate | 1 oz. | 8 | |
| Tab® | 12 oz. | 45 | |
| Tea, black, Amer., 1-min. brew | 5 oz. | 28 | |
| Tea, black, Amer., 3-min. brew | 5 oz. | 42 | |
| Tea, black, Amer., 5-min. brew | 5 oz. | 46 | |
| Tea, black, Imp., 5-min. brew | 5 oz. | 54 | |
| Tea, green, 1-min. brew | 5 oz. | 14 | |
| Tea, green, 3-min. brew | 5 oz. | 27 | |
| Tea, green, 5-min. brew | 5 oz. | 31 | |
| Tea, instant | 5 oz. | 28 | |
| Tea, oolong | 5 oz. | 13 | |

* Range (content) between various products.

| Medications | Portion | Milligrams of Caffeine |
| --- | --- | --- |
| Anacin® | 1 tablet | 32 |
| Aqua-ban® | 1 tablet | 200 |
| Cafergot® Capsules | 1 tablet | 100 |
| Caffedrine® Capsules | 1 tablet | 200 |
| Cope® | 1 tablet | 32 |
| Dristan® | 1 tablet | 16 |
| Excedrin® | 1 tablet | 65 |
| Fiorinal® | 1 tablet | 40 |
| Midol® | 1 tablet | 32 |
| Migralam® | 1 capsule | 100 |
| No Doz® | 1 tablet | 100 |
| Prolamine® | 1 tablet | 140 |
| Sinarest® | 1 tablet | 30 |
| Soma Compound® | 1 tablet | 32 |
| Triaminicin® | 1 tablet | 30 |
| Vanquish® | 1 tablet | 200 |
| Vivarin® | 1 tablet | 200 |

# Poison-Control Centers
# United States

**Alaska**
Providence Hospital Pharmacy
  3200 Providence Dr.
  Anchorage, AK 99508
  Emergency number
    907-261-3139
**Alabama**
Children's Hospital of Alabama
Poison Control Center
  1600 7th Ave. South
  Birmingham, AL 35233
  Emergency numbers
    205-939-9201
    205-933-4050
    800-292-6678
Alabama Poison Center
  809 University Blvd. East
  Tuscaloosa, AL 35401
  Emergency numbers
    205-345-0600
    800-462-0800 (Alabama)
**Arkansas**
Arkansas Poison & Drug
Information Center
  College of Pharmacy-UAMS
  4301 W. Markham St. Slot 522
  Little Rock, AR 72205
  Emergency numbers
    501-666-5532
    800-482-8948
**Arizona**
Samaritan Regional Poison Center
  Good Samaritan Medical Center
  1130 E. McDowell Rd.
  Phoenix, AZ 85006
  Emergency number
    602-253-3334
Arizona Poison & Drug Information Center
  Health Sciences Center Room 3204K
  1501 N. Campbell Ave.
  Tucson, AZ 85724
  Emergency numbers
    602-626-6016
    800-362-0101 (Arizona)
**California**
Fresno Regional Poison Control Center
  Fresno Community Hospital and
  Medical Center
  2823 Fresno St.
  Fresno, CA 93721
  Emergency numbers
    209-445-1222
    800-346-5922
Los Angeles County Medical Association
  Regional Poison Center
  1925 Wilshire Blvd.
  Los Angeles, CA 90057
  Emergency numbers
    213-664-2121  213-484-5151

University of California Irvine Medical Center
  Regional Poison Center
  101 The City Dr.
  Route 78
  Orange, CA 92668
  Emergency numbers
    714-634-5988
    800-544-4404
UC Davis Regional Poison Control Center
  2315 Stockton Blvd.
  Sacramento, CA 95817
  Emergency numbers
    916-453-3692
    800-342-9293
San Diego Regional Poison Center
  UCSD Medical Center
  225 Dickinson St. H925
  San Diego, CA 92103
  Emergency number
    619-542-6000
San Francisco Bay Area Regional
Poison Center
  San Francisco General Hospital
  1001 Potrero Ave.
  San Francisco, CA 94110
  Emergency numbers
    415-476-6600
    800-523-2222 (Northern California)
Santa Clara Valley Medical Center
  Regional Poison Center
  751 S. Bascom Ave.
  San Jose, CA 95128
  Emergency numbers
    408-299-5112
    408-299-5113
    408-299-5114
    800-662-9886
    800-662-9887
**Colorado**
Rocky Mountain Poison & Drug Center
  645 Bannock St.
  Denver, CO 80204-4507
  Emergency numbers
    303-629-1123
    800-332-3073 (Colorado)
    800-525-9083 (Montana)
    800-442-2702 (Wyoming)
**Connecticut**
Connecticut Poison Control Center
  University of Connecticut Health Center
  Farmington Ave.
  Farmington, CT 06032
  Emergency numbers
    203-679-3456
    203-679-3457
    203-679-4039

**District of Columbia**
National Capital Poison Center
  Georgetown University Hospital
  3800 Reservoir Rd. NW
  Washington, DC 20007
  Emergency numbers
    202-625-3333
    202-784-4660 (TTY)
**Florida**
St. Vincent's Medical Center
  1800 Barrs St.
  Jacksonville, FL 32203
  Emergency number
    904-387-7500
University Hospital Clinical Toxicology Service
  655 W. 8th St.
  Jacksonville, FL 32209
  Emergency number
    904-764-7667
Florida Poison Information Center
  The Tampa General Hospital
  Davis Islands
  PO Box 1289
  Tampa, FL 33601
  Emergency numbers
    813-253-4444
    800-282-3171 (Florida)
Winterhaven Hospital Poison-Control Center
  200 Ave. F NE
  Winterhaven, FL 33880
  Emergency number
    813-299-9701
**Georgia**
Georgia Regional Poison Control Center
  80 Butler St. SE
  PO Box 26066
  Atlanta, GA 30335
  Emergency numbers
    800-282-5846
    404-525-3323 (TTY)
**Hawaii**
Hawaii Poison Center
  Kapiolani Women's & Children's
  Medical Center
  1319 Puahou St.
  Honolulu, HI 96826
  Emergency number
    808-941-4411
**Iowa**
Variety Club Poison & Drug Information Center
  Iowa Methodist Medical Center
  1200 Pleasant St.
  Des Moines, IA 50309
  Emergency numbers
    515-283-6254
    515-283-6534
Poison Control Center
  University of Iowa Hospitals and Clinics
  Iowa City, IA 52242
  Emergency numbers
    319-356-2292
    800-272-6477 (Iowa)

St. Luke's Poison Center
  St. Luke's Regional Medical Center
  2720 Stone Park Blvd.
  Sioux City, IA 51104
  Emergency numbers
    800-352-2222 (Iowa)
    800-831-1111 (Nebraska, S. Dakota)
**Illinois**
Chicago & Northeast Illinois Regional
Poison Control Center
  Rush Presbyterian-St. Luke's Medical
  Center
  1753 W. Congress Pky.
  Chicago, IL 60612
  Emergency numbers
    312-942-5969
    800-942-5969 (Illinois)
**Indiana**
Indiana Poison Center
  Methodist Hospital of Indiana
  1701 N. Senate Blvd.
  Indianapolis, IN 46206
  Emergency numbers
    317-929-2323
    800-382-9097 (Indiana)
**Kansas**
Mid-American Poison Control Center
  Kansas University Medical Center
  Department of Pharmacy Room B-400
  39th and Rainbow Blvd.
  Kansas City, KS 66103
  Emergency numbers
    913-588-6633
    800-332-6633
**Kentucky**
Kentucky Regional Poison Center of Kosair
Children's Hospital
  PO Box 35070
  Louisville, KY 40232-5070
  Emergency numbers
    502-589-8222
    800-722-5725 (Kentucky)
**Louisiana**
Louisiana Regional Poison Center
  LSU Medical Center
  PO Box 33932
  Shreveport, LA 71130
  Emergency numbers
    318-425-1524
    800-535-0525
**Massachusetts**
Massachusetts Poison Control System
  300 Longwood Ave.
  Boston, MA 02115
  Emergency numbers
    617-232-2120
    800-682-9211 (Massachusetts)

**Maryland**
Maryland Poison Center
  20 N. Pine St.
  Baltimore, MD 21201
  Emergency numbers
    301-528-7701
    800-492-2414 (Maryland)
**Maine**
Maine Poison Control Center
  Maine Medical Center
  22 Bramhall St.
  Portland, ME 04102
  Emergency numbers
    207-871-2449
    800-442-6305 (Maine)
**Michigan**
Emma L. Bixby Hospital Poison Center
  818 Riverside Ave.
  Adrian, MI 49221
  Emergency number
    517-263-2412
University of Michigan Poison Information Center
  1500 E. Medical Center Dr.
  c/o Emergency Services
  Ann Arbor, MI 48109
  Emergency numbers
    313-764-7667
    313-936-6021
Poison Control Center
  Children's Hospital of Michigan
  3901 Beaubien Blvd.
  Detroit, MI 48201
  Emergency numbers
    313-745-5711
    800-462-6642 (Michigan)
Blodgett Regional Poison Center
  1840 Wealthy SE
  Grand Rapids, MI 49506
  Emergency number
    800-632-2727 (Michigan)
Bronson Poison Information Center
  252 E. Lovell St.
  Kalamazoo, MI 49007
  Emergency numbers
    616-341-6409
    800-442-4112 (Michigan)
Midwest Poison Center
  Borgess Medical Center
  1521 Gull Rd.
  Kalamazoo, MI 49001
  Emergency number
    616-393-7070
Saginaw Regional Poison Center
  Saginaw General Hospital
  1447 N. Harrison
  Saginaw, MI 48602
  Emergency number
    517-755-1111
**Minnesota**
St. Mary's Medical Center Poison
Information Service
  407 E. Third St.
  Duluth, MN 55805

Emergency number
  218-726-4500
Hennepin Regional Poison Center
  Hennepin County Medical Center
  701 Park Ave. South
  Minneapolis, MN 55415
  Emergency number
    612-347-3141
Minnesota Regional Poison
  St. Paul-Ramsey Medical Center
  640 Jackson St.
  St. Paul, MN 55101
  Emergency numbers
    612-221-2113
    800-222-1222 (Minnesota)
**Missouri**
Children's Mercy Hospital Poison-Control Center
  24th at Gillham Road
  Kansas City, MO 64108
  Emergency number
    816-234-3000
Cardinal Glennon Children's Hospital
Regional Poison Center
  1465 S. Grand Blvd.
  St. Louis, MO 63104
  Emergency numbers
    314-577-5200
    800-392-9111
**Mississippi**
Regional Poison Control
  University of Mississippi Medical Center
  2500 N. State St.
  Jackson, MS 39216
  Emergency number
    601-354-7660
**North Carolina**
Western North Carolina Poison
Information Center
  Emergency Care Center
  Memorial Mission Hospital
  509 Biltmore Ave.
  Ashville, NC 28801
  Emergency number
    704-258-9907
Duke Regional Poison Control Center
  Duke University Medical Center
  Box 3007
  Durham, NC 27710
  Emergency numbers
    919-684-8111
    800-672-1697 (North Carolina)
Triad Poison Center
  1200 N. Elm St.
  Greensboro, NC 27401-1020
  Emergency numbers
    919-379-4105
    800-722-2222 (North Carolina)
**North Dakota**
North Dakota Poison Center
  720 N. 4th St.
  Fargo, ND 58122
  Emergency numbers
    701-234-5575  800-732-2200 (North Dakota)

**Nebraska**
Mid-Plains Poison Center
  8301 Dodge St.
  Omaha, NE 68114
  Emergency numbers
    402-390-5400
    800-642-9999 (Nebraska)
    800-228-9515 (Surrounding states)
**New Hampshire**
New Hampshire Poison Information Center
  Dartmouth-Hitchcock Medical Center
  2 Maynard St.
  Hanover, NH 03756
  Emergency numbers
    603-646-5000
    800-523-8236 (New Hampshire)
**New Jersey**
New Jersey Poison Information &
Education System
  201 Lyons Ave.
  Newark, NJ 07112
  Emergency numbers
    201-923-0764
    800-962-1253 (New Jersey)
    201-926-8008 (TTY)
**New Mexico**
New Mexico Poison & Drug Information Center
  University of New Mexico
  Albuquerque, NM 87131
  Emergency numbers
    505-843-2551
    800-432-6866 (New Mexico)
**Nevada**
Washoe Medical Center
  77 Pringle Way
  Reno, NV 89520
  Emergency number
    702-328-4144
**New York**
Center for Community Health
  New York State Department of Health
  Corning Tower Room 621
  Empire State Plaza
  Albany, NY 12237
  Emergency number
    518-473-1143
Western New York Poison Control Center at
Children's Hospital of Buffalo
  219 Bryant St.
  Buffalo, NY 14222
  Emergency number
    716-878-7654
Nassau County Medical Center's Long
Island Regional Poison Control Center
  2201 Hempstead Turnpike
  East Meadow, NY 11554
  Emergency numbers
    516-542-2323
    516-542-2324
    516-542-2325

New York City Poison Center
  455 First Ave. Room 123
  New York, NY 10016
  Emergency numbers
    212-764-7667
    212-POISONS
Hudson Valley Poison Center
  Nyack Hospital
  North Midland Ave.
  Nyack, NY 10960
  Emergency number
    914-353-1000
Finger Lakes Regional Poison-Control Center at
Life Line
  University of Rochester Medical Center
  PO Box 777
  601 Elmwood Ave.
  Rochester, NY 14642
  Emergency numbers
    716-275-5151
    716-275-4354
Ellis Hospital Poison Control Center
  1101 Nott St.
  Schenectady, NY 12308
  Emergency numbers
    518-382-4039
    518-382-4309
Central New York Poison Control Center
  750 E. Adams St.
  Syracuse, NY 13210
  Emergency number
    315-476-4766
**Ohio**
Akron Regional Poison Center
  281 Locust St.
  Akron, OH 44308
  Emergency numbers
    216-379-8562
    800-362-9922 (Ohio)
Stark County Poison Control Center
  1320 Timken Mercy Dr. NW
  Canton, OH 44708
  Emergency number
    800-722-8662
Regional Poison Control System &
Cincinnati Drug & Poison Information Center
  231 Bethesda Ave. ML #144
  Cincinnati, OH 45267-0144
  Emergency numbers
    513-872-5111
    513-872-5112
    513-872-5113
    800-872-5111
Greater Cleveland Poison Control Center
  2101 Adelbert Road
  Cleveland, OH 44106
  Emergency number
    216-231-4455
Central Ohio Poison Center
  700 Children's Dr.
  Columbus, OH 43205
  Emergency numbers
    614-228-1323
    800-682-7625

Western Ohio Regional Poison & Drug
Information Center
Children's Medical Center
One Children's Plaza
Dayton, OH 45404
Emergency numbers
513-222-2227
800-762-0727
Mahoning Valley Poison Center
St. Elizabeth Hospital Medical Center
1044 Belmont Ave.
Youngstown, OH 44501
Emergency numbers
216-746-2222
800-426-2348
216-746-5510 (TTY)
Bethesda Poison-Control Center
Bethesda Hospital
2951 Maple Ave.
Zanesville, OH 43701
Emergency numbers
614-454-4221
614-454-4000

**Oklahoma**
Oklahoma Poison-Control Center
Children's Memorial Hospital
940 NE 13th St.
Oklahoma City, OK 73126
Emergency numbers
405-271-5454
800-522-4611 (Oklahoma)

**Oregon**
Oregon Poison Center
Oregon Health Sciences University
3181 SW Sam Jackson Park Rd.
Portland, OR 97201
Emergency numbers
503-279-8968
800-452-7165 (Oregon)

**Pennsylvania**
Keystone Region Poison Center
Mercy Hospital of Altoona
2500 Seventh Ave.
Altoona, PA 16603
Emergency numbers
814-946-3711
814-946-3700
Susquehanna Poison Center
Geisinger Medical Center
PO Box 273A
Danville, PA 17822
Emergency number
717-275-6116
Northwest Regional Poison Control Center
Saint Vincent Health Center
232 W. 25th St.
Erie, PA 16544
Emergency number
814-452-3232

Hamot Poison Control Center
Hamot Medical Center
201 State St.
Erie, PA 16550
Emergency numbers
814-870-6111
814-870-6112
800-221-5252 (Pennsylvania, Ohio,
New York)
Capital Area Poison Center
University Hospital
The Milton S. Hershey Medical Center
Hershey, PA 17033
Emergency number
717-531-6111
St. Joseph Hospital & Health Care Center
250 College Ave.
PO Box 3509
Lancaster, PA 17604
Emergency number
717-299-4546
Delaware Valley Regional Poison-Control Center
One Children's Center
34th & Civic Center BLvd.
Philadelphia, PA 19104
Emergency number
215-386-2100
Pittsburgh Poison Center
One Children's Place
3705 5th Ave. at DeSoto
Pittsburgh, PA 15213
Emergency number
412-681-6669
The Institution of Education
Communications
Children's Hospital Poison Center
3356 5th Ave.
Pittsburgh, PA 15213
Emergency number
412-647-5315
Williamsport Hospital & Medical Center Poison
Control Center
777 Rural Ave.
Williamsport, PA 17701
Emergency number
717-321-2000

**Rhode Island**
Rhode Island Poison Center
593 Eddy St.
Providence, RI 02902
Emergency number
401-277-5727

**South Carolina**
Palmetto Poison Center
University of South Carolina
College of Pharmacy
Columbia, SC 29208
Emergency numbers
803-765-7359
800-922-1117

## South Dakota

Dakota Midland Poison Center
1400 15th Ave. NW
Aberdeen, SD 57401
Emergency numbers
605-225-1880
800-592-1889

McKennan Poison Center
800 E. 21st St.
Sioux Falls, SD 57117-5045
Emergency numbers
800-952-0123 (South Dakota)
800-843-0505 (Iowa, Minnesota,
Nebraska, North Dakota

## Tennessee

Middle Tennessee Regional Poison Center
1161 21st Ave. South B-101 VUH
Nashville, TN 37232
Emergency number
615-322-6435

## Texas

Montgomery County Poison Information Center
504 Medical Center Blvd.
Conroe, TX 77304
Emergency number
409-539-7700

North Texas Poison Center
PO Box 35926
Dallas, TX 75235
Emergency numbers
214-590-5000
800-441-0040 (Texas)

El Paso Poison Control Center
4815 Alameda Ave.
El Paso, TX 79905
Emergency number
915-533-1244

Texas State Poison Center
University of Texas Medical Branch
Galveston, TX 77550-2780
Emergency numbers
409-765-1420
713-654-1701
512-478-4490
800-392-8548 (Texas)

## Utah

Intermountain Regional Poison Control Center
50 N. Medical Dr.
Salt Lake City, UT 84132
Emergency number
800-662-0062

## Virginia

Southwest Virginia Poison Center
Roanoke Memorial Hospitals
PO Box 13367
Roanoke, VA 24033
Emergency number
703-981-7336

## Washington

Seattle Poison Center
Children's Hospital and Medical Center
4800 Sandpoint Way NE
PO Box C5371
Seattle, WA 98105
Emergency numbers
206-526-2121
800-732-6985 (Washington)

Spokane Poison Center
South 715 Cowley
Spokane, WA 99202
Emergency numbers
509-747-1077
800-572-5842 (Washington)
800-541-5624 (Elsewhere)

Mary Bridge Children's Hospital Poison Center
317 S. K St.
PO Box 5299
Tacoma, WA 98405-0987
Emergency numbers
206-594-1400
206-594-1414
800-542-6319 (Washington)

Central Washington Poison Center
2811 Tieton Dr.
Yakima, WA 98902
Emergency numbers
509-248-4400
800-572-9176 (Washington)

## Wisconsin

Green Bay Poison Control Center
St. Vincent Hospital
835 S. Van Buren
PO Box 13508
Green Bay, WI 54307-3508
Emergency numbers
414-433-8100
414-870-6112

LaCrosse Area Poison Center
700 W. Ave. South
LaCrosse, WI 54601
Emergency number
608-784-3971

Milwaukee Poison Center
1700 W. Wisconsin
Milwaukee, WI 53233
Emergency number
414-931-4114

## West Virginia

West Virginia Poison Center
3110 MacCorkle Ave. SE
Charleston, WV 25304
Emergency numbers
304-348-4211
800-642-3625 (West Virginia)

# Canadian Poison-Control Centres

**British Columbia**

Poison Information Center
  Saint Paul's Hospital
  1081 Burrard St.
  Vancouver, British Columbia V6Z 1Y6

**Manitoba**

Poison Control Centre
  Children's Hospital
  685 Bannatyne Ave.
  Winnipeg, Manitoba R3E 0WI
  Emergency number
    204-787-2444

**Ontario**

Provensial Regional Poison Centre
  Children's Hospital Eastern Ontario
  401 Smyth Road
  Ottawa, Ontario K1H 8L1
  Emergency numbers (French and
  English)
    613-737-1100
    800-267-1373

Poison Centre
  Hospital for the Sick
  555 University Ave.
  Toronto, Ontario M5G 1X8
  Emergency number
    416-598-5900

**Quebec**

Centre Antipoisons
  Hospital Sainte Justine
  3175 Chemin de la Cote Sainte
  Catherine
  Montreal, Quebec H3T 1C5
  Emergency number
    800-463-5060 (French and English)

Centre de Toxicologie du Quebec
  Le Centre Hospitalier de L'Universite
  Laval
  2705 Boulevard Lurier
  Sainte Foy, Quebec G1B 4G2
  Emergency number
    418-656-8326

# Brand Names of Medications, Vitamins, Minerals and Supplements

$C$heck each product you use carefully. Many drugs are combinations of various ingredients. Look up *each* ingredient. You may find the same brand name under several different generic products. If you can't find the ingredients on the label, ask your pharmacist.

Many of these products are available over the counter. Some are available only with a doctor's prescription.

Inclusion of a brand name does *not* imply recommendation or endorsement. Exclusion does *not* imply a brand name is less effective or less safe than those listed.

## Acetaminophen

| | | | |
|---|---|---|---|
| Aceta® | Dapa® | Liquiprin® | Tapar® |
| Acetagesic® | Datril® | Lyteca® | Temetan® |
| Actamin® | Dimindol® | Med-Apap® | Tempra® |
| Aminodyne Elixir® | Dolanex® | Medigesic® | Tenlap® |
| Anapap® | Dularin® | Nebs® | Tussapap® |
| Anelix® | Febrinol® | Nilprin® | Tylenol® |
| Anuphen® | Fendon® | Panadol® | Valadol® |
| Apap® | G-1® | Parten® | Valorin® |
| Capital® | Janupap® | Phenaphen® | |
| Chlor-A-Tyl® | Lestemp® | Proval® | |

## Alumina/Magnesia

| | | | |
|---|---|---|---|
| Algenic Alka Improved® | AntaGel-II® | Kudrox® | Neutralca-S® |
| Algicon® | Camalox® | Liquimint® | Newtrogel II® |
| Alma-Mag 4 Improved® | Creamlin® | Maalox®, 1, 2, Plus, TC | Rulox®, 1, 2 |
| Alma-Mag Improved® | Delcid® | Magmalin® | Silain-Gel®, 2 Gel |
| Almacone® | Di-Gel® | Magnagel® | Simaal Gel® |
| Almacone II® | Diovol®, Ex | Mi-Acid® | Simeco® |
| Aludrox® | Duracid® | Mintox® | Tempo® |
| Alumid® | Gaviscon®, -2 | Mygel® | Univol® |
| Alumid Plus® | Gelamal® | Mygel II® | WinGel® |
| Amphojel® 500, Plus | Gelusil®, Extra Strength,-M | Mylanta®, Mylanta-II® | |
| AntaGel® | Kolantyl® | Mylanta-II Extra Strength® | |

## Aminophylline

| | | | |
|---|---|---|---|
| Aminodur® | Corophyllin® | Phyllocontin® | |
| Aminophyl® | Lixaminol® | Somophyllin Oral | |
| Amphylline® | Panamin® | Liquid® | |

## Ammonium Chloride (Some of these are combination products. Check all ingredients.)

| | | | |
|---|---|---|---|
| Baby Cough Syrup® | Kophane® | Quelidrine® | Twin-K-Cl® |
| Efricon® | Noedma® | Romilar CF® | Zypan® |
| Endotussin-NN® | Noratuss® | Romilar III® | |
| Kiddies Pediatric® | P-V-Tussin® | Tricodene Sugar-Free® | |

## Amoxicillin

| | | | |
|---|---|---|---|
| Amoxil® | Sumox® | Utimox® | |
| Polymox® | Trimox® | Wymox® | |

## Ampicillin

| | | | |
|---|---|---|---|
| Amcap® | D-Amp® | Pensyn® | Roampicillin® |
| Amcill® | Omnipen® | Polycillin® | Supen® |
| Ameril® | Penbritin® | Principen® | Totacillin® |

## Antidiabetic Agents (Oral)

| | | | |
|---|---|---|---|
| Acetohexamide Dymelor® | Chlorpropamide Diabenese® | Glyburide Dia Beta® | Tolinase® |
| | Glucamide® | Micronase® | Tobutamide |
| | Glipizide Glucotral® | Tolazamide Ronan® | Ornaise® |

## Anthraquinone Laxatives (These are combination products. Check all ingredients.)

| | | | |
|---|---|---|---|
| Black Draught® | Garfields Tea® | Modane® | Senokot®, S |
| Dorbane® | Gentlax S® | Nature's Remedy® | Swiss Kriss® |
| Dorbantyl®, Forte | Innerclean Herbal | Pleasant Pellets® | Tonelax® |
| Doxan® | Laxative® | Senokap DSS® | Unilax® |

## Aspirin

| | | | |
|---|---|---|---|
| Aceticyl® | Acetylsal® | Bayer® | Saletin® |
| Acetol® | Anacin® | Buffinol® | St. Joseph® |
| Acetosal® | Aspergum® | Ecotrin® | |
| Acetosalin® | Aspirjen JR® | Empirin® | |
| Acetylin® | BC tablets® | Measurin® | |

## Atropine (Some of these are combination products. Check all ingredients.)

| | | | |
|---|---|---|---|
| Antrocol® | Donnagel®, | Hybephen® | Ocean-A/S® |
| Arco-lase Plus® | Donnagel PG® | Isopto-Atropine® | Ru-Tuss® |
| Atrohist® | Donnatal®, 2 | Kinesed® | Urised® |
| Barbella® | Donnazyme® | Lomotil® | |
| Donnacin® | Enuretol® | Lyopine® | |

## Belladonna (These are all combination products. Check all ingredients.)

| | | | |
|---|---|---|---|
| Accelerase-PB® | Bellophen® | Donnabarb® | |
| Belladenal® | Comhist LA® | Donnatal® | |
| Bellergal® | Coryztime® | Medi-Spas® | |

## Brompheniramine (These are all combination products. Check all ingredients.)

| | | | |
|---|---|---|---|
| Bromepaph® | Bro-Tane® | Dimetane | Expectorant®, DC |
| Brompheniramine | Bro-Tapp® | Decongestant® | Dimetapp® |
| Expectorant® | Cartane® | Dimetane | Eldatapp® |

## Bulk Laxatives (These are all combination products. Check all ingredients.)

| | | | |
|---|---|---|---|
| Afko-Lube Lax® | Dialose Plus® | Disoplex® | Cascara Suspension® |
| Comfolax® | Diothron® | Lane's Pills® | Nature's Remedy® |
| Concentrated® | Disanthrol® | Malsupex® | Peri-Colace® |
| Constiban® | Disolan Forte® | Milk of Magnesia | Syllamalt® |

## Calcium Carbonate

| | | | |
|---|---|---|---|
| Alka-2 Mints® | Calcium | New Potent Calcium | Potent Calcium 600® |
| BioCal® | Carbonate-500® | Plus® | Rolaids® |
| Bisodol® | Calcium Complete® | Os-Cal 250®, Os-Cal | Suplical® |
| Cal Sup® | Calcium Junior— | 500® | Theracal® |
| Calciday-667® | Chewable® | Oyster-Cal® | Titralac® |
| Calcitab® | Caltrate® | Oyster Calcium® | Tums®, Tums EX® |
| | Chooz® | Oyster Shell 500® | |

## Calcium Citrate

| | | | |
|---|---|---|---|
| Citracal® | | | |

## Calcium Glubionate

| | | | |
|---|---|---|---|
| Neo-Calglucon® | | | |

## Calcium/Magnesium Carbonate

| | | | |
|---|---|---|---|
| Noralac® | Spastosed® | | |

## Chlorpheniramine (Some are combination products. Check all ingredients.)

| | | | |
|---|---|---|---|
| A.R.M.® | Atussin® | Chew-Hist® | Chlortab® |
| Al-Ay® | B.M.E.® | Chlo-Amine® | Co-Histine® |
| Alclear Anti-Allergy® | Barachlor T.D.® | Chlo-Niramine® | Co-Tylenol® |
| Alcon Decongestant® | Bellafedrol A-H® | Chlor-4® | Codimal® |
| Alermine® | Bobid® | Chlor-Span® | Colrex® |
| Algetuss® | Breacol® | Chlor-Trimeton | Comtrex® |
| Allercomp® | Brolade® | Decongestant® | Contac® |
| Allerdec® | Bur-Tuss® | Chloraman® | Coricidin® |
| Allerest® | C.D.M.® | Chlormene® | Cosea® |
| Allergesic® | Cenahist® | Chlorodri® | Deconamine® |
| Allergy® | Cenaid® | Chlorophen® | Dristan® |
| Alo-Tuss® | Centuss® | Chlor-pen® | Extendryl® |
| Alumadrine® | Cerose® | Chlorphenade T.D.® | Fedahist® |
| Amohist® | Chestamine® | Chlorphenwol® | |

≫→

| | | | |
|---|---|---|---|
| Histacon® | Novafed A® | Polaramine® | Strength® |
| Histaspan® | Novahistine® | Pyranistan® | Sudafed Plus® |
| Histex® | Oraminic® | Rhinihist® | Teldrin® |
| Midran® | Ornade® | Sinarest® | Triaminicin® |
| Naldecon® | Panahist® | Sine-Off® | Trymegon® |
| Nasahist® | Phenetron® | Sinu-Tab Extra | |

## Chlorpromazine

| | | | |
|---|---|---|---|
| Chloractil® | Promachlor® | Sonazine® | |
| Chlorzine® | Promapar® | Terpium® | |
| Largactil® | Promaz® | Thorazine® | |

## Codeine (These are all combination products. Check all ingredients.)

| | | | |
|---|---|---|---|
| Actifed C® | Coastaldyne® | Histussinol® | w/Codeine® |
| Amaphen 3® | Codalan® | Isoclor® | Poly-histine® |
| Anexsia® | Codap® | Kiddi-Koff® | Proval No. 3® |
| APAP w/Codeine® | Codasa I and II® | Mallergan® | Prunicodeine® |
| A.P.C. w/Codeine® | Codel® | Maxigesic® | Respi-sed® |
| Ascriptin 2, 3® | Colrex® | Naldecon CX® | Robitussin A-C® |
| Asphac-G w/Codeine® | Codimal PH® | Novahistine DH® | Sedapap 3® |
| Aspodyne w/Codeine® | Cosanyl® | Nucofed® | Soma® |
| B.A.C. 3® | Co-Xan® | Partuss AC® | Syrcodate® |
| Bancap w/Codeine® | Dimetane DC® | Pavadon® | Tega-code® |
| Bri-Stan® | Dolprin 3® | Pediacof® | Tolu-sed® |
| Buff-A-Comp® | Drucon® | Percogesic-C® | TSG Croup Liquid® |
| Calcidrine® | Empirin 2, 3, 4® | Phenaphen 2, 3, 4®, | Tussar-2® |
| Capital w/Codeine® | Fedahist-C® | 650 | Tussi-Organidin® |
| Cerose® | Fiorinal 1, 2, 3® | Phenatuss® | Tylenol 1, 2, 3, 4® |
| Cetro-Cirose® | G-3® | Phenergan Expectorant | |
| Cheracol® | Golacol® | w/Codeine® | |
| Chlor-Trimeton Expt® | Guialyn® | Phenodyne | |

## Dextromethorphan

(These are all combination products. Check all ingredients.)

| | | | |
|---|---|---|---|
| Congesprin® | Kolephrin®, GG/DM | Robitussin-DM®, Cough | Tolu-Sed DM® |
| Coricidin® | N-N Cough Syrup® | Calmers®, PE | Triaminic-DM® |
| Coryban® | Naldecon DX® | Romilar CF®, | Tricidene Forte®, |
| Coryzex® | Naldetuss® | Children's,III® | Sugar-Free |
| Cosanyl DM® | Noratuss II® | Silexin Cough Syrup® | Tricodene Pediatric® |
| DayCare® | Novahistine® | Sorbutuss® | Triminacol® |
| Delsym® | NyQuil® | Spec-T Sore | Trind DM® |
| Dimacol® | Nycoff® | Throat/Cough | Tussagesic® |
| Dondril Anticough® | Ornacol® | Suppressant Lozenges® | Tussar DM® |
| Dorcol Children's | Orthoxocol® | Spec-T Sore Throat/ | 2/G-DM® |
| Cough Syrup® | PediaCare 1® | Decongestant | Vicks Cough Silencer |
| Dr. Drake's® | PediaCare 3® | Lozenges® | Lozenges® |
| Dristan Cough | Pertussin® | St. Joseph Cough | Vicks Cough Syrup® |
| Formula® | Pinex® | Syrup® | Viromed® |
| Endotussin-NN® | Quelidrine® | Sucrets Cough Control | |
| Formula 44® | Queltuss® | Formula® | |
| Halls® | Quiet-Nite® | Sudafed Cough Syrup® | |
| Kleer® | REM® | Supercitin® | |

## Dibasic Calcium

| | | | |
|---|---|---|---|
| Dical D® | Dimenate® | Dramamine® | Eldodram® |
| Dical D Wafers® | Dimenest® | Dramocen® | Hydrate® |
| Dicalcium Phosphate® | Dimentabs® | Dymenate® | Trav-Arex® |
| Dimenhydrinate | Dipendrate® | Eldryl® | Traveltabs® |

## Dimethylmethane Laxatives

(These are combination products. Check all ingredients.)

| | | | |
|---|---|---|---|
| Agoral® | Dulcolax® | Evac-U-Gen® | Fleet Bagenema |
| Alopen® | Effersyllium® | Ex-Lax® | 1105® |
| Correctol® | Espotabs® | Extra Gentle Ex-Lax® | Fleet Bisacodyl Enema® |
| Dual Formula | Evac-Q-Kit®, | Feen-A-Mint® | Hydrocil Instant® |
| Feen-A-Mint® | Evac-Q-Kwik® | | |

| Laxative® | L.A. Formula® | Petro-Syllium® No. 1, 2 | Siblin® |
|---|---|---|---|
| Kondremul with | Laxcaps® | Petrogalar with | Syllact® |
| Phenolphthalein® | Metamucil®, | Phenolphthalein® | Syllamalt® |
| Konsyl® | Instant Mix® | Phenolax® | |

**Diphenhydramine** (Some of these are combination products. Check all ingredients.)

| | | | |
|---|---|---|---|
| Baramine® | Bentrac® | Fenylhist® | Rodryl® |
| Bax® | Benylin® | Histine® | Rohydra® |
| Benachlor® | Diphen-Ex® | Hyrexin® | Span-Lanin® |
| Benadryl® | Eladryl® | Nordryl® | Symptrol® |
| Benahist® | Fenylex® | Para-Hist Antitussive® | Tusstat® |

**Docusate** (These are all combination products. Check all ingredients.)

| | | | |
|---|---|---|---|
| Afko-Lube® | Plus® | Dorbantyl Forte® | Laxcaps® |
| Afko-Lube Lax® | Dio Medicone® | Doxan® | Modane Soft® |
| Colace® | Dio-Sul® | Doxidan® | Peri-Colace® |
| Coloctyl® | Diothron® | Doxinate® | Regutol® |
| Comfolax® | Disanthrol® | Dual Formula | Senodap DSS® |
| Comfolax Plus® | Disolan®, Forte | Feen-A-Mint® | Softenex® |
| Constiban® | Disonate® | Extra Gentle Ex-Lax® | Surfax® |
| Correctol® | Disoplex® | Gentlax S® | Unilax® |
| Dialose®, Dialose | Dorbantyl® | Kasof® | |

**Ephedrine** (Some of these are combination products. Check all ingredients.)

| | | | |
|---|---|---|---|
| Amsec® | Bronkaid® | Phedral C.T.® | Theodrine® |
| Azma Aid® | Bronkolizer® | Primatene®M, P | Theofedral® |
| Bofedrol® | Bronkotabs® | T.E.P.® | Theophenyllin® |
| Bronitin® | NyQuil® | Tedral® | Theoral® |

**Epinephrine**

| | | | |
|---|---|---|---|
| Adrenalin® | Asthma Meter® | Epinal® | Primatene Mist® |
| Ana-Kit® | Asthmanefrin® | Epitrate® | Sus-Phrine® |
| Asmolin® | Epifrin® | Medihaler-Epi® | Vaponefrin® |

**Erythromycin**

| | | | |
|---|---|---|---|
| A/T/S® | ERYC® | Ery-Tab® | T-Stat 2.0% Topical |
| Benzamycin Topical | Erycette® | Erythromycin Filmtab® | Solution® |
| Gel® | EryDerm® | Ilotycin® | |
| E-Mycin® | Erymax Topical | Pediamycin® | |
| ETS 2%® | Solution® | Pediazole® | |

**Ferrous Fumurate**

| | | | |
|---|---|---|---|
| Feco-T® | Fersamal® | Hemocyte® | Novofumar® |
| Femiron® | Fumasorb® | Ircon® | Palafer® |
| Feostat® | Fumerin® | Neo-Fer® | Palmiron® |

**Ferrous Gluconate**

| | | | |
|---|---|---|---|
| Apo-Ferrous | Feralet® | Fertinic® | Simron® |
| Gluconate® | Fergon® | Novoferrogluc® | |

**Ferrous Sulfate**

| | | | |
|---|---|---|---|
| Apo-Ferrous Sulfate® | Fero-Grad® | Hematinic® | Slow Fe® |
| Feosol® | Fero-Gradumet® | Mol-Iron® | |
| Fer-In-Sol® | Ferralyn® | Novoferrosulfa® | |
| Fer-Iron® | Fesofor® | PMS Ferrous Sulfate® | |

**Folate**

| | | | |
|---|---|---|---|
| Apo-Folic® | Folvite® | Novofolacid® | Vitamin B-9® |

**Guiafenesin** (Some of these are combination products. Check all ingredients.)

| | | | |
|---|---|---|---|
| Actifed C Expectorant® | Coricidin® | Mudrane GG® | 2/G® |
| Ambenyl® | DM Plus® | Novahistine Products® | 2/G-DM® |
| Anti-tuss D.M.® | Dextro-Tuss GG® | PMP Expectorant® | Vicks Cough Formula® |
| Bronkilixir® | Dilor-G® | Quibron® | Vicks Formula 44D |
| C.D.M® | Dimetane Expectorant® | Robitussin® | Decongestant Cough |
| Cheracol-D® | Entex® | Sudafed Cough Syrup® | Mixture® |
| Chlor-Trimeton | G-100® | Tolu-Sed® | |
| Expectorant® | GG-Cen® | Trind® | |

**Hydrocodone** (These are all combination products. Check all ingredients.)

| | | | |
|---|---|---|---|
| Amacodone® | Citra Forte® | Tussend® | |
| Bancap® | Codimal® | Tussionex® | |

**Ibuprofen**

| | | | |
|---|---|---|---|
| Advil® | Motrin® | Rufen® | |
| Mediprin® | Nuprin® | Tendar® | |

**Indomethacin**

| | | | |
|---|---|---|---|
| Indocid®, Indocin® | Indo-Lemmon® | Novomethacin® | |
| Indocin SR® | Indomed® | | |

**Insulin**

| | | | |
|---|---|---|---|
| Humulin L, N, R® | Lente® | Novulin N® | Ultralente® |
| Iletin Regular I, II® | Mixtard® | R, 70/30® | Velosulin® |
| Insulatard NPH® | NPH Iletin, I® | Semilente® | |

**Iron Polysaccharide**

| | | | |
|---|---|---|---|
| Hytinic® | Niferex® | Nu-Iron® | |

**Isoniazid**

| | | | |
|---|---|---|---|
| INH® | Niconyl® | Rolazid® | Trinaid® |
| Laniazid® | Panzid® | Teebaconin® | Uniad® |

**Isoproterenol**

| | | | |
|---|---|---|---|
| Aerolene® | Iso-Asminyl® | Medihaler-Iso® | Vapo-Iso® |
| Asminorel® | Isophed® | Norisodrine Aerotrol® | |
| Duo-Medhaler® | Isuprel® | Proternol® | |

**Magnesium Hydroxide**

| | | | |
|---|---|---|---|
| Haley's M-O® | Milk of Magnesia® | M.O.M.® | Phillips' Milk of Magnesia® |

**Magnesium Oxide**

| | | | |
|---|---|---|---|
| Mag-Ox 400® | Maox® | Par-Mag® | Uro-Mag® |

**Magnesium Trisilicate/Alumina/Magnesia**

| | | | |
|---|---|---|---|
| Escot® | Magnatril® | | |

**Manganese**

| | | | |
|---|---|---|---|
| Mn-Plus® | | | |

**Metronidazole**

| | | | |
|---|---|---|---|
| Flagyl® | Metronid® | Prostat® | |
| Metric 21® | Metryl® | Satric® | |

**Mineral oil** (These are all combination products. Check all ingredients.)

| | | | |
|---|---|---|---|
| Agoral® | with Cascara, | Neo-Cultol® | Petrogalar with |
| Agoral Plain® | with Phenolphthalein | Petro-Syllium® 1, 2 | Phenolphthalein® |
| Krondremul® | Milkinol® | Petrogalar® | |

**Niacin**

| | | | |
|---|---|---|---|
| Diacin® | Nico-400® | Nicolar® | Tega-Span® |
| Niac® | Nico-Span® | Nicotex® | |
| Niacin Capsules® | Nicobid® | Span-Niacin® | |

**Nitrofurantoin**

| | | | |
|---|---|---|---|
| Furadantin® | Macrodantin® | Sarodant® | |
| Furalan® | Nitrex® | Trantoin® | |
| Furantoin® | Nitrofor® | Urotoin® | |

**Omega-3 Polyunsaturated Fatty Acids**

| | | | |
|---|---|---|---|
| Cardi-Omega 3® | Marine 1000® | Promega® | Sea-Omega 50® |
| Marine 500® | Max-EPA® | Proto-Chol® | |

**Oral contraceptives**

| | | | |
|---|---|---|---|
| Brevicon® | Micronor® | Norlestrin® | Ovrette® |
| Demulin® | Modicon® | Ortho Novum® | Ovulen® |
| Enovid® | Nor Q.D.® | Ortho Novum 7-7-7® | Tri-Norinyl® |
| Lo-Ovulen® | Nordette® | Ovcon® | Triphasil® |
| Loestrin® | Norinyl® | Ovral® | |

## Penicillin G

| | | | |
|---|---|---|---|
| Acrocillin® | G-Recillin-T® | Lanacillin® | Pensorb® |
| Biotic T® | Hyasorb® | Palocillin-S® | Pentids® |
| Cryspen® | L-Cillin® | Palocillin-5® | Pfizerpen® |
| Deltapen® | K-Pen® | Parcillin® | SK-Penicillin® |

## Penicillin VK

| | | | |
|---|---|---|---|
| Beepen® | Lanacillin® | Phenethicillin | SuspenUticillin VK® |
| Betapen® | Ledercillin® | Potassium® | V-Cillin K® |
| Biotic V® | LV Tabs® | Repen VK® | V-Pen® |
| Bopen® | Penapar® | Robicillin-VK® | Veetids® |
| Cocillin® | Penagen-VK® | Ro-Cillin VK® | |
| Compocillin® | Pen-Vee-K® | SaroPen VK® | |
| Dowpen® | Pfizerpen VK® | SK-Penicillin VK® | |

## Pheniramine (Some of these are combination products. Check all ingredients.)

| | | | |
|---|---|---|---|
| Allerstat® | Fiogesic® | Robitussin-AC® | Tritussin® |
| Corizahist® | Inhiston® | Triaminic® | Tussagesic® |
| Decobel® | Poly-Histine® | Triminacol® | Tussar-2® |

## Phenobarbital

| | | | |
|---|---|---|---|
| Barbipil® | Hypnette® | Phenonyl® | SK-Phenobarbital® |
| Barbita® | Luminal® | Pheno-square® | Solu-barb® |
| Henomint® | Orprine® | Sedadrops® | Somonal® |

## Phenylephrine (Some of these are combination products. Check all ingredients.)

| | | | |
|---|---|---|---|
| Alcon-Efrin® | Demazin® | Prefrein-A® | Spectab® |
| Allerest Nasal Spray® | Dimetane | Prefrein-Z® | Sucrets Cold |
| C.D.M.® | Decongestant® | Prefrin® | Decongestant |
| Chlor-Trimeton | Dimetane Expectorant® | Pyracort-D® | Lozenge® |
| Expectorant® | Dimetane | Sinarest Nasal Spray® | Tearfrin® |
| Clistin-D® | Expectorant-DC® | Sinex® | Trind® |
| Conar® | Entex® | Singlet® | Trind DM® |
| Congesprin® | Ephrine® | Spec-T Sore Throat- | Vasodidin® |
| Coricidin® | Neo-Synephrine® | Decongestant | |
| Dimetapp® | Pediacof® | Lozenges® | |

## Phenytoin

| | | | |
|---|---|---|---|
| Dihycon® | Di-phenyl® | Diphenytion® | |
| Dilantin® | Diphenylan® | Ekko® | |
| Di-Phen® | Diphenylan Sodium® | Toin® | |

## Potassium Bicarbonate

| | | | |
|---|---|---|---|
| Klor-Con/EF® | K-Lyte® | | |

## Potassium Bicarbonate/Potassium Chloride

| | | | |
|---|---|---|---|
| K-Lyte/Cl® | Klorvess® | Neo-K® | Potassium—Sandoz® |

## Potassium Bicarbonate/Potassium Citrate

| | | | |
|---|---|---|---|
| K-Lyte DS® | | | |

## Potassium Chloride

| | | | |
|---|---|---|---|
| Apo-K® | Kalium Durules® | Klorvess® | Roychlor® |
| Cena-K® | Kaochlor® | Klotrix® | Rum-K® |
| K-10® | Kaochlor S-F® | Micro-K® | SK-Potassium Chloride® |
| KCL® | Kaon-Cl® | Novo-Lente-K® | Slo-Pot® |
| K-Dur® | Kato® | Potachlor® | Slow-K® |
| K-Long® | Kay Ciel® | Potage® | |
| K-Lor® | Klor-10%® | Potasalan® | |
| K-Tab® | Klor-Con® | Potassine® | |

## Potassium Gluconate

| | | | |
|---|---|---|---|
| Bayon® | Kao-Nor® | Kaylixir® | Royonate® |
| K-G Elixir® | Kaon® | Potassium-Rougier® | |

## Prednisone

| | | | |
|---|---|---|---|
| Delta-Dome® | Keysone® | Meticort® | Pan-sone® |
| Deltasone® | Liquid Pred® | Meticorten® | Pred-5® |
| Fernisone® | Lisacort® | Orasone® | |

## Prenatal vitamins

| | | | |
|---|---|---|---|
| Berocca Plus® | Furonatal FA Tablets® | Natafort Filmseal® | Pramet F.A.® |
| Bonacal Plus Tablets® | Iromin-G® | Natalins Rx® | Pramilet F.A.® |
| Chromagen® | Materna Tablets® | Natalins Tablets® | Prenate 90 Tablets® |
| Filibon F.A.® | Mission Prenatal F.A.® | Nestabs® | Stuart Prenatal Tablets® |
| Filibon Forte® | Mission Prenatal H.P.® | Niferex PN® | Stuartnatal 1 + 1® |
| Filibon Prenatal | Mission Prenatal Rx® | Niferex-PN Forte® | Zenate® |
|   Vitamin Tablets® | Natabec Rx Kapsules® | Norlac Rx® | |

## Promethazine (Some of these are combination products. Check all ingredients.)

| | | | |
|---|---|---|---|
| Mallergan® | Phenergan® | Pediatric, VC | Rolamethazine® |
| Maxigesic® | Phenergan |   Expectorant® | Synalgos® |
| Mepergan® |   Compound-D® | Phenerhist® | Synalgos DC® |
| Pentazine® | | Remsed® | |

## Pseudoephedrine

| | | | |
|---|---|---|---|
| Actifed® | Dimacol® | Novahistine Sinus | Robitussin PE® |
| Ambenyl-D® | Drixoral® |   Tablets® | Robutussin DAC® |
| Cenafed® | Eldafed® | Phenergan Compound® | Rondec D, C, S, T, DM® |
| Chlor-Trimeton® | Fedahist® | Phenergan-D® | Sinufed® |
| Co-Tylenol® | Kronofed-A® | Polaramine | Sudafed® |
| D-Feda® | Novafed® |   Expectorant® | Sudafed Plus® |
| Deconamine® | Novafed A® | Ro-Fedrin® | Sudahist® |

## Pyridoxine (B6) Hydrochloride

| | | | |
|---|---|---|---|
| Hexa-Betalin® | Pyroxin® | Rodex® | TexSix T.R.® |

## Pyrilamine (Some of these are combination products. Check all ingredients.)

| | | | |
|---|---|---|---|
| Allergine® | Corizahist® | Prefrin-A Ophthalmic | |
| Antihistamine Cream® | MSC Triaminic® |   Solution® | |
| C.P.C. Cough Syrup® | Nervine® | Pyristan® | |

## Riboflavin (Vitamin B2)  Riobin-50®

## Selenium Sulfide

| | | | |
|---|---|---|---|
| Selenium Sulfide | | | |
|   Tablets®—200mcg | | | |

## Selenium Sulfide topical preparations

| | | | |
|---|---|---|---|
| Excel® | Selsun® | Selsun Blue® | Sul-Blue® |

## Simethicone (These are all combination products. Check all ingredients.)

| | | | |
|---|---|---|---|
| Amphojel Plus® | Mylanta® | Phazyme® | |
| Di-Gel® | Mylanta II® | Silain® | |
| Maalox Plus® | Mylicon® | Silain-Gel® | |

## Sodium Fluoride

| | | | |
|---|---|---|---|
| Denta-FL® | Fluoritab® | Luride® | Pediaflor® |
| Flo-Tab® | Fluorodex® | Luride-SF® | Solu-Flur® |
| Fluor-A-Day® | Flura® | Nafeen® | Stay-Flo® |
| Fluorident® | Karidium® | Pedi-Dent® | Studaflor® |

## Spermicides

| | | | |
|---|---|---|---|
| Because® | Delfen® | Gynol II® | Ortho-Creme® |
| Conceptrol® | Emko® | Intercept® | Ramses 10 Hour® |
| Dalkon® | Encare® | Koromex® | Semicid® |

## Terpin Hydrate (Some of these are combination products. Check all ingredients.)

| | | | |
|---|---|---|---|
| Cerose Compound® | Histogesic® | Lozenges® | Terpichlor® |
| Creoterp® | Ipaterp® | SK-Terpin Hydrate | Tussagesic® |
| Dicodethal® | Palodyne® |   and Codeine® | Tussaminic® |
| Gylanphen® | S.A.C. Throat | Terp® | |

## Tetracycline

| | | | |
|---|---|---|---|
| Achromycin® | Desamycin® | Retet® | Tet-cy® |
| Amer-Tet® | Fed-Mycin® | Robitet® | Tetra-C® |
| Anacel® | G-Mycin® | SK-Tetracycline® | Tetra-Co® |
| Bicycline® | Maso-Cycline® | Sarcocycline® | Tetracap® |
| Centet® | Nor-Tet® | Scotrex® | Tetrachel® |
| Cyclopar® | Partrex® | Sumycin® | Tetrachor® |

| | | | |
|---|---|---|---|
| Tetracyn® | Tetram® | Tetramax® | Trexin® |
| Tetralan® | Tetram-S® | Topicycline® | |

**Theophylline**

| | | | |
|---|---|---|---|
| Aerolate® | Lodrane® | Sustaire® | Theolair® |
| Aquaphyllin® | Optiphyllin® | Theo-II® | Theolair SR® |
| Bronkodyl® | Oralphyllin® | Theobid® | Theolixir® |
| Duraphyl® | Quibron T® | Theobron® | Theon® |
| Elixicon® | Quibron T SR® | Theocap® | Theospan-SR® |
| Elixophyllin® | Slo-Bid® | Theoclear 80® | Theostat 80® |
| Elixophyllin SR® | Slo-Phyllin® | Theoclear L. A.® | Theovent Long Acting® |
| Lanophyllin® | Somophyllin® | Theo-dur® | |

**Thiamine (B₁) Hydrochloride**

| | | | |
|---|---|---|---|
| Betalin® | Bewon® | Pan-B-1® | |
| Betalin S® | Biamine® | | |

**Thyroid Medications**

| | | | |
|---|---|---|---|
| Arco® | Delcoid® | Thermoloid® | |
| Armour® | Maroin® | Thyrocrine® | |
| Dathroid® | S-P-T® | Thyro-Teric® | |

**Tribasic Calcium Phosphate**

| | | | |
|---|---|---|---|
| Posture® | | | |

**Tryptophan**

| | | | |
|---|---|---|---|
| Pacitron® | Trofan® | Tryptacin® | |

**Vitamin A**

| | | | |
|---|---|---|---|
| Afaxin® | Alphalin® | Aquasol A® | |

**Vitamin B₁₂**

| | | | |
|---|---|---|---|
| Acti-B12® | Betalin 12® | Droxomin® | Redisol® |
| alphaREDISOL® | Codroxomin® | Ener B intranasal B₁₂ | Rubion® |
| Anacobin® | Cyanabin® | Gel® | Rubramin® |
| Bedoz® | Cyanocobalamin | Kaybovite® | Rubramin PC® |
| Berubigen® | Injection® | Kaybovite-1000® | |

**Vitamin C (Ascorbic Acid)**

| | | | |
|---|---|---|---|
| Apo-C® | Cecon® | Cevalin® | Redoxon® |
| Arco-Cee® | Cee-1000 T.D. Tablets® | Cevi-Bid® | |
| Ascorbicap® | Cemill® | Cevita® | |
| Ce-Vi-So® | Cetane® | Flavorcee® | |

**Vitamin D**

| | | | |
|---|---|---|---|
| Calciferol® | DHT Intensol® | Hytakerol® | Radiostol Forte® |
| Calderol® | Deltalin® | Ostoforte® | Rocaltrol® |
| DHT® | Drisdol® | Radiostol® | |

**Vitamin E**

| | | | |
|---|---|---|---|
| Aquasol E® | E-Ferol® | Epsilan-M® | Viterra E® |
| Chew-E® | Eprolin® | Pheryl-E® | |

**Vitamin K**

| | | | |
|---|---|---|---|
| Mephyton® | Synkavite Injection® | Synkavite Tablets® | |

**Zinc**

| | | | |
|---|---|---|---|
| Medizinc® | Verazinc® | Zincate® | ZinKaps-220® |
| Orazinc® | Zinc-220® | ZinKaps-110® | |

BRAND NAMES

397

# Glossary

**Abruptio placenta**—Premature detachment of the placenta, often associated with shock.

**Accessory nipple**—Extra nipple.

**Acidosis**—Dangerous condition caused by the accumulation of acid in the blood.

**Acute**—Having a short, relatively severe course.

**Adrenal insufficiency**—Reduced functioning of the adrenal glands. One gland is attached to each kidney, which produces steroid hormones and adrenalin.

**Agenesis corpus callosum**—Absence of part of the brain.

**Alkalosis**—Dangerous condition caused by acid loss and accumulation of base in the blood.

**Amniocentesis**—Surgical insertion of a needle into the uterus to obtain amniotic fluid.

**Amniotic fluid**—Fluid contained in the sac in which the fetus grows and develops.

**Anaphylaxis**—Unusual or exaggerated allergic reaction to a foreign substance.

**Anemia**—Condition in which the blood is low in red blood cells or hemoglobin.

**Angina**—Severe but temporary heart pain causing a sensation of suffocation or constriction. Results from decreased oxygen supply to the heart.

**Angiomas**—Non-malignant tumor of blood vessels. Sometimes called *spiders.*

**Ankylosing spondylitis**—rheumatoid arthritis of the spine, causing spinal rigidity.

**Anophthalmia**—Developmental defect characterized by complete absence of the eye or by the presence of eye remnants.

**Antiasthmatic**—Substance that prevents or treats asthma attacks. See *Asthma.*

**Anticholinergic**—Blocks activity of the parasympathetic nervous system. Your pharmacist can tell you which medications are anticholinergic.

**Antiemetic**—Substance that prevents or treats nausea and vomiting.

**Antioxidant**—Substance that prevents oxidation. Oxidation can cause substances to break down and damage cells.

**Antiprotozoal**—Anti-infective agent that treats infections caused by microorganisms of the protozoan group.

**Antiserotonin**—Substance that blocks the activity of serotonin in the body.

**Antispasmodic**—Agent that relieves muscle spasm.

**Antitussive**—Substance that prevents or treats cough.

**Apgar score**—Numerical expression of the condition of a newborn infant. Usually determined at 1 minute and 5 minutes after birth. It is the sum of points gained on assessment of the heart rate, respiratory effort, muscle tone, reflex, irritability and baby's color.

**Aplasia**—Lack of development of an organ or tissue. Cellular components of the organ of tissue.

**Apnea**—Transitory absence of breathing.

**Arrhythmia**—Deviation from normal heart rhythm.

**Arthritis**—Inflammation of a joint.

**Asthma**—Attack of breathlessness from constriction of bronchiols.

**Ataxia**—Staggering.

**Benign**—Doing little or no harm. Not malignant. See *Malignant.*

**Beriberi**—Disease caused by a deficiency of thiamine. Characterized by nerve damage, heart disease and edema. The epidemic form is found primarily in areas in which white (polished) rice is the staple food, such as Japan, China, the Phillipines, India and other Southeast Asian countries.

**Beta-adrenergic blocker**—Inhibits activity of some sympathetic-nervous-system receptors. Your pharmacist can tell you which medications have this property.

**Breaking of the waters**—Rupture of the amniotic fluid sac that holds the fetus.

**Bronchitis**—Inflammation or swelling of the airway leading to the lung.

**Bronchodilator**—Agent that causes expansion in the size of the airways leading to the lungs.

**Bursitis**—Inflammation or swelling of a sac-like cavity, called a *bursa,* located in the tissue at places where friction might build up. For example, the achilles tendon has a bursa. Swelling is occasionally accompanied by calcium deposits.

**Carcinogen**—Any cancer-producing substance.

**Carminative**—Medicine that relieves flatulence (stomach or intestinal gas) and decreases intestinal pain.

**Cataracts**—Condition that turns eye lens opaque.

**Cerebral palsy**—Muscle disorder that appears before age 3. Due to non-progressive damage to the brain.

**Cesarean section**—Incision through the abdominal and uterine walls for delivery of a fetus.

**Cholesterol**—Fatty substance in the blood. It is obtained from animal foods in the diet, and it is manufactured in the liver. High blood-cholesterol levels are associated with an increased risk for heart disease.

**Chronic**—Persisting over a long period of time.

**Cleft lip**—Elongated opening in the lip.

**Cleft palate**—Elongated opening in the bone in the top of the mouth.

**Club foot**—Congenital deformity of the foot. Foot is twisted out of shape or position.

**Colic**—Pain in the lower intestine of an infant that occurs intermittently not continuously. Infant draws its legs up to the chest and cries.

**Colitis**—Inflammation of the colon or lower portion of the intestine.

**Colon cancer**—Cancer in the colon or lower portion of the intestine.

**Congenital malformation**—Referring to a defective formation present at birth, regardless of cause.

**Cortical blindness**—Blindness due to a problem of the external part of the eye lens.

**Cushing's disease (Cushing's syndrome)**—Condition in which the adrenal gland is overactive. Symptoms may include fattening of the face, neck and trunk, softening of the spine, loss of menstrual periods, extra hair, impotence, purple marks on complexion, high blood pressure, pain in stomach and back, and muscle weakness.

**Cyanosis**—Bluish discoloration of the skin due to a reduced delivery of oxygen in the blood.

**Cyclopia**—Abnormal development resulting in child having only one eye. Nose may be absent or located above the eye.

**Cystic fibrosis**—Hereditary disorder characterized by chronic lung disease, dysfunction of the pancreas and high electrolyte content in the sweat.

**Dandy-Walker syndrome**—Type of water on the brain due to the obstruction of the vessels draining the fluid around the brain.

**Decreased sperm motility**—Reduction in the ability of sperm cells to move through the vagina and uterus and fertilize an egg. This is one cause of infertility.

**Delirium**—Mental disturbance marked by illusions, hallucinations, physical restlessness and inability to make sense. Usually it results from a toxic state and lasts a short time.

**Ebstein's anomaly**—Malformation of heart and heart valve.

**Diabetes**—Disease characterized by increased urination. Usually refers to diabetes mellitus. See *Diabetes mellitus.*

**Diabetes mellitus**—Condition characterized by abnormally high blood sugar due to insufficient insulin activity.

**Diaphoretic**—Sweating.

**Diuretic**—Agent that promotes urine secretion.

**DNA**—Deoxyribonucleic acid.

**Down's syndrome**—Type of congenital mental retardation due to abnormality of chromosomes.

**Ductus arteriosus**—Blood vessel that connects the pulmonary artery directly to the artery leaving the heart.

**Dwarfism**—Stunted growth.

**Dysplasia**—Abnormality in development.

**Eclampsia**—Convulsions and coma (rarely coma alone) that occur in the last half of pregnancy and in the first week after birth. It is associated with high blood pressure, edema and/or loss of protein in the urine.

**Edema**—Swelling of tissue due to accumulation of fluid.

**Emetic**—Agent that causes vomiting.

**Emmenagogue**—Agent that induces menstruation.

**Emphysema**—Distension of lung's air sacs.

**Encephalopathy**—Any degenerative disease of the brain.

**Endometriosis**—Presence of uterine-lining tissue in abnormal sites, such as the abdominal cavity.

**Enzyme**—Protein capable of accelerating or producing a reaction.

**Epicanthal folds**—Vertical skin folds on either side of the nose. Folds are present as a normal characteristic in people of certain races. Sometimes occurs as a congenital abnormality in other races.

**Epilepsy**—Episodes of disordered activity in the brain. Usually causes loss of consciousness.

**Epileptic seizure**—Episode of disordered activity in the brain. Causes loss of consciousness and convulsions.

**Extrapyramidal symptoms**—Abnormal movements, rigidity or uncontrollable twitching.

**FDA (Food and Drug Administration)**—U.S. federal agency responsible for evaluating safety and effectiveness of medications.

**Fetal hydantoin syndrome**—Group of malformations that occur after exposure to hydantoin medications, including barbiturates and phenytoin.

**Fibrocystic breast disease**—Benign disease characterized by many benign lumps in the breasts.

**Fibrosing alveolitis**—Inflammation of lung air sacs causing formation of excessive tissue.

**Fluorosis**—Mottled discoloration of tooth enamel resulting from ingestion of excess amounts of fluorine during fetal tooth development.

**Fontanel**—Membrane space between bones of the skull; they form a soft area.

**Forceps delivery**—Vaginal delivery of an infant using surgical instruments.

**G6PD deficiency**—Hereditary deficiency of Glucose-6-phosphate dehydrogenase. Seen in people of Mediterranean decent. Associated with destruction of red blood cells.

**Genital herpes**—Blistered skin lesions due to infection with herpes virus.

**Goiter**—Enlargement of the thyroid gland, causing a swelling in the front part of the neck.

**Gonorrhea**—Infectious sexually transmitted disease.

**Gout**—Hereditary form of arthritis characterized by an excess of uric acid in the blood and by recurrent attacks of acute arthritis usually involving a single joint.

**Growth retardation**—Growth at a slower-than-expected rate.

**Grand mal**—Form of an epiletic attack with or without coma.

**Hallucinations**—False perception occurring without true sensory stimulus. Common in some psychiatric diseases, during some types of intoxication and after head injury.

**Heartburn**—Burning acid sensation in the stomach.

**Heme**—Oxygen-carrying component of red blood cells.

**Hemolytic anemia**—Anemia caused by excessive destruction of red blood cells.

**Hemorrhagic newborn**—Self-limited bleeding disorder in the first days of life. Caused by vitamin-K deficiency.

**Hemorrhoids**—Varicose veins in the rectum.

**Hernia**—Protrusion of a loop or knuckle of an organ or tissue through an abnormal opening.

**Hip dislocation**—Displacement of hip bone away from its normal position in hip socket.

**Hives**—Allergic skin rash that itches intensely.

**Hyaline membrane disease**—Difficulty breathing in newborns, especially premature infants; due to failure to secrete a protein-lipid complex in the lung. Also called *respiratory-distress syndrome.*

**Hydrocele**—Swelling due to accumulation of fluid in the testes.

**Hydrocephalus**—Condition characterized by abnormal accumulation of fluid in the skull. Accompanied by enlargement of the head, prominence of the forehead, slow growth of the brain, mental deterioration and convulsions.

**Hydrops fetalis**—Accumulation of fluid throughout the entire body of a newborn.

**Hyperbilirubinemia**—Excessive bilirubin in the blood.

**Hypertension**—High blood pressure.

**Hyperthyroidism**—Excessive activity of the thyroid gland. Causes rapid pulse, sleeplessness and weight loss.

**Hypoplasia left-heart syndrome**—Incomplete development of the left ventricle of the heart.

**Hypothyroidism**—Deficient activity of the thyroid gland. Causes sluggishness, decreased mental capacity and goiter.

**Hysteria**—Psychiatric condition characterized by excitability and anxiety.

**Imperforate anus**—Absence of the opening into the rectum.

**Impotence**—Inability of a man to have sexual intercourse. Unable to have and maintain an erection.

**Infantile beriberi**—Disease of breast-fed infants whose mothers have thiamine deficiency. Characterized by diminished urine secretion, progressive edema and often by acute heart failure, which may end in sudden death of the infant.

**Inflammatory bowel disease (Crohn's disease)**—Regional inflammation of the intestine.

**Inguinal hernia**—Protrusion of a loop or knuckle of an organ or tissue through an abnormal opening between the abdomen and thigh.

**Insomnia**—Sleeplessness.

**Intercranial hemorrhage**—Bleeding in or around the brain.

**Intercranial hypertension**—Abnormally high pressures in and around the brain. Causes brain damage.

**Intestinal motility**—Rhythmic movement of the intestine to move its contents.

**Intestinal perforation**—Rupture of the intestinal wall.

**Intestinal ulceration**—Formation of sores on the surface of the lining of the intestine.

**Intrauterine death**—Death of the fetus inside the uterus before birth.

**Intravenous**—Into a vein.

**Iron-deficiency anemia**—Most common type of anemia. Caused by insufficient iron intake and/or stores.

**Jaundice**—Symptom of liver damage, gallbladder disease or red-blood-cell damage. Whites of eyes and skin are yellow, urine is dark and stools are light color.

**Kernicterus**—Bile accumulates, staining brain structures. May result in mental retardation.

**Kidney stones**—Small, solid stones of calcium, cholesterol or other body chemicals that develop in the kidney of some people.

**Laxative**—Medications that stimulate evacuation of the bowel.

**Letdown reflex (Ejection reflex)**—Reflex initiated by the suckling of the infant at the breast. Triggers pituitary gland to release oxytocin into the bloodstream. Oxytocin causes cells in the breast to contract and release milk from ducts.

**Lymph**—Fluid derived from tissue fluids.

**Lymph glands**—Gathering of cells specialized to secrete or excrete lymph. See *Lymph.*

**Malabsorption**—Poor nutrient absorption from the digestive tract.

**Malaise**—Feeling of illness and discomfort.

**Malignant**—Very dangerous; likely to cause death.

**Manic episodes**—Prevailing mood of elation, without cause. Often accompanied by overactivity and excessive excitement.

**Meconium staining**—Staining of the amniotic fluid with fetal stool. Meconium is usually passed after birth. Its presence in amniotic fluid usually indicates fetal distress.

**Megaloblastic anemia**—Anemia characterized by presence of large, immature red blood cells in bone marrow.

**Melancholia**—Severe depression.

**Meningocele**—Protrusion of membranes, which line the brain and spinal cord, through a defect in the skull.

**Meningomyelocele**—Protrusion of a portion of the spinal cord and its enclosing membranes through a defect in spinal bone.

**Metabolic**—Product of a series of chemical changes in the body.

**Metered-dose-inhaler**—Device for inhaling precisely measured dose of medication.

**Migraine headache**—Periodic throbbing headache involving one side of the head.

**Myocardial infarction**—Damage to the heart muscle due to inadequate oxygen supply. Commonly called *heart attack.*

**Nebulizer**—Device for converting liquids to a fine spray for inhalation.

**Neonatal depression**—Decrease in functional activity during early newborn period.

**Neonatal goiter**—Enlargement of thyroid gland in a newborn.

**Normotensive**—Blood pressure within normal limits.

**Oligohydraminios**—Insufficient amount of amniotic fluid.

**Oral clefts**—Elongated opening in the mouth

area. See *Cleft lip; cleft palate.*

**Osteoarthritis**—Arthritis caused by degeneration of joint cartilage.

**Osteomalacia**—Abnormal patterns of mineral deposits in mature bone. Causes pain and softening of the bone.

**Osteoporosis**—Loss of bone mineral and strength from excess loss of calcium, phosphorus and protein.

**Ovarian cysts**—Non-specific term applied to various types of fluid-filled sacs on the ovary.

**Oxytocin**—Hormone that causes the letdown reflex and contractions of the uterus. See *Letdown reflex.*

**Pancreatitis**—Inflammation of the pancreas.

**Paralytic ileus**—Paralysis of intestinal muscle.

**Parasiticide**—Agent that destroys parasites.

**Parenteral**—Not passing through the gastrointestinal tract. Injected through some other route.

**Pellegra**—Syndrome due to deficiency of niacin (or failure to convert tryptophan to niacin). Characterized by skin inflammation, inflammation of mucous membranes, diarrhea and psychic disturbances.

**Peripheral neuropathy**—Functional disturbance of the nervous system outside the brain and spinal cord.

**Perineal**—Pertaining to the area around the pelvic region.

**Persistent fetal circulation**—Failure of newborn's circulatory system to make the transition from fetal circulation.

**Petit mal epilepsy**—Disturbance in brain function in which there is a sudden momentary loss of consciousness with minor jerks. Seen especially in children.

**Phenothiazine tranquilizers**—One category of tranquilizers that have similar chemical structure. Phenothiazine group has 3 subgroups; each has a characteristic group of effects.

**Phenylketonuria**—Inborn error of metabolism. Enzyme that changes phenylalanine to tyrosine is not present. Accumulation of phenylalanine occurs, which results in mental retardation.

**Placental hemorrhage**—Bleeding of placenta.

**Pneumonia**—Inflammation of lung caused by infection.

**Pre-eclampsia**—Loss of protein in the urine. High blood pressure and swelling in pregnancy may precede eclampsia. It is a form of toxemia of pregnancy. See *Toxemia.*

**Pre-eruptive phase**—Time just before the teeth emerge from gums.

**Pulmonary embolism**—Obstruction of blood vessels in the lung by blood clot or other material.

**Radius**—Bone on outer side of forearm or lower arm.

**Rebound acid secretion**—Return of acid secretion when the effect of antacid is gone. Rebound effect may be more severe than before treatment.

**Rebound congestion**—Return of congestion when the effect of medication is gone. Rebound effect may be more severe than before treatment.

**Rebound scurvy**—Condition due to overactivation of breakdown enzymes for vitamin C. Marked by weakness, anemia, spongy gums and a tendency to hemorrhage just below the skin.

**Reflux**—Backward flow.

**Reproductive failure**—Inability to conceive or carry a pregnancy.

**Respiratory distress syndrome**—Difficulty breathing in newborns, especially premature infants. Caused by failure to secrete a protein-lipid complex. Also called *hyaline membrane disease.*

**Retrolental fibroplasia**—Presence of fibrous tissue in the eye between the retina and the lens. Causes blindness. Seen most commonly in premature infants who require high concentrations of oxygen.

**Reye's syndrome**—Disease of the brain and other organs that may cause permanent brain damage. Associated with aspirin use in viral illness in children and young adults (to age 19).

**Rh incompatibility**—Rh-negative mother's development of antibodies against her Rh-positive baby.

**Rheumatic syndrome**—Symptoms resembling a rheumatic disease, such as arthritis.

**Rheumatoid arthritis**—Disease involving joints and other tissues. Results in crippling joint deformities.

**Rickets**—Condition caused by deficiency of vitamin D, especially in infancy and childhood, with disturbance of normal bone development.

**RNA**—Ribonucleic acid .

**Scabies**—Parasitic skin disease caused by the itchmite.

**Scoliosis**—Curvature of the spine.

**Scurvy**—Vitamin-C deficiency disease.

**Seborrhea**—Long-term inflammatory disease of skin. Cause is unknown. Characterized by moderate redness and swelling, dry, moist or greasy scaling, and yellow-crusted patches on various areas.

**SIDS**—Sudden infant death syndrome. Sudden, unexplained death of an apparently healthy child. Cause is unknown.

**Single nasopharynx**—Congenital malformation of the nose and throat.

**Sitz bath**—Bath in which you sit in the tub with hips and buttocks immersed.

**Skin tags**—Excess skin, usually growing from a stalk.

**Sodium overload**—Excessive intake and retention of sodium.

**Sonography**—Graphic recording of soundwaves as they pass through tissue.
Used as a test to diagnose some medical conditions. Especially useful in pregnancy to determine dates.

**Spasticity**—Condition of rigidity or spasm.

**Spina bifida**—Defective closure of the bony encasement of the spinal cord. The cord and lining may or may not protrude.

**Sternum**—Long plate of bone forming the middle of the front wall of the chest.

**Stevens-Johnson syndrome**—Severe allergic reaction involving skin, mucous membranes and other tissues.

**Stool softener**—Laxative that softens feces by increasing moisture content.

**Stroke**—Usually sudden paralysis from injury to the brain or spinal cord. Caused by a blood clot or hemorrhage in the brain.

**Sympathetic nervous system**—Portion of the nervous system that regulates activity of heart muscle, smooth muscle and glands.

**Syndactyly**—Webbed fingers or toes.

**Systemic lupus erythematosus syndrome**—Generalized connectivetissue disorder characterized by skin changes, joint pain, fever and other symptoms.

**T's and Blues**—Street name for tripelenamine and pentazocin.

**Tendonitis**—Inflammation of a tendon.

**Thrombophlebitis**—Inflammation of a vein associated with clot formations.

**Thrush**—Infection with yeast *candida albicans.*

**Thyroid storm**—Severe manifestations of hyperthyroidism that have sudden onset and may be fatal.

**Thyrotoxicosis**—Serious condition resulting from overactive thyroid gland.

**Tibia**—Shin bone. It is the larger of two bones in the lower leg.

**Toxemia**—See *Pre-eclampsia; eclampsia.*

**Tremor**—Involuntary trembling.

**Tuberculosis**—Infection caused by mycobacterium tuberculosis. May cause lung, kidney or other tissue damage.

**Tumors**—Mass of abnormal tissue that resembles the normal tissue but has no useful function. May be benign or malignant. See *Benign; malignant.*

**Ulcer disease**—Open sore occurring in the stomach or duodenum.

**Ulcerative colitis**—Inflammatory condition of the colon.

**Ulcers**—Open sores on a body surface.

**Uremia**—Retention of excessive by-products of protein metabolism in the blood and the toxic condition produced. Marked by nausea, vomiting, headache, vertigo, dimness of vision, coma or convulsions.

**Ureter**—Tube through which urine passes from the kidney to the bladder.

**Urogenitial**—Pertaining to urinary and genital organs.

**Uterine fibroids**—Benign tumors of the uterus. See *Benign.*

**Vertigo**—Illusion of movement, as if the external world were revolving around the person.

**Wernicke-Korsafoff's syndrome**—Syndrome caused by thiamine deficiency. Characterized by eye-muscle instability and difficulty maintaining balance.

**Wheezing**—Making a whistling, breathy sound, such as in asthma. See *Asthma.*

**Wilson's disease**—Degeneration of part of the liver.

**Xerophthalmia**—Dryness of the eye due to vitamin-A deficiency. Condition begins with night blindness.

# Index

**A**

A.P.C. w/Codeine® 392
A-Poxide® 64
A.R.M.® 391
A-200® 231
A/T/S® 393
Abnormal heart rhythm 25, 208, 229, 239
Abruptio placenta 294, 328, 354, 398
Accelerase-PB® 391
Accessory nipple 124, 398
Accutane® 2, 5, 154, 328, 329
Aceta® 390
Acetagesic® 390
Acetaldehyde 347
Acetaminophen 16-17, 45, 47, 83, 99, 137, 175, 197, 348, 390
Acetazolamide 117, 213
Aceticyl® 391
Acetohexamide 18, 38, 390
Acetol® 391
Acetosal® 391
Acetosalin® 391
Acetylin® 391
Acetylsal® 391
Acetylsalicylic acid 40
Achromycin® 396
Acidosis 26-27, 40, 102, 252, 398
Acidulated phosphate fluoride 292
Acrocillin® 395
Actamin® 390
Acti-B12® 397
Actifed® 392, 396, 396
Acyclovir 18-19
Adapin® 112
Adenosylcobalamin 331
Adrenal corticosteroids 296, 319, 334, 337
Adrenal insufficiency 398
Adrenal-gland activity 216
Adrenalin® 393
Adrenalin insufficiency 398
Adrenergic stimulants 21, 149, 153, 173, 253
Advil® 394
Aerolate® 397
Aerolene® 394
Afaxin® 397
Afko-Lube® 391, 393
African yohimbe bark 359
Agenesis corpus callosum 398
Agoral® 392, 394
Al-Ay® 391
Albuterol 20-21, 172
Alclear Anti-Allergy® 391
Alcohol 2, 5-7, 13-14, 130, 346-347
Alcon® Decongestant 391, 395
Alermine® 391
Algenic Alka Improved® 390
Algetuss® 391
Algicon® 390
Alginate 366-367
Alka-2® 379, 391
Alkalosis 32-33, 102, 324, 398
Allercomp® 391
Allerdec® 391
Allerest® 391, 395
Allergesic® 391
Allergine® 396
Allergy® 391
Allerstat® 395
Allopurinol 280
Alma-Mag 4 Improved® 390
Alma-Mag Improved® 390
Almacone® 390

Alo-Tuss® 391
Aloe 36
Aloin 36
Alopen® 392
Alpha tocopherol 338, 339, 366
Alphalin® 397
alphaREDISOL® 397
Aludrox® 380, 390
Alumadrine® 391
Alumid® 390
Alumid Plus® 390
Alumina/Magnesia 390
Alupent® 172
Amacodone® 394
Amantadine 45, 47
Amaphen 3® 392
Ambenyl® 393
Amcap® 390
Amcill® 390
Amer-Tet® 396
American Academy of Pediatrics 6
Ameril® 390
Amiloride 313
Aminodur® 390
Aminodyne Elixir® 390
Aminoglycosides 101
Aminophyl® 390
Aminophylline 22-23, 121, 353, 355, 362, 390
Aminopterin 294, 296
Aminosalicylic acid 237, 280
Amiodarone 280
Amitriptyline 24-25, 321
Ammonium chloride 26-27, 42, 117, 229, 390
Amniocentesis 107, 277, 398
Amniotic fluid 398
Amohist® 391
Amoxicillin 28-29, 390
Amoxil® 390
Amphetamines 25, 73, 91, 113, 141, 189, 334
Amphojel® 390, 396
Amphylline® 390
Ampicillin 28, 30-31, 60, 62, 96, 193, 390
Amsec® 393
Ana-Kit® 393
Anacel® 396
Anacin® 382, 391
Anacobin® 397
Analgesics iii
Anapap® 390
Anaphylaxis 118, 398
Anaprox® 184
Anatomic malformations 4
Anelix® 390
Anemia 12, 14, 28, 30, 38, 40, 42, 68, 98, 126, 128, 132, 138, 166, 186, 187, 221, 224, 226, 240, 246, 248, 250, 260, 262, 266, 268, 290, 294-296, 299, 315, 340, 342-343, 348, 398, 400-401
iron-deficiency 12, 14, 299, 400
Anexsia® 392
Angina 398
Angiomas 398
Animal studies 6-7
Anithistamines 275
Ankylosing spondylitis 184, 398
Anophthalmia 328, 398
Anspor® 62
Antacids 32-34, 42, 65, 73, 75, 99, 115, 129, 151, 193, 200, 213, 217, 223, 225, 257, 261, 269, 286, 293, 301, 310

AntaGel® 390
Anthraquinone laxatives 37, 110, 391
Anti-infectives iii
Anti-inflammatory agents iii, 248
Anti-tuss D.M.® 393
Antianxiety agent 49, 64, 67, 75, 87, 89, 94, 101, 105, 165, 194, 203, 233, 275
Antiasthmatic 84, 398
Antibacterial 122, 178, 186-187, 246, 272
Antibiotic 28, 30, 56, 58, 60, 62, 76, 96, 150, 200, 236, 244, 256
Anticholinergic agents 25, 73, 91, 113, 141, 188, 223, 261, 269
Anticoagulant iii, 134, 278, 341
Anticonvulsant iii, 52-53, 78-79, 94, 106, 108, 124-125, 168-169, 199, 204, 206, 211, 213, 218, 220, 270, 271, 276, 277, 341
Antidepressant 24, 25, 45, 49, 65, 67, 75, 83, 87, 89, 90, 95, 101, 105, 112, 137, 140, 165, 175, 177, 195, 197, 203, 208, 213, 223, 225, 233, 275
Antidiabetic agents, oral iii, 18, 38-39, 42, 73, 119, 157, 161, 193, 217, 237, 261, 265, 269, 349, 390
Antidiarrhea medications 46, 77
Antiemetic 86, 100, 164, 214, 224, 398
Antiepilepsy medication, see Anticonvulsant
Antifungal 80, 180, 190
Antihistamine 5, 45, 47-49, 66-67, 74-75, 83, 86-89, 100-101, 104-105, 135, 137, 164-165, 175, 177, 202-203, 224, 232-233, 274-275, 348
Antihistamine Cream® 396
Antihypertensive medication 119
Antinauseants 348
Antioxidant 322, 398
Antiprotozoal 178, 398
Antiseizure medication, see Anticonvulsant
Antiserotonin 88, 398
Antispasmodic 44, 46, 94, 359, 398
Antithrombin K® 278
Antithyroid agent 226
Antitussive 82, 92, 136, 398
Antiviral 18
Antivert® 164
Antrocol® 391
Anuphen® 390
Apap® 390, 392
Apgar score 398
Aplasia 398
Apnea 22, 258, 352, 398
Apo-C® 397
Apo-Ferrous Gluconate® 393
Apo-Ferrous Sulfate® 393
Apo-Folic® 393
Apo-K® 395
Aqua-ban® 382
Aquaphyllin® 397
Aquasol® 397
Arco® 397, 391
Armour® 397
Arrhythmias 398
Arthritis 5, 139, 185, 241, 398-399, 401
Artifical heart valves 134
Artificial flavoring 366
Artificial sweetener 350
ASA 40
Ascorbic acid, see also Vitamin C, 9, 42, 169, 206, 220, 366, 397
Ascorbicap® 333, 397
Ascriptin 2, 3® 392

INDEX

Asminorel® 394
Asmolin® 393
Aspartame 350-351, 366
Aspergum® 391
Asphac-G® 392
Aspirin 5, 27, 34, 40-41, 83, 98, 126, 135, 137-139, 166, 175, 184, 197, 217, 240-241, 250, 266, 280, 301, 348, 353, 391
Aspirjen JR® 391
Aspodyne® 392
Asthma iv, 4, 20-23, 44-45, 84-85, 116, 118, 119, 148-149, 152-153, 172-173, 216, 252-253, 258-259, 398, 402
Asthma Meter® 393
Asthmanefrin® 393
Astringent 359
Ataxia 398
Atenolol 29, 31
Atrohist® 391
Atropine 44-46, 391
Atussin® 391
Avidin 283
Azma Aid® 393
Azulfidine® 248

**B**

B.A.C. 3® 392
B.M.E.® 391
Baby Cough Syrup® 390
Bactrim® 246
Bancap® 392, 394
Barachlor T.D.® 391
Baramine® 393
Barbella® 391
Barbipil® 395
Barbita® 395
Barbiturates 23, 25, 53, 91, 113, 189, 213, 217, 223, 259, 296, 332, 334, 337, 348
Bax® 393
Bayer® 391
Bayon® 395
BC tablets® 391
Because® 396
Bedoz® 397
Bee pollen 363
Beepen® 395
Belladenal® 391
Belladonna 46-47, 391
Bellafedrol A-H® 391
Bellergal® 391
Bellophen® 391
Benachlor® 393
Benadryl® 393
Bisacodyl 102-103, 392
Bismuth subsalicylate 257
Bisodol® 391
Bisulfite, sodium 369
Black Draught® 391
Blessed thistle 359-361
Blood pressure 3, 25, 39, 73, 91, 93, 117, 129, 133, 141, 151, 179, 208, 223, 229, 232, 238-239, 261, 263, 269, 348-349, 359-360
Blood sugar 39, 42, 57, 73, 129, 147, 223, 225, 237, 261, 269, 348-349
Blue No. 1 366
Blue No. 2 366
Bobid® 391
Body temperature 65, 95, 163, 359
Bofedrol® 393
Bonacal Plus Tablets® 396
Bone meal 285
Bonine® 164
Bopen® 395
Borage leaf 359

Brand names of medications, vitamins, minerals and supplements 390-397
Breacol® 391
Breaking of the waters 398
Breast-feeding 5-6, 13-14
Brethaire® 252
Brethine® 252
Brevicon® 394
Bri-Stan® 392
Bricanyl® 252
Brigen-G® 64
Bro-Tane® 391
Bro-Tapp® 391
Broccoli 363
Brolade® 391
Bromepaph® 391
Brominated vegetable oil (BVO) 366
Brompheniramine 48-49, 228, 391
Brompheniramine Expectorant® 391
Bronchitis 116, 354, 398
Bronchodilator 20, 22, 44, 116, 148, 152, 172, 252, 258, 398
Bronitin® 393
Bronkaid® 393
Bronkilixir® 393
Bronkodyl® 397
Bronkolizer® 393
Bronkosol® 148
Bronkotabs® 393
Brussels sprouts 363
Buff-A-Comp® 392
Buffinol® 391
Bulk laxatives 50, 316, 357, 391
Bur-Tuss® 391
Bursitis 184, 398
Butylated hydroxyanisole 366
Butylated hydroxytoluene (BHT) 366

**C**

C.D.M.® 391, 393, 395
C.P.C. Cough Syrup® 396
Ca-Plus® 379
Cabbage 363
Cadmium 291
Cafergot® Capsules 382
Caffedrine® Capsules 382
Caffeine 6, 22, 210, 258, 286, 352, 355, 381
Cal Sup® 391
Calcet® 379
Calcicaps Tablets® 379
Calciday-667® 379, 391
Calcidrine® 392
Calciferol® 397
Calcitab® 379, 391
Calcium 32, 169, 204, 206, 211, 213, 220, 256-257, 284-286, 293, 302, 304, 310, 311, 316, 336, 343, 353, 357-358, 366, 375, 379, 380, 391-392, 401
Calcium carbonate 284-285, 379, 391
Calcium Carbonate-500® 391
Calcium Complete® 379, 391
Calcium content of selected supplements 380
Calcium Junior® 379, 391
Calcium Orotate® 379
Calcium with Vitamin D® 379
Calciwafers® 379
Calderol® 397
Calorie intake 371
Caltrate® 379, 391
Camalox® 380, 390
Cancer therapy 176
Cannibis 362
Capital® 390, 392
Captopril 42, 144, 313

Carbamazepine 23, 52-53, 115, 121, 151, 163, 169, 193, 206, 213, 220, 259
Carbohydrates 214, 372
Carboxyhemoglobin levels 354
Carboxymethyl cellulose 50, 369
Carcinogen 178, 360, 398
Cardi-Omega 3® 394
Carminative 398
Carotenoids 328
Carrageenan 366
Cartane® 391
Casanthranol 36
Cascara sagrada 36
Casein 367
Caseinate, sodium 367
Castor oil 54-55
Cataracts 26, 209, 216, 398
Catnip 359, 361
Cauliflower 363
Cayenne 359-360
Ce-Vi-So® 397
Cecon® 397
Cee-1000 T.D. Tablets® 397
Cefoxitin 56-57, 60, 63
Ceftriaxone 58-59
Cemill® 397
Cena-K® 395
Cenafed® 396
Cenahist® 391
Cenaid® 391
Centet® 396
Central-nervous-system, adverse effects 133, 151, 158
Central-nervous-system stimulant 352
Centuss® 391
Cephalexin 56, 58, 60-62
Cephalosporin 58, 348
Cephalosporin class of antibiotics 56, 58, 60, 62
Cephalothin 245
Cephradine 62-63
Cerebral palsy 138, 398
Cerose® 391-392, 396
Cesarean delivery 19, 40, 44, 74, 106, 116, 124, 146-147, 162, 205, 212, 218, 234, 276, 398
Cetane® 397
Cetro-Cirose® 392
Cevalin® 397
Cevi-Bid® 397
Cevita® 397
Chamomile 359, 360
Chelated calcium 379
Chelated zinc 342-343
Cheracol® 392
Cheracol-D® 393
Chestamine® 391
Chew-E® 397
Chew-Hist® 391
Chewable Biocal® 379
Chicken 365
Chlo-Amine® 391
Chlo-Niramine® 391
Chlor-A-Tyl® 390
Chlor-4® 391
Chlor-pen® 391
Chlor-Span® 391
Chlor-Trimeton® 391, 392, 393, 395, 396
Chloractil® 392
Chloral hydrate 193
Chloraman® 391
Chlorambucil 294, 296
Chloramphenicol 29, 169, 193, 201, 206, 213, 220, 341
Chlordiazepoxide 64-65, 193
Chlormene® 391

Chlorodri® 391
Chlorophen® 391
Chloroquine 34
Chlorphenade T.D.® 391
Chlorpheniramine 66-67, 210, 391
Chlorphenwol® 391
Chlorpromazine 34, 68, 70, 73, 75, 112,
    221, 260, 268, 321, 392
Chlorpropamide 27, 38, 74, 280, 390
Chlortab® 391
Chlorthalidone 217
Chlorzine® 392
Chocolate 353, 363
Cholesterol 154, 343, 372, 398
Cholestyramine 157, 161, 265, 286, 301,
    330, 332, 337
Cholramphenicol 31
Chooz® 379, 391
Chromagen® 316, 396
Chromium 288, 290
Chronic 398
Cibalith® 162
Cigarettes 9, 13, 354-355
Cimetidine 23, 25, 34, 42, 65, 73-75, 91,
    95, 113, 195, 234, 259, 261, 269, 280,
    141, 189, 348
Cinnamon 359, 361
Cis-retinoic acid 154
Citra Forte® 394
Citracal® 391
Citrate, sodium 324, 367
Citric acid 367
Citrus red No. 2 367
Cleft, oral 398, 400, 401
Cleft palate 398, 400, 401
Clemastine 74-75
Cleocin® 76
Clindamycin 76-77
Clinitest® 57
Clinoril® 250
Clistin-D® 395
Clofibrate 193, 280
Clonazepam 78-79
Clonidine 25, 39, 91, 113, 141, 189
Clotrimazole 80
Club foot 398
Co-Histine® 391
Co-Tylenol® 391, 396
Co-Xan® 392
Coastaldyne® 392
Cobalamin 331
Cocaine 7, 356
Cocillin® 395
Codalan® 392
Codap® 392
Codasa® 392
Codeine 82-83, 136, 353, 392
Codel® 392
Codimal® 391, 392, 394
Codroxomin® 397
Coenzyme 318, 326
Coenzyme A 308
Cohosh 359-361
Coke 356
Cola drinks 286
Colace® 393
Cold products iv
Colic 36, 102, 360, 398
Colitis 76-77, 398, 402
Coloctyl® 393
Colon cancer 357, 398
Colrex® 391-392
Coltsfoot 359, 361
Comfolax® 391, 393
Comfrey 359, 360-361
Comhist LA® 391
Compazine® 221

Compocillin® 395
Comtrex® 391
Conar® 395
Concentrated® 391
Conceptrol® 396
Congesprin® 392, 395
Congestion 207, 401
Constiban® 391, 393
Constipation 2, 372
Contac® 391
Contraceptives iv, 14, 29, 31, 53, 57,
    65, 95, 125, 151, 169, 179, 183, 188,
    191-193, 195, 201, 206, 213, 220, 237,
    247, 257, 286, 291, 296, 307, 318, 319,
    330, 331, 334, 355, 394
Cope® 382
Copper 169, 206, 213, 220, 290, 305,
    343, 334, 357-358
Coriander seed 359
Coricidin® 391-393, 395
Corizahist® 395-396
Corn sugar 367
Corn syrup 367
Corophyllin® 390
Corpus callosum 278
Correctol® 392-393
Cortical blindness 398
Corticosteroids 34, 85, 216, 237, 239,
    286
Cortisone 343
Coryban® 392
Coryzex® 392
Coryztime® 391
Cosanyl® 392
Cosea® 391
Coumadin® 278, 339
Crack 356
Creamlin® 390
Creoterp® 396
Crohn's disease 400
Cromoglycate, sodium 84
Cromolyn 84-85
Cryspen® 395
Cushing's disease 88, 399
Cyanabin® 397
Cyanocobalamin 169, 191, 206, 213,
    220, 294, 295, 331
Cyanocobalamin Injection® 397
Cyanosis 399
Cyclizine 86-87
Cyclopar® 396
Cyclophosphamide 247
Cyclopia 399
Cyproheptadine 88-89
Cystic fibrosis 341, 399
Cytolen® 156
Cytomel® 160

D
D-alpha-tocopherol 338, 339
D-Amp® 390, 338, 339
DHT Intensol® 397
D-Feda® 396
DM Plus® 393
DMSO 251
DNA 399
D1-alpha-tocopherol acetate Dairy
    products 338-339, 364
Dalkon® 396
Dandy-Walker syndrome 278, 399
Danthron 36-37, 110-111
Dapa® 390
Dathroid® 397
Datril® 390
DayCare® 392
Debrisoquin 25, 91, 113, 141, 188, 208
Decobel® 395

Deconamine® 392, 396
Decongestant 44, 46, 116, 119, 207,
    209, 228, 213, 280
Deep-vein thrombosis 134, 279
Dehydroascorbic acid 333
Delcid® 380, 390
Delcoid® 397
Delfen® 396
Delirium 399
Delsym® 392
Delta-Dome® 395
Deltalin® 397
Deltapen® 395
Deltasone® 395
Demazin® 395
Demulin® 394
Denta-FL® 396
Dental disease 318
Depakene® 276
Depakote® 106
Desamycin® 396
Desipramine 90-91, 140
Dexatrim® 382
Dexamethasone 117
Dextran 280
Dextro-Tuss GG® 393
Dextromethorphan 92-93, 392
Dextrose 367
Di-Cal D® 379
Di-Gel® 390, 396
Di-Gel® 380
Di-Phen® 395
Di-phenyl® 395
Dia Beta® 390
Diabenese® 390
Diabetes 3, 4, 38-39, 130, 147, 176,
    214, 288-289, 318, 399
Diacin® 394
Dialose® 393
Dialose Plus® 391, 393
Diaphoretic 399
Diazepam 78, 94-95, 108, 151, 163,
    193, 194, 237, 277
Dical D® 392
Dical D Wafers® 392
Dicalcium Phosphate® 379, 93
Disonate® 393
Disoplex® 391, 393
Disopyramide 237
Disulfiram 151, 179, 213, 280
Diuretics 163, 257, 359, 399
Divalporex 106-108
Docusate 36-37, 103, 110-111, 183, 393
    calcium 110
    potassium 110
    sodium 110
Dolanex® 390
Dolomite 285, 302, 303
Dolophine® 174
Dolprin 3® 392
Dondril Anticough® 392
Donnabarb® 391
Donnacin® 391
Donnagel® 391
Donnatal® 391
Donnazyme® 391
Dorbane® 391
Dorbantyl® 391, 393
Dorcol Children's Cough
    Syrup® 392
Down's syndrome 399
Dowpen®112-113, 395
Doxan® 391, 393
Doxidan® 393
Doxinate® 393
Doxycycline 53, 114-115, 206
Dr. Drake's® 392

Dramine® 392
Dramocen® 392
Drisdol® 397
Dristan® 382, 392
Drixoral® 396
Droxomin® 397
Drucon® 392
Dual Formula Feen-A-Mint® 392-393
Ductus arteriosus 399
Dularin® 390
Dulcolax® 392
Duo-Medhaler® 394
Duracid® 390
Duraphyl® 397
Dwarfism 297, 342, 399
Dycill® 96
Dymenate® 392
Dynapen® 96
Dysplasia 399

**E**

EDTA 367
E.E.S.® 120
E-Ferol® 397
E-Mycin® 120, 393
ERYC® 393
ETS 2%® 393
Ebstein's anomaly 162, 399
Eclampsia 33, 146-147, 227, 284, 324, 399, 402
Ecotrin® 391
Ectopic pregnancy 192
Edema 290, 399
Ebstein's anomaly 399
Effersyllium® 392
Efricon® 390
Eggs 364
Ekko® 395
Eladryl® 393
Elavil® 24
Eldafed® 396
Eldaryl® 392
Eldatapp® 391
Eldodram® 392
Electrolyte imbalance 186
Electrolyte solution 324
Elegen-G® 24
Elixicon® 397
Elixophyllin® 397
Emergency Ana-Kit® 393
Emeside® 124
Emetic 399
Emetrol® 214
Emko® 396
Emmenagogue 399
Emphysema 116, 399
Empirin® 391, 392
Emulsoil® 54
Encare® 396
Encephalopathy 150, 399
Endep® 24
Endometriosis 191, 399
Endotussin-NN® 390, 392
Ener B intranasal B12 Gel® 397
Energy requirements and weight gain 370
Enovid® 394
Entex® 393, 395
Enuretol® 391
Enzyme 399
Ephedrine 23, 27, 34, 48, 116-117, 259, 393
Ephrine® 395
Epicanthal folds 399
Epifrin® 393
Epilepsy 107, 205, 219, 277, 294, 399

Epinal® 393
Epinephrine 25, 91, 113, 118-119, 141, 189, 393
Epitrate® 393
Eprolin® 397
Epsilan-M® 397
Equal® 350
Erthrocin Lactobionate® 120
Erthrocin Stearate Filmtab® 120
Ery-Tab® 393
Erycette® 393
EryDerm® 393
Erymax Topical Solution® 393
EryPed® 120
Erythorbic acid 367
Erythromycin 23, 53, 120-121, 259, 321, 393
Escot® 394
Eskacef® 62
Eskalith® 162
Espotabs® 392
Estriol excretion 28, 30
Estrogen-progestogen pills 318
Ethacrynic acid 217, 280
Ethambutol 122-123
Ethanol 346
Ethosuximide 124-125, 193, 319
Ethril® 120
Ethyl vanillin 369
Evac-Q-Kit® 392
Evac-Q-Kwik® 392
Evac-U-Gen® 392
Ex-Lax® 392
Excedrin® 382
Excel® 396
Expectorant 26, 130, 254
Extendryl® 392
Extra Gentle Ex-Lax® 392-393

Extrapura middle symptoms 399
Extrapyramidal symptoms 68, 72, 128, 129, 176, 221, 224, 260-261, 268-269, 399

**F**

FDA (Food and Drug Administration) 399
False unicorn 359-360
Fat requirements 372
Fat-soluble vitamins 182-183
Febrinol® 390
Feco-T® 393
Fed-Mycin® 396
Fedahist® 392, 396
Fedahist-C® 392
Feen-A-Mint® 392
FEMCAL Powder® 379
Femiron® 393
Fendon® 390
Fennel seed 359
Fenoprofen 42, 126-127, 280
Fenylex® 393
Fenylhist® 393
Feosol® 393
Feostat® 393
Fer-In-Sol® 393
Fer-Iron® 393
Feralet® 393
Fergon® 393
Fernisone® 395
Fero-Grad® 393
Fero-Gradumet® 393
Ferralyn® 393
Ferrous fumerate 299, 393
Ferrous gluconate 299, 367, 393
Ferrous sulfate 299-300, 393
Fersamal® 393

Fertility 10, 13, 221, 352-353
decreased 128
Fertinic® 393
Fesofor® 393
Fetal alcohol syndrome 130, 342, 346-347, 362
Fetal death 3, 105, 138, 142
Fetal goiter 162, 226
Fetal hydantoin syndrome 399
Fetal tooth formation 292
Fetal warfarin syndrome 278
Fiber 291, 301, 303, 316, 343, 357-358, 372, 375
Fibrocystic breast disease 191, 352, 399
Fibrosing alveolitis 248, 399
Filibon F.A.® 316, 396
Filibon Forte® 316, 396
Filibon O.T. Prenatals® 316
Filibon Prenatal Vitamin Tablets® 396
Fiogesic® 395
Fiorinal® 382, 392
Fish 365
Fish-oil pills 363
Flagyl® 394
Flavoproteins 320
Flavorcee® 397
Fleet Bagenema 1105® 393
Flo-Tab® 396
Fluid in lungs 239
Fluor-A-Day® 396
Fluoride 34, 286, 292-293, 303, 324, 396
Fluorident® 396
Fluoritab® 396
Fluorodex® 396
Fluorosis 292, 399
Fluphenazine 128-129
Flura® 396
Folacin 294
Folate 12, 151, 169, 204, 206, 211, 213, 218, 220, 246, 249, 271, 273, 294, 296, 315, 321, 348, 375, 393
Folic acid 272
Folvite® 393
Fontanel 399
Fontanel bulging 256
Food allergies 6
Forceps delivery 40, 399
Formula 44® 392
Fragula 36
Fructose intolerance 214
Fumaric acid 367
Fumasorb® 393
Fumerin® 393
Furadantin® 394
Furalan® 394
Furantoin® 394
Furonatal FA Tablets® 396
Furosemide 42, 139, 144, 185, 213, 217, 251

**G**

GG-Cen® 393
G-Mycin® 396
G-1® 390
G-100® 393
G6PD deficiency 186, 246, 399
G-3® 392
Gamma benzene hexachloride 158
Gantanol® 246
Garfields Tea® 391
Garlic pills 363
Gastric defoaming agent 242
Gastric-acid secretion 234
Gaviscon® 390
Gelamal® 390
Gelatin 367

Gelusil®380, 390
Genital herpes 18-19, 399
Gentlax S® 391, 393
Glipizide 38, 130, 390
Glucamide® 390
Glucose 236, 367
Glucose-6-phosphate
    dehydrogenase 156, 246, 399
Glucotral® 390
Glyburide 38, 130, 390
Glycerin 367
Glycerol 367
Glyceryl guaiacolate 130
Goiter 297, 399
Goiter, fetal 162, 226
Golacol® 392
Gonadal immaturity 342
Gonorrhea 56, 58, 399
Gotu kola 359
Gout 184, 399
Green No. 3 367
Growth retardation 399
Guaifenesin 130-131, 393
Guanethidine 25, 73, 91, 113, 117, 129,
    133, 141, 189, 208, 223, 225, 261, 263,
    269
Guialyn® 392
Gums 367
Gylanphen® 396
Gyne-Lotrimin® 80
Gynol II® 396

**H**
HDL cholesterol 154, 343
Haldol® 132
Haley's M-O® 394
Halls® 392
Hallucinations 24, 44, 46, 64, 74, 86,
    88, 90, 94, 112, 140, 188, 194, 228,
    234, 248, 359, 399
Haloperidol 132-133, 163
Heart arrythmias 312, see also
    Abnormal heart rythm
Heart attack 302, 400
Heart disease 193, 302, 311, 343, 347,
    354, 398
Heart rate 21, 24, 39, 149, 151, 153,
    173, 179, 253, 348-349, 360
Heart-rhythm disturbances 20, 22, 24,
    128, 132, 260, 268
Heart valves, artificial 279
Heartbeat 352
Heartbeat irregularities 18, 20, 22
Heartburn 2, 32-33, 40, 62, 98, 126,
    138, 142, 176, 236, 240, 250, 266, 399
Heat intolerance 132
Hematinic® 393
Heme 399
Hemocyte® 393
Hemolytic anemia 399
Hemorrhages 13, 209, 210
Hemorrhagic newborn 399
Hemorrhoidal preparations 4
Hemorrhoids 360, 372, 357, 399
Henomint® 395
Heparin 42, 134-135, 279, 337
Heptyl paraben 367
Herbs 359-361
Hernia 400
Heroin 174
Hexa-Betalin® 396
High-blood-pressure medication 117,
    208, 229
Hip dislocation 400
Histacon® 392
Histapp® 48
Histaspan® 392

Histex® 392
Histine® 393
Histogesic® 396
Histussinol® 392
Hives 400
Homoatropine methylbromide 46
Hormone 156, 160, 264
Horsetail 359-360
Humulin L, N, R® 394
Hyaline membrane disease 258, 400-401
Hyasorb® 395
Hybephen® 391
Hydralazine 144, 319
Hydrate® 392
Hydrocele 400
Hydrocephalus 124, 302, 400
Hydrocil Instant® 393
Hydrocodone 136-137, 394
Hydrogenated vegetable oil 367
Hydrolyzed vegetable protein (HVP)
    368
Hydrops fetalis 142, 400
Hydroxazine 73
Hydroxycobalamin 331
Hydroxyzine 261, 269
Hyoscine 46
Hyoscyamine 46
Hyperbilirubinemia 341, 400
Hyperemesis gravidarum 70, 86, 100,
    133, 165, 177, 214, 222, 225, 269
Hypertension 148, 318, 400, see also
    High blood pressure
Hyperthyroidism 160, 227, 264, 400, 402
Hypnette® 395
Hypoplasia left-heart syndrome 400
Hypothyroidism 226, 297, 400
Hyrexin® 393
Hysteria 360, 400
Hytakerol® 397
Hytinic® 394

**I**
INH® 394
IUD 2
Ibuprofen 5, 138-139, 280, 394
Iletin Regular I, II® 394
Ilosone® 120
Ilotycin® 393
Imipramine 24, 90, 140-141, 188, 321
Imperforate anus 400
Impotence 128, 221, 260, 400
In-vitro-fertilization 352
Indo-Lemmon® 394
Indocid® 394
Indocin SR® 394
Indomed® 394
Indomethacin 34, 98, 117, 126, 138,
    142-144, 163, 166, 184, 208, 217, 229,
    240, 250, 266, 280, 348, 394
Infantile beriberi 400
Infertility 290, 297, 346
Inflammatory bowel disease 249, 400
Inguinal hernia 400
Inhiston® 395
Innerclean Herbal Laxative® 391, 393
Insoluble fiber 357
Insomnia 400
Insulatard NPH® 394
Insulin 38, 39, 73, 129, 146-147, 157,
    161, 193, 223, 225, 261, 265, 269, 289,
    348, 394
Intal® 84
Intercept® 396
Intestinal complaint products v
Intestinal motility 46, 400
Intestinal perforation 142, 400
Intestinal ulceration 400

Intracranial hemorrhage 209-210, 400
Intracranial hypertension 400
Intracranial pressure 154
Intrauterine death 400
Iodine 297-298
Iodized salt 297
Ipaterp® 396
Ircon® 393
Iromin-G® 396
Iron 12, 14, 257, 286, 299-301, 303,
    304, 316, 321, 334, 339, 343, 348,
    357-358, 375-376, 400
Iron-deficiency anemia 12, 14, 299, 400
Iron overload 348
Iron polysaccharide 394
Iron preparations 34
Iso-Asminyl® 394
Isoclor® 392
Isoetharine 148-149, 152
Isoniazid (INH) 34, 53, 55, 65, 95, 150-
    151, 193, 195, 213, 217, 237, 296, 307,
    319, 348, 394
Isophed® 394
Isoproterenol 25, 148, 152-153, 193, 394
Isopto-Atropine® 391
Isotretinoin 2, 154-155, 328, 329
Isuprel® 394

**J**
Janupap® 390
Jaundice 400

**K**
KCL® 395
K-Dur® 395
K-G Elixir® 395
K-Long® 395
K-Lor® 395
K-Lyte® 395
K-Pen® 395
K-Tab® 395
K-10® 395
Kalium Durules® 395
Kao-Nor® 395
Kaochlor® 395
Kaolin 229
Kaon® 395
Karidium® 396
Kasof® 393
Kato® 395
Kava-kava 359
Kay Ciel® 395
Kaybovite® 397
Kaylixir® 395
Keflex® 60
Kellogg's Tasteless Castor Oil® 54
Kernicterus 246, 248, 341, 400
Ketoconazole 75
Ketone bodies 372
Keysone® 395
Kiddi-Koff® 392
Kiddies Pediatric® 390
Kidney damage 244-245, 257
Kidney failure 200
Kidney stones 32, 285, 400
Kidney toxicity 257
Kinesed® 391
Kleer® 392
Klonopin® 78
Klor-Con® 395
Klor-10%® 395
Klorvess® 395
Klotrix® 395
Kola nut 359
Kolantyl® 390
Kolantyl Liquid® 380
Kolantyl Tablets® 380

Kolantyl Wafers® 380
Kolephrin® 392
Kolephrin GG/DM® 392
Kondremul with Phenolphthalein® 393
Konsyl® 393
Kophane® 390
Koromex® 396
Krondremul® 394
Kronofed-A® 396
Kudrox® 390
Kwell® 158

**L**

L-Cillin® 395
L.A. Formula® 393
LV Tabs® 395
Laboratory tests 28, 30
Lactic acid 368
Lactose 368
Lanacillin® 395
Lane's Pills® 391
Laniazid® 394
Lanophyllin® 397
Largactil® 392
Lasix 313
Laxative 36, 50, 54, 102, 103, 151, 182, 302, 359, 400, 402
Laxcaps® 393
Lecithin 368
Ledercillin® 395
Lente® 394
Lestemp® 390
Letdown reflex 346, 353, 355, 400, 401
Levoid® 156
Levothyroxine 156-157, 226
Libritabs® 64
Librium® 64
Licorice 364
Lidocaine 75
Lindane 158
Linoleic acid 339
Liothyronine 160-161
Liquid Pred® 395
Liquimint® 390
Liquiprin® 390
Lisacort® 395
Lithane® 162
Lithium 23, 53, 65, 73, 95, 129, 133, 144, 162-163, 185, 195, 223, 257, 259, 261, 269, 286, 298, 325
Lithobid® 162
Liver damage 17, 37, 111, 151, 182, 183, 237, 348
Liver toxicity 17, 111, 151, 183, 237, 348
Lixaminol® 390
Lo-Ovulen® 394
Lobelia 359-360
Local anesthetics 247
Lodrane® 397
Loestrin® 394
Lomotil® 391
Lotrimin® 80
Luminal® 395
Lung cancer 354
Luride® 396
Luride-SF® 396
Lymph 400
Lymph glands 400
Lyopine® 391
Lysine 364
Lyteca® 390

**M**

MAO, see Monoamine oxidase inhibitor
M.O.M.® 394
MSC Triaminic® 396
Maalox® 380, 390, 396

Macrodantin® 394
Mag-Ox 400® 394
Magmalin® 390
Magnagel® 390
Magnatril® 394
Magnesium 32, 33, 38, 169, 206, 213, 220, 239, 257, 293, 302-303, 304, 311, 316, 337, 348, 357-358, 375, 394
Malabsorption 400
Malaise 400
Malformation 3, 8, 398
Malignant 398, 400, 402
Mallergan® 392, 396
Malsupex® 391
Malt-soup extract 50
Mandrake 359
Manganese 286, 304-305, 311, 394
Manic episodes 400
Mannitol 368
Maox® 394
Marevan® 278
Marijuana 7, 343, 362
Marine 500, 1000® 394
Maroin® 397
Marzine® 86
Maso-Cycline® 396
Mate 359
Materna Tablets® 316, 396
Max-EPA® 394
Maxigesic® 392, 396
Maxigesic® 391
Measurin® 391
Mebaral® 168
Meclizine 164-165
Meclofenamate 166-167
Meclomen® 166
Meconium staining 400
Med-Apap® 390
Medi-Spas® 391
Medications for psychiatric disease iv
Medicinal creams 4
Medicinal herbs 4-5
Medigesic® 390
Medihaler-Epi® 393
Medihaler-Iso® 394
Mediprin® 394
Medizinc® 397
Mefenamic acid 280
Mefoxin® 56
Melancholia 360, 400
Mellaril® 260
Menadione 341
Meningocele 106, 276, 400
Meningomyelocele 52, 400
Menrium® 64
Menstruation 13, 359-360
Mepergan® 396
Meperidine 73, 169, 206, 220, 239
Mephobarbital 168, 170
Mephyton® 397
Metamucil® 393
Metaprel® 172
Metaproterenol 172-173
Metered-dose-inhaler 400
Methadone 27, 136, 174-175, 196, 213
Metharbital 341
Methemoglobinemia 176
Methotrexate 29, 31, 42, 97, 144, 185, 201, 247, 294, 296, 331
Methscopolamine bromide 46
Methylatropine nitrate 46
Methylcellulose 50
Methylcobalamin 331
Methyldopa 25, 73, 91, 113, 117, 129, 133, 141, 163, 189, 193, 223, 225, 261, 269, 280
Methyl xanthine 352

Meticort® 395
Meticorten® 395
Metoclopramide 17, 176-177
Metoprolol 237, 253
Metric 21® 394
Metronid® 394
Metronidazole 169, 178-179, 193, 206, 220, 280, 348, 394
hydrochloride 178
Metryl® 394
Mi-Acid® 390
Miconazole 180-181
Micro-K® 395
Micronase® 390
Micronor® 394
Midol® 382
Midran® 392
Migraine headache 252, 400
Migralam® 382
Milk 365
Milk let-down, see Letdown reflex
Milk of Magnesia® 380, 394
Milk of Magnesia-Cascara Suspension® 391
Milk-alkali syndrome 32
Milkinol® 394
Mineral oil 110-111, 182, 337, 339, 341, 394
Minerals iv
Mintox® 390
Miscarriage 3, 88, 107, 134, 138, 191, 192, 227, 249, 278, 282, 294, 296, 322, 333, 342, 352, 354, 360
Mission Prenatal® 396
Mistletoe 359, 361
Mixtard® 394
Mn-Plus® 394
Modane® 391, 393
Modicon® 394
Mol-Iron® 393
Molybdenum 305, 291
Monistat® 180
Mono-Gesic® 240
Monoamine oxidase (MAO) inhibitors 25, 39, 45, 47, 53, 91, 113, 117, 119, 141, 169, 189, 206, 220, 280, 229
Monofluorophosphate, sodium 292
Monoglycerides 368
Monosodium glutamate (MSG) 368
Mood elevation 359, 362
Mormon tea 359
Morning sickness 3, 357, 372
Motion sickness 164
Motrin® 394
Mudrane GG® 393
Muscle relaxant 238
Myambutol® 122
Mycelex® 80
Mycostatin® 190
Mygel® 390
Mylanta® 380, 390, 396
Mylicon® 396
Myocardial infarction 134, 191, 193, 400
Mysoline® 218

**N**

N-N Cough Syrup® 392
NPH Iletin, I® 394
Nafeen® 396
Naldecon® 392
Naldetuss® 392
Nalfon® 126
Nalidixic acid 187, 280

Naprosyn® 184
Naproxen 34, 184-185, 280
Narcotics 73, 75, 82, 83, 136, 137, 174,
    175, 177, 196, 261, 348
Nasahist® 392
Nasal decongestant 44
Nasal sprays 4
Nasalcrom® 84
Natabec Rx Kapsules® 396
Natafort Filmseal® 396
Natalins® 316, 396
National Institute of Health 372
Nature's Remedy® 391
Navane® 262
Nebs® 390
Nebulizer 400
Neo-Calglucon® 379, 391
Neo-Cultol® 394
Neo-Fer® 393
Neo-K® 395
Neo-Synephrine® 395
Neomycin 193, 301, 331, 341
Neonatal depression 302, 400
Neonatal goiter 226, 400
Nervine® 396
Nestabs® 396
Neural-tube defects 12, 146,
    294-295, 315, 347
Neutralca-S® 390
New Biocal-500® 379
New Potent Calcium Plus® 379, 391
Newtrogel II® 390
Niac® 394
Niacin 306-307, 319, 394
Nibustat® 180
Nico-400® 394
Nico-Span® 394
Nicobid® 394
Nicolar® 394
Niconyl® 394
Nicotex® 394
Nicotine 6, 355
Nifedipine 75
Niferex® 316, 394
Nilprin® 390
Nilstat® 190
Nitrate 369
Nitrex® 394
Nitrofor® 394
Nitrofurantoin 34, 186-187, 193, 213,
    296, 394
    macrocrystals 186-187
No Doz® 382
Noedma® 390
Non-acetylated salicylates
    (salsalates) 348
Nonoxynol-9 243
Nor Q.D.® 394
Nor-Tet® 396
Noralac® 391
Noratuss® 390, 392
Nordette® 394
Nordryl® 393
Norinyl® 394
Norisodrine Aerotrol® 394
Norlac Rx® 396
Norlestrin® 394
Normotensive 400
Noroxine® 156
Norpramin® 90
Nortriptyline 24, 140, 188-189
Novafed® 392, 396
Novahistine® 392, 393, 396
Novo-Lente-K® 395
Novoferrogluc® 393
Novoferrosulfa® 393
Novofolacid® 393

Novofumar® 393
Novomethacin® 394
Novulin N® 394
Nu-Iron® 394
Nucofed® 392
Nuprin® 394
Nutmeg 359
Nutrasweet® 350
Nutrient analysis 373
Nycoff® 392
NyQuil® 392-393
Nystatin 190
Nystex® 190

O
O-V Statin® 190
Oatstraw 359
Ocean-A/S® 391
Octamide® 176
Oligohydraminios 400
Omega-3 polyunsaturated fatty acids
    394
Omnipen® 390
Opticrom 4%® 84
Optiphyllin® 397
Oralphyllin® 397
Oraminic® 392
Orasone® 395
Orazinc® 397
Organogenesis 4
Ornacol® 392
Ornade® 392
Ornaise® 390
Orphenadrine 73, 129, 223, 225, 261,
    269
Orprine® 395
Ortho Novum® 394
Ortho-Creme® 396
Orthoxocol® 392
Os-Cal® 379, 391
Osmotic laxatives 313
Osteoarthritis 166, 401, 184
Osteomalacia 335, 401
Osteoporosis 126, 134, 216, 284, 302,
    401
Ostoforte® 397
Ovarian cysts 401
Ovcon® 394
Ovral® 394
Ovrette® 394
Ovulen® 394
Oxazepam 95, 193, 194-195
Oxytocin 207, 401
Oyster Cal® 379, 391
Oxycodone 196-197

P
PBZ-SR® 274
PMP Expectorant® 393
PMS Ferrous Sulfate® 393
P-V-Tussin® 390
Pacitron® 397
Palafer® 393
Palmiron® 393
Palocillin-5® 395
Palodyne® 396
Pamelor® 188
Pan-B-1® 397
Pan-sone® 395
Panadol® 390
Panahist® 392
Panamin® 390
Pancreatitis 114 256, 401
Pantothenic acid 308-309
Panwarfin® 278
Panzid® 394
Par-Mag® 394

Para-aminobenzoic acid (PABA) 247
Para-aminosalicylic acid (PAS) 27, 42,
    105, 213
Para-Hist Antitussive® 393
Paralytic ileus 401
Paramethadione 198-199
Parasiticide 401
Parcillin® 395
Parenteral 401
Parten® 390
Partrex® 396
Partuss AC® 392
Passion flower 359
Pathocil® 96
Pavadon® 392
Pedi-Dent® 396
PediaCare® 392
Pediacof® 392, 395
Pediaflor® 396
Pediamycin® 393
Pediatric, VC Expectorant® 396
Pediazole® 393
Pellegra 401
Pen-Vee-K® 395
Penagen-VK® 395
Penapar® 395
Penbritin® 390
Pencillamine 34
Penicillin 28, 30, 96, 121, 193, 200-201,
    257, 395
Pennyroyal 359-361
Pensorb® 395
Pensyn® 390
Pentazine® 396
Pentazocin 274, 402
Pentids® 395
Pentoxifylline 280
Peppermint 359-360
Peptic ulcer 217
Percogesic-C® 392
Peri-Colace® 391, 393
Periactin® 88
Perineal 401
Peripheral neuropathy 401
Periwinkle 359-360
Permitil® 128
Phenaphen® 392
Phenatuss® 392
Phenelzine 93
Phenergan® 396
Phenerhist® 396
Phenethicillin Potassium® 395
Phenetron® 392
Pheniramine 202-203, 395
Pheno-square® 395
Phenobarbital 9-10, 13, 73, 75, 108,
    115, 127, 129, 133, 168-169, 193, 204-
    206, 218-219, 249, 261, 269, 277, 286,
    291, 294, 295, 303, 319, 341, 395
Phenodyne w/Codeine® 392
Phenolax® 393
Phenolphthalein 102-103, 111, 337
Phenonyl® 395
Phenothiazine 25, 34, 45, 47, 91, 113,
    141, 163, 170, 189, 206, 220, 260, 268,
    349, 401
Phenylalanine 350-351, 401
Phenylephrine 25, 207-208, 395
    intravenous 91, 113, 141, 189
Phenylketonuria 350-351, 401
Phenylpropanolamine 27, 209-210
Phenytoin 23, 25, 34, 42, 53, 65, 67, 91,
    95, 108, 115, 133, 141, 151, 157, 161,
    163, 170, 175, 187, 189, 193, 195, 206,
    211-213, 217, 220, 223, 225, 259, 265,
    280, 286, 291, 294-296, 303, 319, 331,
    341, 349, 395

INDEX

409

Pheryl-E® 397
Phillips' Milk of Magnesia® 394
Phosphates 293, 304
Phosphorated carbohydrate 214-215
Phosphoric acid 368
Phosphorus 34, 214, 286, 310-311, 401
Phyllocontin® 390
Pinex® 392
Piperonyl butoxide 231
Piroxicam 163
Placenta previa 354
Placental hemorrhage 401
Placental tears 13
Pleasant Pellets® 391
Pneumonia 182, 354-355, 401
Poison-Control Centers,
　Canada 389
　United States 383
Polaramine® 392
Polaramine Expectorant® 396
Poly-histine® 392, 395
Polycarbophil 50
Polycillin® 390
Polymox® 390
Polysaccharide-iron complex 299
Polysorbate 60 368
Posture® 379, 397
Potachlor® 395
Potage® 395
Potasalan® 395
Potassine® 395
Potassium 45, 47, 163, 217, 312-313,
　324, 349, 369, 395
Potatoes 364
Potent Calcium 600® 379, 391
Potter's face 142
Povidone-iodine 298
Pramet F.A.® 396
Pramilet F.A.® 396
Prazosin 144
Pre-eclampsia 22, 33, 40, 146-147, 227,
　258, 284, 294, 302, 401-402
Pred-5® 395
Prednisone 216-217, 395
Prefrein-A® 395
Prefrein-Z® 395
Prefrin® 395, 396
Pregnancy test 2, 268
Pregnancy-induced
　hypertension, see also
　Hypertension, 40, 284, 342,
　352
Premature birth 333, 362
Premature closure of the ductus
　arteriosus 142, 399
Premature delivery 16, 21, 23, 38, 41,
　85, 114, 134, 143, 146, 148, 152, 173,
　185, 216, 238-239, 253, 256, 259, 346
Premature infants 299
Premature labor 20-21, 40-41, 54, 142-
　143, 146-147, 172, 184, 185, 204, 227,
　238-239, 252-253, 352, 356, 360
Premenstrual syndrome (PMS) 319
Prenatal vitamins 5, 6, 110, 314-316, 396
Prenate 90 Tablets® 396
Presamine® 140
Primatene® 393
Primidone 13, 151, 193, 218-220, 341
Principen® 390
Probenecid 19, 42, 56-57
Procainamide 75
Prochloperazine 221-223
Prolamine® 382
Prolixin® 128
Proloprim® 272
Promachlor® 392
Promapar® 392

Promaz® 392
Promega® 394
Promethazine 224-226, 396
Propacil® 226
Propranolol 39, 73, 129, 133, 144, 147
Propyl gallate 368
Propylthiouracil 226-227
Prostat® 394
Protein 375-376, 401
Protein requirements 372
Proternol® 394
Proto-Chol® 394
Proval® 390
Proval No. 3® 392
Proventil® 20
Proxyphene 113
Prunicodeine® 392
Pseudoephedrine 27, 228-229, 396
Psyllium seeds 50
Pteroylglutamic acid (PGA) 294
Pulmonary embolism 134, 279, 401
Pyracort-D® 395
Pyranistan® 392
Pyrethrins 232
Pyribenzamine® 274
Pyridoxine, also see Vitamin B₆, 125,
　150-151, 170, 191, 206, 213, 220, 307,
　321, 327, 349, 355, 375
　hydrochloride 318-319, 396
Pyrilamine 232, 396
Pyristan® 396
Pyrithione 342-343
Pyroxin® 396

**Q**

Quelidrine® 390, 392
Queltuss® 392
Quibron® 393
Quibron T® 397
Quibron T SR® 397
Quiet-Nite® 392
Quinidine 34, 75, 111, 170, 206, 213,
　220, 237, 280
Quinine 280, 368
Quinine water 364

**R**

R 70/30® 394
REM® 392
RNA 401
Radiostol® 397
Radius 401
Ragweed alergy 231
Ramses 10 Hour® 396
Ranitidine 23, 34, 234-235, 259
Rebound acid secretion 285,
　401
Rebound congestion 207, 401
Rebound scurvy 401
Recommended diet during
　pregnancy and lactation 370
Red No. 3 368
Red No. 40 368
Red raspberry 359-361
Redisol® 397
Redoxon® 397
Reflux 401
Reglan® 176
Regutol® 393
Remsed® 396
Repen VK® 395
Reproductive failure 401
Reserpine 117
Respi-sed® 392
Respiratory diseases 354
Respiratory-distress syndrome 142, 400,
　401

Retet® 396
Retin-A® 328
Retinoic 328
Retinol 328
Retinoid 154
Retrolental fibroplasia 401
Reye's syndrome 41, 401
Rh-incompatible pregnancies 224
Rheumatic syndrome 150, 401
Rheumatoid arthritis 41, 98, 126, 139,
　143, 166, 184, 240-241, 250-251, 266-
　267, 296, 398, 401
Rhinihist® 392
Rhubarb 36
Riboflavin 121, 191, 245, 257, 319, 320-
　321, 327, 396
Rickets 335, 401
Rid® 231
Rifadin® 236
Rifampin 23, 39, 95, 151, 175, 193, 217,
　235, 237, 259
Rifomycin® 236
Rimactane® 236
Riobin-50® 396
Riopan® 380
Ritodrine 20, 142-143, 172, 238-239, 302
Ro-Cillin VK® 395
Ro-Fedrin® 396
Ro-Hist® 274
Roampicillin® 390
Robicillin-VK® 395
Robitet® 396
Robitussin® 393
Robitussin AC® 392, 392, 395, 396
Rocaltrol® 397
Rocephin® 58
Rodex® 396
Rodryl® 393
Rohydra® 393
Rolabromophen® 48
Rolaids® 379, 391
Rolamethazine® 396
Rolazid® 394
Rolox® 390
Romilar® 390, 392
Ronan® 390
Rondec® 396
Roychlor® 395
Royonate® 395
Ru-Tuss® 391
Rubion® 397
Rubramin® 397
Rue 359, 361
Rufen® 394
Rulox® 390
Rum-K® 395

**S**

S.A.C. Throat Lozenges® 396
S-P-T® 397
SIDS, see Sudden infant
　death syndrome
Saccharin 368
Safrole 360
St. Joseph® 391, 392
Salbutamol 20
Saletin® 391
Salicylates 40, 296, 334
Salicylazosulfapyridine 296
Salsalate 240-241
Sarcocycline® 396
Sarodant® 394
SaroPen VK® 395
Sassafras 359-361
Satric® 394
Scabies 401
Scoliosis 401

410

Scotrex® 396
Scullcap 359-360
Scurvy 401
Sea-Omega 50® 394
Searle Pharmaceuticals, Inc. 350
Seborrhea 282, 401
Sedadrops® 395
Sedapap 3® 392
Sedative 359
Seizure medication, see
    Anti-convulsant
Seizures 10
Selenium 322-323, 334, 396
Selenium Sulfide Tablets® 396
Selsun® 396
Selsun Blue® 396
Semicid® 396
Semilente® 394
Senna 36, 359-361
Senokap DSS® 391, 393
Senokot® 391
Sertan® 218
Shepherd's purse 359-360
Siblin® 393
Silain® 380, 390, 396
Silexin Cough Syrup® 392
Simaal Gel® 390
Simatin® 124
Simeco® 390
Simeco Suspension® 380
Simethicone 242, 396
Simplesse 369
Simron® 393
Sinarest® 382, 392, 395
Sine-Off® 392
Sinex® 395
Single nasopharynx 401
Singlet® 395
Sinequan® 112
Sinu-Tab Extra Strength® 392
Sinufed® 396
Sitz bath 401
SK-Erythromycine® 120
SK-Penicillin® 395
SK-Penicillin VK® 395
SK-Phenobarbital® 395
SK-Potassium Chloride® 395
SK-Terpin Hydrate and Codeine®
    396
SK-Tetracycline® 396
Skin tags 401
Skin wrinkling 354
Sleep aids 5, 177
Slo-Bid® 397
Slo-Phyllin® 397
Slo-Pot® 395
Slow Fe® 393
Slow-K® 395
Snakeroot 359
Sodium 32, 38, 313, 324-325
    benzoate 369
    bicarbonate 33, 117, 163, 229, 324
    bisulfite 369
    carboxylmethylcellulose 369
    caseinate 367
    chloride 163, 324
    citrate 324, 367
    cromoglycate 84
    fluoride 292, 324, 396
    monofluorophosphate 292
    nitrite 369
Sodium overload 401
Softenex® 393
Solu-barb® 395
Solu-Flur® 396
Soma® 382, 392
Somonal® 395

Somophyllin® 397
Somophyllin Oral Liquid® 390
Sonazine® 392
Sonography 107, 277, 401
Sorbic acid 369
Sorbitan monostearate 369
Sorbitol 369
Sorbutuss® 392
Soy 364
Span-Lanin® 393
Span-Niacin® 394
Spasticity 401
Spastosed® 391
Spec-T Sore Throat Lozenges® 392, 395
Spectab® 395
Sperm motility, decreased 399
Spermicides 243, 396
Spiders 398
Spiknard 359
Spina bifida 106-107, 276-277, 402
Spironolactone 27, 313
Squaw vine 359
St. John's wort 359-361
Stannous fluoride 292
Starch, modified 369
Starvation 372
Stay-Flo® 396
Sterility 294
Sternum 402
Steroids 42, 144, 151, 170, 206, 213,
    220, 257, 398
Stevens-Johnson syndrome 186, 187,
    246, 402
Stillbirths 114, 134, 152, 256
Stomach complaint products v
Stool softener 110, 316, 402
Streptomycin 244-245, 321
Stroke 134, 191, 193, 402
Stuart Prenatal Tablets® 396
Stuartnatal 1 + 1® 396
Studaflor® 396
Sucralfate 34
Sucrets®392, 395
Sucrets Cough Control Formula® 392
Sudafed® 392-393, 396
Sudahist® 396
Sudden infant death syndrome 13, 354,
    401
Sugar 368
Sul-Blue® 396
Sulfamethoxazole 246-248, 272-273
Sulfapyridine 248
Sulfasalazine 248-249
Sulfisoxazole 39, 183
Sulfites 369
Sulfonamides 55, 103, 193, 280, 296
Sulfur dioxide 369
Sulfur-containing vitamin 282
Sulindac 250-251
Sulphonamides 341
Sumox® 390
Sumycin® 396
Supen® 390
Supercitin® 392
Suplical® 379, 391
Surfax® 393
Sus-Phrine® 393
Sushi 365
Sustaire® 397
Swiss Kriss® 391
Syllact® 393
Syllamalt® 391, 393
Sympathetic nervous system 402
Symptom 3® 48
Symptrol® 393
Synalgos® 396
Syndactyly 402

Synkavite® 397
Synthroid® 156
Syrcodate® 392
Systemic lupus erythematosus
    syndrome 150, 402

T

T's and Blues 274, 402
T.E.P.® 393
THC 362
T-Quil® 94
TSG Croup Liquid® 392
T-Stat 2.0% Topical Solution® 393
Tagamet® 74
Tanimine® 140
Tansy 359, 361
Tapar® 390
Tardive dyskinesia 128, 132, 176, 221,
    260, 262, 268
Tavist® 74
Tearfrin® 395
Tedral® 393
Teebaconin® 394
Tega-code® 392
Tega-Span® 394
Tegretol® 52
Teldrin® 392
Temaril® 268
Temazepam 105
Temetan® 390
Tempo® 390
Tempra® 390
Tendar® 394
Tendonitis 184, 402
Tenlap® 390
Terbutaline 20, 142-143, 148, 152, 172,
    238, 252-253
Terp® 396
Terpichlor® 396
Terpin hydrate 254-255, 396
Terpium® 392
Tet-cy® 396
Tetra-C® 396
Tetra-Co® 396
Tetracap® 396
Tetrachel® 396
Tetrachor® 396
Tetracycline 4, 29, 31, 34, 97-98, 113,
    135, 163, 190, 193, 201, 256-257, 286,
    301, 303, 321, 343, 396
Tetracyn® 397
Tetralan® 397
Tetram® 397
Tetramax® 397
TexSix T.R.® 396
Thalidomide 3
Theo-dur® 397
Theo-II® 397
Theobid® 397
Theobromine 353
Theobron® 397
Theocap® 397
Theoclear® 397
Theodrine® 393
Theofedral® 393
Theolair® 397
Theolixir® 397
Theon® 397
Theophenyllin® 393
Theophylline 4, 22-23, 53, 75, 117, 121,
    163, 170, 206, 220, 258-259, 352-353,
    355, 362, 397
Theoral® 393
Theospan-SR® 397
Theostat 80® 397
Theovent Long Acting® 397
Theracal® 391

Thermoloid® 397
Thiamine 326-327, 349, 397, 398, 400, 402
Thiazide diuretics 42, 99, 144, 185, 217, 313
Thiocynate levels 354
Thioridazine 260-261
Thorazine® 392
Thiothixine 262-263
Thorn apple 359
Thrombophlebitis 338, 402
Thrush 28, 30, 60, 62, 96, 402
Thyro-Teric® 397
Thyrocrine® 397
Thyroid v, 160, 264-265, 280, 397
    damage 163
    hormone levels 211-212
    storm 227, 402
Thyrotoxicosis 297, 402
Tibia 402
Titralac® 379, 391
Tobacco 5, 7, 354
Tobutamide 390
Tocoterienols 338
Tofranil® 140
Toin® 395
Tolazamide 38, 266, 390
Tolbutamide 38, 266, 280
Tolectin® 266
Tolinase® 390
Tolmetin 266-267
Tolu-Sed® 392-393
Tonelax® 391
Tooth discoloration 114-115, 257
Tooth staining 256
Topicycline® 397
Totacillin® 390
Toxemia 401-402
Trace element 342
Tranquilizers 49, 67, 69, 75, 83, 87, 89, 101, 105, 132, 137, 165, 175, 177, 197, 203, 221, 233, 260, 262, 268, 275, 359, 401
Trantoin® 394
Trav-Arex® 392
Traveltabs® 392
Tremor 402
Tretinoin 328
Trexin® 397
Tri-Norinyl® 394
Triaminic® 392, 395
Triaminicin® 382, 392
Triamterene 144, 313
Tribasic calcium phosphate 397
Tricidene® 392
Tricodenei® 390, 392
Tricyclic antidepressants 47, 73, 75, 119, 170, 206, 220, 261, 321, 349
Tridione® 270
Trifluperazine 268-270
Triglycerides 154, 338
Trimethadione 270-271, 296
Trimethoprim 246, 272-273, 296
Triminacol® 392, 395
Trimox® 390
Trimpex® 272
Trinaid® 394
Trind® 392, 393, 395
Tripelennamine 274-275, 402
Triphasil® 394
Tritussin® 395
Trobicin® 244
Trofan® 397
Troxidone® 270

Trymegon® 392
Tryptacin® 397
Tryptophan 307, 365, 397, 401
Tuberculosis 402
Tumors 402
Tums® 379, 391
Tussagesic® 392, 395-396
Tussaminic® 396
Tussapap® 390
Tussar® 392, 395
Tussend® 394
Tussi-Organidin® 392
Tussionex® 394
Tusstat® 393
Twin-K-Cl® 390
2/G® 392, 393
Tylenol® 390, 392
Tyrosine 401

U
Ulcerative colitis 402
Ulcer 217, 234, 402
Ultralente® 394
Uniad® 394
Unilax® 391, 393
Univol® 390
Uremia 402
Ureter 402
Urethane 346
Uric-acid levels 99
Urine acidifier 26
Urised® 391
Uro-Mag® 394
Urogenital 402
Urotoin® 394
Uterine contractions 359
Uterine fibroids 190, 402
Utimox® 390

V
V-Cillin K® 395
V-Pen® 395
Vaginal yeast infections 180
Valadol® 390
Valcaps® 94
Valerian 359-360
Valium® 94
Valoid® 86
Valorin® 390
Valproate 106-107, 276, 277
Valproic acid 65, 95, 106-107, 170, 195, 206, 213, 220, 276-277, 343
Valrelease® 94
Vanillin 369
Vanquish® 382
Vapo-Iso® 394
Vaponefrin® 393
Varicose veins 400
Vasodidin® 395
Veetids® 395
Vegetables 363
Vegetarian 331, 332
Velocef® 62
Velosulin® 394
Veltane® 48
Ventolin® 20
Veracillin® 96
Verapamil 23, 259
Verazinc® 397
Vertigo 164, 402
Vibra-Tabs® 114
Vibramycin® 114
Vicks Cough Formula® 392, 393
Viromed® 392

Vitamins v, 124
Vitamin A 5, 154, 217, 316, 328-330, 331, 334, 335, 337, 339, 355, 366, 375, 397, 402
Vitamin B1 326
Vitamin B2, see Riboflavin
Vitamin B2® 320, 396
Vitamin B6, see also Pyridoxine, 125, 150-151, 170, 191, 206, 213, 220, 307, 321, 327, 349 355, 375
Vitamin B-9® 393
Vitamin B12 169, 191, 206, 213,294-295, 331-332, 334, 397
Vitamin C 9, 42, 169, 200, 206, 291, 301, 323, 330, 333-334, 355, 375, 397, 401
Vitamin D 204, 206, 211, 213, 218, 220, 285-286, 303, 316, 331, 335-337, 339, 349, 397, 401
Vitamin D2 335
Vitamin D3 335
Vitamin E 330, 338-339, 397
Vitamin H 282
Vitamin K 12, 182, 247, 330, 339, 340-341, 397, 399
Vitamin K1 340
Vitamin K2 340
Vitamin-K3 341
Viterra E® 397
Vivarin® 382
Vivox® 114

W
Warfarin 25, 37, 42, 50, 53, 55, 75, 99, 103, 121, 127, 134, 144, 151, 157, 161, 167, 179, 181, 183, 185, 189, 06, 217, 220, 237, 242, 245, 251, 265, 267, 278-280
Water on the brain 399
Weight, desirable 371
Weight-loss aids 4
Wernicke-Korsakoff's syndrome 326, 402
Wheat 364
Wheezing 402
Wilson's Disease 291, 402
WinGel® 390
WinGel Liquid®66 380
Wormwood 359
Wymox® 390

X
Xerophthalmia 328, 402

Y
Yarrow 360-361
Yeast infections 80, 178, 190
Yellow No. 5 369
Yellow No. 6 369

Z
Zantac® 234
Zarontin® 124
Zenate® 396
Zinc 107, 257, 277, 286, 291, 296, 301, 342, 343, 349, 355, 357-358, 362, 366, 375, 378, 397
Zinc-220® 397
Zincate® 397
ZinKaps® 397
Zovirax® 18
Zypan® 390